Sleisenger and Fordtran's
GASTROINTESTINAL
AND LIVER DISEASE
REVIEW AND ASSESSMENT

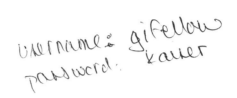

Sleisenger and Fordtran's
GASTROINTESTINAL AND LIVER DISEASE
REVIEW AND ASSESSMENT

8th EDITION

Editor

Anthony J. DiMarino, Jr., MD

William Rorer Professor of Medicine and Chief
Division of Gastroenterology and Hepatology
Department of Medicine
Thomas Jefferson University
Philadelphia, Pennsylvania

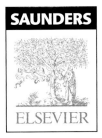

SAUNDERS

ELSEVIER

SAUNDERS
ELSEVIER

1600 John F. Kennedy Blvd.
Ste. 1800
Philadelphia, PA 19103-2899

Sleisenger and Fordtran's GASTROINTESTINAL AND LIVER
DISEASE REVIEW AND ASSESSMENT

ISBN: 978-1-4160-3366-0

Notice

Knowledge and best practice in this field are constantly changing. As new research and experience broaden our knowledge, changes in practice, treatment, and drug therapy may become necessary or appropriate. Readers are advised to check the most current information provided (i) on procedures featured or (ii) by the manufacturer of each product to be administered, to verify the recommended dose or formula, the method and duration of administration, and contraindications. It is the responsibility of the practitioner, relying on his or her experience and knowledge of the patient, to make diagnoses, to determine dosages and the best treatment for each individual patient, and to take all appropriate safety precautions. To the fullest extent of the law, neither the Publisher nor the Editor assumes any liability for any injury and/or damage to persons or property arising out of or related to any use of the material contained in this book.

The Publisher

Previous editions copyrighted 1999, 1996

Library of Congress Cataloging-in-Publication Data

DiMarino, Anthony J.
    Sleisenger and Fordtran's gastrointestinal and liver disease review and assessment / Anthony J. DiMarino.—8th ed.
        p. cm.
    ISBN 978-1-4160-3366-0
    1. Gastrointestinal system—Diseases—Examinations, questions, etc.   I. Sleisenger and Fordtran's gastrointestinal and liver disease.   II. Title.
RC801.G384 2006 Suppl.
616.3'30076—dc22

2007009832

Acquisitions Editor: Rolla Couchman
Developmental Editor: Melissa Dudlick
Publishing Services Manager: Frank Polizzano
Project Manager: Jeff Gunning
Design Direction: Steve Stave

Printed in China

Working together to grow
libraries in developing countries

www.elsevier.com | www.bookaid.org | www.sabre.org

ELSEVIER   BOOK AID International   Sabre Foundation

Last digit is the print number: 9   8   7   6   5   4   3   2   1

Dedicated to medical students, residents, fellows and faculty, Division of Gastroenterology and Hepatology, Jefferson Medical College and Thomas Jefferson University Hospital.

Special dedication is given to the section leaders—Sidney Cohen, Steven K. Herrine, Anthony Infantolino, David Kastenberg, Howard S. Kroop, David Loren, and Ivan Rudolph—who helped coordinate this effort.

Anthony J. DiMarino, Jr., MD

Contributors

Jeffrey A. Abrams, MD
Clinical Assistant Professor of Medicine, Division of Gastroenterology and Hepatology, Department of Medicine, Thomas Jefferson University, Philadelphia, Pennsylvania

Monica Awsare, MD
Fellow, Division of Gastroenterology and Hepatology, Department of Medicine, Thomas Jefferson University, Philadelphia, Pennsylvania

Kuldip Banwait, MD
Fellow, Division of Gastroenterology and Hepatology, Department of Medicine, Thomas Jefferson University, Philadelphia, Pennsylvania

Cuckoo Choudhary, MD
Clinical Assistant Professor of Medicine, Division of Gastroenterology and Hepatology, Department of Medicine, Thomas Jefferson University, Philadelphia, Pennsylvania

Robert M. Coben, MD
Clinical Assistant Professor of Medicine and Academic Coordinator, Fellowship Program, Division of Gastroenterology and Hepatology, Department of Medicine, Thomas Jefferson University, Philadelphia, Pennsylvania

Matthew S. Cohen, MD
Fellow, Division of Gastroenterology and Hepatology, Department of Medicine, Thomas Jefferson University, Philadelphia, Pennsylvania

Sidney Cohen, MD
Professor of Medicine, Division of Gastroenterology and Hepatology, Department of Medicine, Thomas Jefferson University; Director, Research Programs, Division of Gastroenterology and Hepatology, Department of Medicine, Thomas Jefferson University, Philadelphia, Pennsylvania

Mitchell Conn, MD, MBA
Clinical Associate Professor of Medicine; Co-Director of Gastrointestinal Bleeding Center and Director of Endoscopic Training, Division of Gastroenterology and Hepatology, Department of Medicine, Thomas Jefferson University, Philadelphia, Pennsylvania

Anthony J. DiMarino, Jr., MD
William Rorer Professor of Medicine and Chief, Division of Gastroenterology and Hepatology, Department of Medicine, Thomas Jefferson University, Philadelphia, Pennsylvania

Michael DiMarino, MMS, MD
Clinical Assistant Professor of Medicine, Division of Gastroenterology and Hepatology, Department of Medicine, Thomas Jefferson University, Philadelphia, Pennsylvania

Gregg S. Gagliardi, MD
Fellow, Division of Gastroenterology and Hepatology, Department of Medicine, Thomas Jefferson University, Philadelphia, Pennsylvania

Steven Greenfield, MD
Clinical Assistant Professor of Medicine, Division of Gastroenterology and Hepatology, Department of Medicine, Thomas Jefferson University, Philadelphia, Pennsylvania

Hie-Won Hann, MD
Professor of Medicine; Director, Liver Disease Prevention Center, Division of Gastroenterology and Hepatology, Department of Medicine, Thomas Jefferson University, Philadelphia, Pennsylvania

Nikroo Hashemi, MD
Fellow, Division of Gastroenterology and Hepatology, Department of Medicine, Thomas Jefferson University, Philadelphia, Pennsylvania

Steven K. Herrine, MD
Associate Medical Director, Liver Transplant Program; Associate Director, Fellowship Program; Professor of Medicine, Division of Gastroenterology and Hepatology, Department of Medicine, Thomas Jefferson University; Assistant Dean, Academic Affairs, Jefferson Medical College, Philadelphia, Pennsylvania

Anthony Infantolino, MD
Clinical Associate Professor of Medicine; Director of Endoscopic Ultrasound; Director of Photodynamic Therapy; Chairman, Clinical Practice Committee; CME Coordinator for Division, Division of Gastroenterology and Hepatology, Department of Medicine, Thomas Jefferson University, Philadelphia, Pennsylvania

David Kastenberg, MD, FACP, AGAF
Clinical Assistant Professor of Medicine and Co-Director, Nutrition and Metabolic Disease Center, Division of Gastroenterology and Hepatology, Department of Medicine, Thomas Jefferson University, Philadelphia, Pennsylvania

Leo C. Katz, MD
Clinical Assistant Professor of Medicine; Co-Director, Center for Nutrition and Metabolic Disease, Department of Gastroenterology and Hepatology, Department of Medicine, Thomas Jefferson University, Philadelphia, Pennsylvania

Thomas Kowalski, MD
Clinical Associate Professor of Medicine; Director of GI Endoscopy, Department of Gastroenterology and Hepatology, Department of Medicine, Thomas Jefferson University, Philadelphia, Pennsylvania

Howard S. Kroop, MD
Clinical Associate Professor of Medicine, Division of Gastroenterology and Hepatology, Department of Medicine, Thomas Jefferson University, Philadelphia, Pennsylvania; Chairman, Department of Medicine, Underwood Memorial Hospital, Woodbury, New Jersey

Michael Lipcan, MD
Fellow, Division of Gastroenterology and Hepatology, Department of Medicine, Thomas Jefferson University, Philadelphia, Pennsylvania

David Loren, MD
Clinical Assistant Professor of Medicine; Director, GI Endoscopic Research Program, Division of Gastroenterology and Hepatology, Department of Medicine, Thomas Jefferson University, Philadelphia, Pennsylvania

Pradnya Mitroo, MD
Fellow, Division of Gastroenterology and Hepatology, Department of Medicine, Thomas Jefferson University, Philadelphia, Pennsylvania

Victor Navarro, MD
Clinical Associate Professor of Medicine; Medical Director, Liver Transplantation, Division of Gastroenterology and Hepatology, Department of Medicine, Thomas Jefferson University, Philadelphia, Pennsylvania

Joseph Palascak, MD
Fellow, Division of Gastroenterology and Hepatology, Department of Medicine, Thomas Jefferson University, Philadelphia, Pennsylvania

Jorge A. Prieto, MD
Clinical Assistant Professor of Medicine, Division of Gastroenterology and Hepatology, Department of Medicine, Thomas Jefferson University, Philadelphia, Pennsylvania

Satish Rattan, DVM
Professor of Medicine; Director of Basic Research, Division of Gastroenterology and Hepatology, Department of Medicine, Thomas Jefferson University, Philadelphia, Pennsylvania

Susie Rivera, MD
Division of Gastroenterology and Hepatology, Department of Medicine, Thomas Jefferson University, Philadelphia, Pennsylvania

Simona Rossi, MD
Clinical Assistant Professor of Medicine, Division of Gastroenterology and Hepatology, Department of Medicine, Thomas Jefferson University, Philadelphia, Pennsylvania

Emily Rubin, RD, LDN
Registered Dietitian, Division of Gastroenterology and Hepatology, Department of Medicine, Thomas Jefferson University, Philadelphia, Pennsylvania

Ivan Rudolph, MD
Clinical Assistant Professor of Medicine; Director, Gastroenterologic Clinic, Division of Gastroenterology and Hepatology, Department of Medicine, Thomas Jefferson University, Philadelphia, Pennsylvania

Ashish Shah, MD
Fellow, Division of Gastroenterology and Hepatology, Department of Medicine, Thomas Jefferson University, Philadelphia, Pennsylvania

Ali Siddiqui, MD
Fellow, Division of Gastroenterology and Hepatology, Department of Medicine, Thomas Jefferson University, Philadelphia, Pennsylvania

Kuntal Thaker, MD
Fellow, Division of Gastroenterology and Hepatology, Department of Medicine, Thomas Jefferson University, Philadelphia, Pennsylvania

Preface

The members of the Division of Gastroenterology and Hepatology at Jefferson Medical College and Thomas Jefferson University Hospital have prepared this self-assessment text that accompanies the eighth edition of *Sleisenger and Fordtran's Gastrointestinal and Liver Disease.* Doctors Mark Feldman, Lawrence S. Friedman, and Lawrence J. Brandt, along with the publisher, Saunders, have somehow improved upon an already outstanding textbook of gastroenterology and hepatology. We are pleased to have worked with them to update the self-assessment companion text. The questions were designed to follow the text of the parent book, and the answers to the questions are included with references to the original text for further elucidation of the covered topics.

We also are pleased to acknowledge the interest and valuable assistance of our fellows in training in gastroenterology at Jefferson. Many important questions and topics were raised by the fellows who have participated in this project. We hope that the readers of this companion text will find the questions stimulating. William Osler stated in 1900 that the profession of medicine is "a lifelong process of obtaining new knowledge and applying it for the improvement of patients." We hope that this text contributes in a small way to this lifelong commitment and improves the care of patients with gastrointestinal and liver disease.

Contents

(Section Editors are listed in boldface)

SECTION

1

Nutrition and Biliary Tract

QUESTIONS

1 Which of the following is the rate-limiting step in the hepatic transport of bile acids from blood into bile?

A. Sinusoidal bile acid uptake
B. Canalicular secretion
C. Intestinal absorption
D. Gallbladder contraction

2 Which groups of foods will provoke oral symptoms in 50% of patients with ragweed-induced allergic rhinitis?

A. Apples, hazelnuts, kiwi
B. Carrots, celery, apples, kiwi
C. Raw potatoes, carrots, celery
D. Watermelon, cantaloupe, honeydew, bananas

3 When planning potentially curative surgery for cholangiocarcinoma, which of the following would have the greatest influence on the choice of surgical procedure?

A. Absence of lymph node involvement on magnetic resonance imaging (MRI)
B. Encasement of the hepatic artery
C. Location of tumor within the extrahepatic biliary system
D. Presence of a solitary liver metastasis < 3 cm in diameter

4 A 42-year-old woman with a history of biliary colic and gallstone disease presents with right upper quadrant (RUQ) abdominal pain, nausea, and vomiting. The patient does not have a fever, and vital signs are stable. On abdominal exam, she has RUQ tenderness. An ultrasound demonstrates multiple gallstones and a nonobstructing gallstone in a normal-sized common bile duct (CBD). Choledocholithiasis is diagnosed. Which of the following is most applicable in this case?

A. The efficacy and safety of precholecystectomy endoscopic sphincterotomy is equivalent to intraoperative CBD exploration.
B. The efficacy of precholecystectomy endoscopic sphincterotomy is inferior to laparoscopic CBD exploration.
C. The efficacy of precholecystectomy endoscopic sphincterotomy is inferior to open CBD exploration.
D. The efficacy of precholecystectomy endoscopic sphincterotomy is superior to laparoscopic CBD exploration.
E. The efficacy of precholecystectomy endoscopic sphincterotomy is superior to open CBD exploration.

5 Which of the following patients is at risk for essential fatty acid deficiency?

A. A patient receiving enteral feedings
B. A patient receiving long-term total parenteral nutrition (TPN) with parenteral lipids
C. A patient with irritable bowel syndrome
D. A patient who has short gut syndrome

6 A 43-year-old woman presents with jaundice, and laboratory evaluation reveals an elevated bilirubin level. Nine months earlier she had a laparoscopic cholecystectomy. An ultrasound demonstrates bile duct dilatation; what is the most likely site of stricture formation?

A. Common bile duct
B. Common hepatic duct
C. Left hepatic duct
D. Right hepatic duct

7 Which of the following is the most important determinant of crystal formation in the human gallbladder?

A. Degree of cholesterol saturation
B. Gallbladder motility
C. Degree of bile acid synthesis

8 A 30-year-old woman with short bowel syndrome and insulin-dependent diabetes mellitus complains of diarrhea. She takes a calcium and magnesium supplement. Her food preferences include milk, sugar-free candy, pasta, cereal, chicken, and fruit. Which recommendation will decrease her diarrhea?

A. She should consume 4 servings of dairy per day.
B. She should continue magnesium supplementation.
C. She should increase the fiber content of her diet.
D. She should decrease her intake of sugar-free candy.

9 A 42-year-old woman undergoes lithotripsy for gallstone disease. What is the 5-year recurrence rate for gallstones after this treatment?

A. 7%
B. 23%
C. 44%
D. 75%
E. 84%

10 A 37-year-old woman with a stone in the common bile duct undergoes endoscopic retrograde cholangiopancreatography (ERCP) and endoscopic sphincterotomy. What is the recommended technique for performing a sphincterotomy?

A. Continuous application of bipolar current
B. Continuous application of monopolar blended current
C. Short bursts of bipolar current
D. Short bursts of monopolar blended current

11 A 20-year-old man presents with a several-year history of large-volume, greasy stools and a 3-month history of weakness and poor coordination. The weakness and decrease in coordination developed gradually but progressed more rapidly over the last 4 weeks. His medical

history is otherwise significant for cystic fibrosis. He denies starting any new medication, change in diet, or recent travel. On physical exam he appears thin but in no acute distress. His height is 5'8" and his weight is 130 lbs. The neurologic exam reveals mild ataxia, decreased vibratory sense, and bilateral hyporeflexia. The remainder of his exam findings are unremarkable. What nutritional deficiency is most likely present in this patient?

A. Vitamin A
B. Vitamin C
C. Vitamin D
D. Vitamin E
E. Zinc

12 Bile acid therapy has been approved by the Food and Drug Administration (FDA) for gallstone dissolution and for the treatment of primary biliary cirrhosis (PBC). In patients with PBC, bile acid therapy has been shown to do which of the following?

A. Decrease the incidence of hepatocellular carcinoma
B. Have no influence on progression of liver fibrosis but improve survival
C. Improve liver enzymes without effect on survival
D. Decrease progression of liver fibrosis and improve survival

13 Which of the following is a true statement regarding risk factors for cholangiocarcinoma?

A. Approximately 5% of patients with primary sclerosing cholangitis are found to have cholangiocarcinoma at autopsy.
B. Chronic infection with *Clonorchis sinensis* reduces the risk for cholangiocarcinoma.
C. Exposure to thorium dioxide (Thorotrast) increases the lifetime risk of cholangiocarcinoma.
D. The low risk for cholangiocarcinoma associated with a choledochal cyst does not warrant surgical evaluation.

14 The levels of what group of serum proteins evaluated in a rapid screen for protein-energy malnutrition (PEM) most accurately indicate a change in an inpatient's nutritional status?

A. Albumin, prealbumin, retinol binding protein
B. Albumin, prealbumin
C. Prealbumin, retinol binding protein, transferrin
D. Prealbumin, transferrin, albumin

15 A 40-year-old woman presents with painless jaundice. She underwent a proctocolectomy with ileal pouch anal anastomosis 20 years ago for familial adenomatous polyposis (FAP). An abdominal ultrasound demonstrates dilatation of the biliary tree and a normal pancreatic duct. The most likely diagnosis is:

A. Ampullary carcinoma
B. Cholangiocarcinoma
C. Duodenal carcinoid
D. Gallbladder cancer
E. Pancreatic cancer

16 A 62-year-old woman with a 25-year history of type I diabetes mellitus presents to the emergency department with a 3-month history of frequent nausea and vomiting. The patient is admitted for intravenous hydration and a thorough evaluation, which results in a diagnosis of diabetic gastroparesis. After all accepted medical treatments have failed to promote adequate oral nutritional intake, the decision is made to place an enteral feeding tube. The need for enteral feeding is expected to last for more than 6 months.

Which surgery/type of enteral feeding tube would be most appropriate in this patient?

A. Direct percutaneous jejunostomy (DPJ)
B. Nasogastric tube (NGT)
C. Nasojejunal tube (NJT)
D. Percutaneous endoscopic gastrojejunostomy (PEG/J)
E. Percutaneous endoscopic gastrostomy (PEG)

17 A 38-year-old woman presents to the emergency department with a 3-hour history of RUQ pain, nausea, vomiting, and fever. Nothing in her past medical history is considered relevant to the current problem. She is alert and oriented and complaining of mild distress. She has a temperature of 100.3°F, a heart rate of 82, a blood pressure of 122/78 mmHg, and a positive Murphy's sign, but no peritoneal signs. Her white blood cell count is 13,000 cells/dL. An ultrasound demonstrates multiple gallstones, a thickened gallbladder wall, pericholecystic fluid, and a positive Murphy's sign. What antibiotic regimen is appropriate for this patient?

A. Intravenous cefoxitin
B. Intravenous piperacillin-tazobactam
C. Intravenous vancomycin
D. Oral amoxicillin-clavulanic acid
E. No antibiotics are needed

18 A 65-year-old man presents to the emergency department with evidence of septic shock and multi-organ failure. The patient is hypotensive and is treated with a vasopressor. Early examination by ultrasound demonstrates the presence of pericholecystic fluid, gallbladder wall

thickening, and Murphy's sign. Acute cholecystitis is diagnosed, and the patient is scheduled for percutaneous cholecystostomy (PC). Which of the following is true regarding PC?

A. Locking the pigtail catheter does not decrease the incidence of bile leak.
B. The overall complication rate of PC is 15% to 20%.
C. PC has no role in managing acalculous cholecystitis.
D. PC is successful in 75% to 80% of cases.
E. Sepsis can be prevented by not overdistending the gallbladder during PC catheter placement.

19 A 40-year-old man with a 4-year history of ulcerative colitis involving the entire colon undergoes ERCP. Based on the results of ERCP (see figure), which of the following interventions is most likely to benefit this patient?

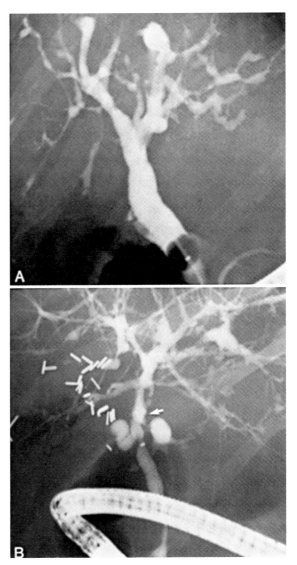

Figure for question **19**

A. Antibiotic prophylaxis
B. Cancer antigen (CA) 19-9 testing every 6 months
C. Colonoscopy with numerous biopsies every 1 to 2 years, beginning in 6 years
D. Dual energy x-ray absorptiometry (DEXA) scan
E. Ursodeoxycholic acid (13 to 15 mg/kg/day)

20 Anorexia nervosa and bulimia nervosa are examples of serious eating disorders. During what period of life do these disorders typically have their onset?

A. Middle age (40 to 65 years)
B. Adolescence
C. Childhood
D. After age 65

21 Which of the following is true about the metabolic response to short-term starvation (1 to 14 days of fasting)?

A. Muscle protein breakdown decreases to less than 30 g/day, causing a marked decrease in urea nitrogen production and excretion.
B. The body relies on obtaining more than 90% of its daily energy requirements from adipose tissue.
C. The decrease in osmotic load decreases urine volume to 200 mL/day, thereby reducing fluid requirements.
D. Overall, glucose production decreases by more than half because of a marked reduction in hepatic glucose output.

22 A 72-year-old man presents with a complaint of persistent abdominal pain and distention, nausea, and vomiting for the last 5 hours. The patient reports similar episodes during the last 5 days, but each of these previous episodes lasted only 15 to 20 minutes and resolved spontaneously. An abdominal obstruction series demonstrates multiple dilated loops of small bowel and pneumobilia. Where is the most likely site of obstruction?

A. Cecum
B. Duodenum
C. Ileum
D. Jejunum
E. Rectum

23 Which of the following pharmacologic agents should be recommended for patients with anorexia nervosa to promote weight gain?

A. None
B. Zinc gluconate
C. Cyproheptadine
D. Risperidone

24 A 41-year-old woman experiences continued abdominal pain after laparoscopic cholecystectomy. The pain is out of proportion to that expected after this procedure. A computed tomography (CT) scan of the abdomen demonstrates an intra-abdominal collection of fluid, and a nuclear medicine scan confirms the suspicion that there is a bile leak. The patient's abdomen is soft and nondistended. What is the best treatment?

A. Bring the patient back to the operating room for bile duct repair.
B. Drain the biloma, then perform an ERCP and place a biliary stent.
C. Observe the patient for spontaneous resolution of signs and symptoms.
D. Perform transcatheter occlusion of the bile duct (e.g., sclerosis with tetracycline).
E. Place a percutaneous transhepatic drainage catheter.

25 Several gastrointestinal malignancies occur more frequently in overweight and obese patients. The obesity-related increase in relative risk is highest for cancer in which of the following organs?

A. Pancreas
B. Stomach
C. Gallbladder
D. Liver
E. Colon

26 Defective bile acid conjugation can cause:

A. Fluid overload
B. Ascites
C. Fat-soluble vitamin deficiency
D. Vitamin B_{12} deficiency

27 A 44-year-old woman presents with abdominal pain and jaundice 3 months after an

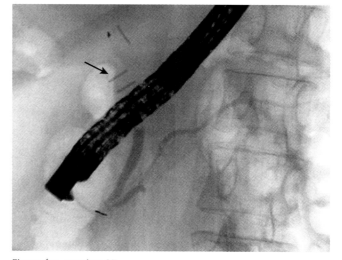

Figure for question **27**

uncomplicated cholecystectomy. She is afebrile and her other vital signs are within normal ranges. Alkaline phosphatase and bilirubin levels are significantly elevated and aspartate aminotransferase (AST) and alanine aminotransferase (ALT) levels are slightly elevated. An ERCP is performed. Based on the results of ERCP (see figure), what is the best long-term management strategy in this case?

A. Endoscopic dilatation
B. Endoscopic metal stent placement
C. Percutaneous drainage
D. Surgery

28 Which one of the following forms of psychotherapy is the treatment of choice for young patients with anorexia nervosa?

A. Cognitive behavioral therapy
B. Psychodynamic psychotherapy
C. Supportive psychotherapy
D. Family therapy

29 A 58-year-old man who recently underwent "long" Roux-en-Y choledochojejunostomy presents to the emergency department with a 1-day history of fever, abdominal pain, and jaundice. His temperature is 102°F, and his blood pressure is 92/40 mmHg. He is deeply jaundiced and has severe RUQ tenderness. He is started on intravenous (IV) antibiotics and scheduled for which of the following procedures?

A. Endoscopic retrograde cholangiopancreatography (ERCP)
B. Exploratory laparotomy
C. Magnetic resonance cholangiopancreatography (MRCP)
D. Percutaneous transhepatic biliary drainage (PTBD)

30 Which is true about the exclusive use of breast milk for infants and its relationship to food allergies?

A. It contains prolactin, which may induce earlier maturation of the gut barrier and thereby promote tolerance to ingested antigens.
B. It contains S-IgA, which does not provide passive protection against foreign proteins and pathogens.
C. It may cause atopic dermatitis.
D. The effect of breast milk on infant immunity is unknown.

31 Biliary manometry is most necessary before sphincterotomy for:

A. Type I sphincter of Oddi dysfunction
B. Type II sphincter of Oddi dysfunction

C. Type III sphincter of Oddi dysfunction
D. Type IV sphincter of Oddi dysfunction

32 A 42-year-old woman arrives in the emergency department with acute-onset RUQ pain. The pain is sharp and radiates to her back. The pain resolves spontaneously approximately 90 minutes after her arrival. She is afebrile and has no abdominal tenderness. Laboratory studies show a total bilirubin concentration of 2.4 mg/dL, alkaline phosphatase level of 202 IU/L, AST of 110 U/L, and ALT of 155 U/L. An ultrasound examination reveals multiple gallstones within the gallbladder and a CBD diameter of 9 mm. Which of the following is the least invasive procedure for accurate diagnosis of choledocholithiasis?

A. Computed tomography (CT)
B. Endoscopic retrograde cholangiopancreatography (ERCP)
C. Laparoscopic cholecystectomy with intraoperative cholangiography (IOC)
D. Magnetic resonance cholangiopancreatography (MRCP)
E. Percutaneous transhepatic cholangiography (THC)

33 A 4-month-old girl presents with protracted diarrhea, vomiting, and failure to thrive. A stool evaluation reveals increased fecal fat, and the results of a D-xylose test are abnormal. Endoscopic biopsies of the intestinal wall show patchy villous atrophy. Cow's milk is eliminated from the infant's diet, and the symptoms resolve. What is the diagnosis?

A. Celiac disease
B. Dietary protein–induced enterocolitis proctocolitis
C. Dietary protein–induced enterocolitis syndrome
D. Dietary protein–induced enteropathy

34 A 20-day-old girl is referred for evaluation of jaundice. The infant was born at 40 weeks' gestation and weighed 7 lbs., 10 oz. at birth. The mother had no complications during the pregnancy. In the postnatal period weight gain has been normal. Upon examination the infant is notably jaundiced. The liver is palpable at 4 cm below the right costal margin. No splenomegaly or ascites is noted. Laboratory studies demonstrate a total bilirubin concentration of 10 mg/dL and a direct bilirubin concentration of 7.5 mg/dL. AST and ALT levels are 50 U/L and 62 U/L respectively, and the alkaline phosphatase concentration is 155 mU/L. Based on the appearance of a liver biopsy specimen (see figure), what is the likely cause of this infant's jaundice?

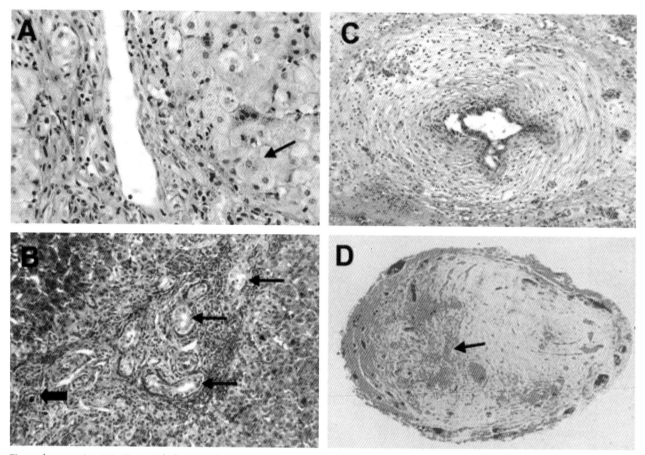

Figure for question **34**. (From Sokol RJ, Mack C, Narkewicz MR, Karrer FM: Pathogenesis and outcome of biliary atresia: Current concepts. J Pediatr Gastroenterol Nutr 37:4, 2003; used with permission.)

A. Alagille's syndrome
B. Caroli's syndrome
C. Choledochal cyst
D. Extrahepatic biliary atresia
E. Neonatal sclerosing cholangitis

35 Which of the following statements is true regarding celiac disease?

A. Celiac disease is strongly associated with human leukocyte antigen (HLA)-DQ2, which is present in 20% of patients.
B. Extensive lymphocytic infiltrate is associated with sensitivity to lactose.
C. Immunoglobulin A (IgA) antibodies specific for celiac disease are present in 80% of adults and children with treated celiac disease.
D. Lifetime elimination of gluten is necessary to control symptoms and reduce the risk for malignancy.

36 A 52-year-old man presents with severe jaundice approximately 5 months after undergoing a liver transplant for cirrhosis due to primary sclerosing cholangitis. Based on the results of ERCP (see figure), what is the most likely cause of this stricture?

A. Chronic graft rejection
B. Cytomegalovirus (CMV) infection
C. Ischemia
D. Postoperative scarring or technical complications of surgery
E. Recurrent primary sclerosing cholangitis

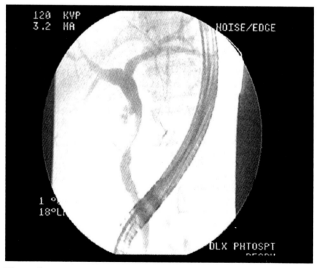

Figure for question **36**

37 A 42-year-old woman arrives in the emergency department with an 8-hour history of severe abdominal pain. The pain is epigastric and radiates to her back. Based on the results of laboratory tests and radiologic examinations, acute pancreatitis is diagnosed. The patient is ordered nothing by mouth and started on IV fluids and IV analgesic medication. Over the next several days the patient's condition worsens. Hypotension develops that is treated by frequent boluses of IV fluid. Subsequently, respiratory failure develops, necessitating intubation and ventilator support. A decision is made to start TPN. The patient's height is 168 cm, and her weight is 75 kg.

What is this patient's daily caloric requirement?

A. 1858 kcal/day
B. 2043.8 kcal/day
C. 2322.5 kcal/day
D. 2787 kcal/day

38 A 50-year-old man with long-standing primary sclerosing cholangitis (PSC) presents with pruritus. Liver enzyme levels are elevated above baseline. On ultrasound, new dilation of the proximal biliary tree to the level of the common bile duct (CBD) is noted. ERCP shows a tight stricture midway along the CBD and proximal dilation of the duct; no malignant cells are seen in the bile duct brush cytology or biopsy specimens. The next step(s) in treating this patient should be:

A. ERCP, repeat cytology, and balloon dilation
B. High-dose ursodeoxycholic acid
C. Surgical consultation
D. Oncology and radiation oncology consultations

39 A 6-week-old boy is brought for evaluation of jaundice and increasing abdominal girth. At birth the infant was healthy and weighed 8 lbs., 1 oz. The mother's pregnancy was uncomplicated, as was the birth. The infant was healthy until 1 week ago when he started to vomit and his appetite decreased. The parents also report noticing a gradual increase in abdominal girth during the last week and that the baby's stools are clay-colored and his urine dark. Laboratory studies demonstrate a total bilirubin concentration of 4 mg/dL and a direct bilirubin concentration of 3 mg/dL. Ultrasound confirms the presence of fluid in the abdomen. A sample obtained by paracentesis is bile-stained but sterile. Based on these findings, bile duct perforation is suspected.

What is the most likely location of this perforation?

A. Junction of the cystic duct and common bile duct

B. Junction of the left and right hepatic ducts and common hepatic duct
C. Cystic duct
D. Distal common bile duct
E. Gallbladder

40 Which of the following is considered an immunoglobulin E (IgE)–mediated, food-induced gastrointestinal hypersensitivity?

A. Celiac disease
B. Dietary protein–induced enterocolitis syndrome
C. Dietary protein–induced eosinophilic proctocolitis
D. Gastrointestinal anaphylaxis

41 Cholangiography results indistinguishable from primary sclerosing cholangitis (PSC) are *least* likely in:

A. A 33-year-old man with AIDS
B. A 45-year-old woman with antithrombin III deficiency and a hepatic artery thrombosis
C. A 50-year-old woman with primary biliary cirrhosis
D. A 60-year-old man with cholangiocarcinoma
E. A 70-year-old man with long-standing choledocholithiasis

42 Total parenteral nutrition (TPN) is most closely associated with the development of which one of the following conditions?

A. Peptic ulcers
B. Inflammatory bowel disease (IBD)
C. Gastroesophageal reflux disease (GERD)
D. Cholelithiasis

43 A 1-year-old boy is brought for evaluation of jaundice and intense pruritus. In addition to generalized jaundice, he has xanthomata on the extensor surfaces of the fingers and in the creases of his palms and hepatosplenomegaly. He has a broad forehead, deeply set and widely spaced eyes, a pointed mandible, a flattened malar eminence, and prominent ears. Laboratory tests demonstrate a total bilirubin level of 7.2 mg/dL and a direct bilirubin level of 5.8 mg/dL. Serum alkaline phosphatase is 500. The findings suggest Alagille's syndrome.

What findings on examination of a liver biopsy specimen would be diagnostic of this condition?

A. Concentric periductal fibrosis ("onion skin" appearance)
B. Expanded portal tract with portal fibrosis, bile duct proliferation, and bile plugs within the bile duct
C. Paucity of interlobular bile ducts
D. Portal tract edema and fibrosis

44 Which of the following psychiatric illnesses have the highest mortality?

A. Depression
B. Schizophrenia
C. Borderline personality disorder
D. Eating disorders

45 A 40-year-old woman has had two episodes of RUQ pain in the 6 months since laparoscopic cholecystectomy. Each episode lasted between 30 and 60 minutes, and a serum sample obtained during each episode showed an ALT level 2.5 to 3.0 times the upper limit of normal. An ultrasound examination revealed that the diameter of the CBD is 13 mm, and MRCP shows no evidence of a stricture or filling defect within the biliary tree. The recommended next step is:

A. A trial of nitrates or a calcium channel blocker
B. Biliary manometry
C. Endoscopic sphincterotomy
D. Initiation of treatment with an anticholinergic medication
E. Noninvasive testing

46 A 5-year-old boy with a history of Kawasaki's disease presents with acute onset of crampy abdominal pain, nausea, and vomiting. On exam, he is afebrile, and the RUQ is tender with a palpable gallbladder. A complete blood count (CBC) reveals a normal white cell count. Ultrasonography demonstrates enlargement and distention of the gallbladder but no evidence of stones, sludge, or acute cholecystitis. What is the most likely diagnosis?

A. Acalculous cholecystitis
B. Acute cholecystitis
C. Acute hydrops of the gallbladder
D. Biliary dyskinesia
E. Mesenteric ischemia

47 Of the following, which medication is most likely to increase the basal sphincter of Oddi pressure:

A. Diazepam
B. Meperidine
C. Midazolam
D. Morphine
E. Verapamil

48 Which of the following complications of gallstone disease is most rapidly fatal?

A. Cholecystitis
B. Pancreatitis
C. Cholangitis
D. Biliary colic

49 The daily volume of bile secreted by the liver ranges from:

A. 200 to 300 mL
B. 500 to 600 mL
C. 750 to 900 mL
D. 900 to 1000 mL

50 A 7-week-old girl is brought for evaluation of increased irritability, vomiting, poor appetite, a 1-week history of worsening jaundice, and the development of clay-colored stools. On physical exam, there is moderate hepatomegaly and a palpable abdominal mass. Laboratory studies demonstrate a total bilirubin concentration of 8.3 mg/dL and a direct bilirubin concentration of 6.7 mg/dL. Alkaline phosphatase and aminotransferase levels are only mildly elevated. An ultrasound examination is performed (see figure).

What is the most likely diagnosis?

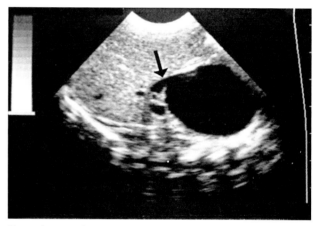

Figure for question **50**

A. Alagille's syndrome
B. Bile plug syndrome
C. Biliary atresia
D. Choledochal cyst
E. Primary sclerosing cholangitis

51 Which of the following statements is true regarding bile storage in patients without a gallbladder (postcholecystectomy)?

A. Bile acids are stored in the distal small intestine.
B. Bile acids are stored in the proximal small intestine.
C. Bile acids are stored in the biliary tree.
D. Bile acids are not stored within the gastrointestinal tract.

52 A 42-year-old man presents to his primary care physician for a routine physical examination. He has no specific complaints, and his medical history is significant only for mild hypertension. He is 68 inches (173 cm) tall and weighs 220 lbs. (100 kg).

What is this patient's body mass index (BMI) and weight classification?

A. 33.3/overweight
B. 33.3/obese
C. 33.3/super obese
D. 57.8/obese
E. 57.8/super obese

53 A 12-year-old boy is brought for outpatient evaluation of chronic abdominal pain. According to the parents, episodes of abdominal pain of varying degree have occurred for 2 years. On several occasions the patient has had fever and mild jaundice associated with the abdominal pain. All episodes resolved spontaneously. The physical examination reveals hepatosplenomegaly. The results of laboratory tests, including total and direct bilirubin, alkaline phosphatase, and aminotransferase levels, are within normal limits. An ultrasound demonstrates multiple bilateral renal cysts and cystic dilatation of the intrahepatic ducts.

What is the most likely diagnosis in this case?

A. Alagille's syndrome
B. Caroli's syndrome
C. Choledochal cyst
D. Extrahepatic biliary atresia
E. Primary sclerosing cholangitis

54 In the United States, what gastrointestinal disorder most often leads to hospitalization?

A. Peptic ulcer disease
B. Gallstone disease
C. Diverticular disease
D. Gastrointestinal bleeding

55 Which of the following has been used to support a theory regarding the etiology and pathogenesis of primary sclerosing cholangitis (PSC)?

A. *Cryptosporidium* and cytomegalovirus have been cultured from the bile of patients with PSC who test negative for human immunodeficiency virus (HIV) infection.
B. Microscopic arterial thromboses are present in explanted livers from PSC patients, supporting a non–immune-mediated etiology.
C. Positive results of serologic testing for anti-neutrophil cytoplasmic antibody (pANCA) have been associated with increased risk of disease progression, supporting an immune-mediated etiology.

D. Several HLA haplotypes conferring increased risk for PSC have been identified, supporting an immune-mediated etiology.

56 Physical activity is important in managing obesity and obesity-related medical problems. Which of the following statements regarding obesity and weight loss is most accurate?

A. Physical activity is not effective for achieving initial weight loss.
B. Physical activity alone usually results in significant weight loss.
C. Moderate endurance exercise, four times per week for up to a year, usually results in significant weight loss.
D. Physical activity may *not* ameliorate or prevent specific obesity-related complications such as coronary disease and diabetes.

57 An 11-year-old boy with recently diagnosed ulcerative colitis is brought for outpatient evaluation of fatigue and jaundice. The patient has been having intermittent abdominal pain for the last 8 weeks and has been jaundiced for the last 3 days. There is no family history of liver disease, and the patient has not been exposed recently to any hepatotoxic chemicals. The family denies any recent travel or contact with sick individuals. The physical examination reveals the presence of scleral icterus and mild hepatosplenomegaly. Laboratory tests show a total bilirubin level of 4.0 mg/dL with a direct fraction of 3.2 mg/dL. The alkaline phosphatase level is 420 (IU/L). On ERCP alternating areas of intrahepatic stricture and dilatation are seen. The diagnosis is primary sclerosing cholangitis (PSC).

Which of the following statements is correct with regard to PSC in children?

A. There are no reported cases of hepatocellular carcinoma in children with PSC.
B. Liver biopsy is often diagnostic.
C. Inflammatory bowel disease always precedes the diagnosis of PSC in the pediatric population.
D. Recurrent PSC often occurs in those who have received a liver transplant.
E. There have been no reported cases of cholangiocarcinoma in children with PSC.

58 Which of the following has been attributed to treatment with octreotide?

A. Decreased gallbladder motility and bile stasis
B. Increased gallbladder motility and bile stasis
C. Decreased gallbladder motility and decreased cholesterol secretion
D. Increased gallbladder motility and decreased cholesterol secretion

59 Bulimia nervosa may be very difficult to diagnose, probably because:

A. Patients with bulimia may be of low body weight.
B. Patients with bulimia may deny the medical seriousness of their condition.
C. Patients with bulimia may have normal results on a physical examination.
D. Patients with bulimia often seek medical care.

60 Which of the following antibiotics has been known to promote biliary sludge formation?

A. Gentamicin
B. Metronidazole
C. Erythromycin
D. Ceftriaxone

61 An 8-year-old girl with a history of sickle cell disease was discovered to have gallstones when CT of the chest was performed to evaluate shortness of breath and chest pain. An ultrasound confirmed the presence of several small gallstones.

The most likely composition of these gallstones is:

A. Calcium bilirubinate
B. Calcium phosphate
C. Calcium palmitate
D. Cholesterol

62 A 52-year-old man who has a history of alcohol abuse presents for evaluation of diarrhea for the last 4 weeks. In addition, he describes significant hair loss and impaired taste. The examination reveals a superficial scaling eruption most notable in the groin and periorally. What is the likely nutrient deficiency?

A. Vitamin A
B. Vitamin B_{12}
C. Vitamin C
D. Magnesium
E. Zinc

63 Elderly patients require larger quantities of which vitamin?

A. Vitamin A
B. Vitamin B_{12}
C. Vitamin C
D. Vitamin E

64 Which of the following conditions poses the greatest risk for gallbladder cancer?

A. Cholelithiasis
B. Choledocholithiasis
C. Cholecystitis
D. Porcelain gallbladder

65 A 37-year-old woman has intermittent, mild biliary colic due to gallstone disease. What is the optimal gallstone diameter for treatment with an oral stone dissolution agent?

A. Less than 2 mm
B. Less than 5 mm
C. Between 6 and 10 mm
D. Less than 10 mm

66 A 48-year-old man with cancer of the head and neck is scheduled to undergo chemotherapy and radiation therapy. The decision is made to place a percutaneous endoscopic gastrostomy (PEG) tube prior to his cancer therapy.

Which of the following is the most common complication of PEG tube placement?

A. Buried "bumper" (embedded PEG tube flange)
B. Colocutaneous fistula
C. Hematoma
D. Peristomal wound infection
E. Peritonitis

67 A 42-year-old burn victim develops RUQ abdominal pain and tenderness. Acalculous cholecystitis is suspected. Which of the following statements is true regarding this condition?

A. Cholecystectomy should be avoided.
B. Gangrene and perforation occur more frequently than with acute cholecystitis caused by gallstones.
C. Sludge is usually absent.
D. Young women are most often affected.

68 Which of the following is most important to assess when evaluating for a serious eating disorder?

A. Appropriateness of weight for height
B. Serum chemistry profile
C. Electrocardiogram
D. Daily food diary

69 A 16-day-old girl is admitted to the hospital for evaluation of persistent hyperbilirubinemia. Initial evaluation demonstrates a total bilirubin concentration of 9.3 mg/dL and a direct bilirubin concentration of 6.1 mg/dL. Serum aminotransferases and alkaline phosphatase levels are mildly elevated. Based on a suspicion of biliary atresia, an ultrasound is ordered.

What ultrasound findings would be most suggestive of this diagnosis?

A. A cone-shaped fibrotic mass, cranial to the portal vein
B. Gallbladder length of 2.5 cm
C. Large cystic mass in the right upper quadrant
D. Massive hepatosplenomegaly

70 Black pigment stone formation is *most* typically associated with which of the following?

A. Chronic hemolysis
B. Chronic gastrointestinal blood loss
C. Chronic hepatitis (without cirrhosis)
D. Chronic biliary infection

71 A 25-year-old woman presents with complaints of intermittent RUQ pain for 2 years. The pain typically follows a meal, radiates to the right shoulder, lasts nearly an hour, and is associated with nausea and vomiting. Other than being overweight, her exam reveals no abnormalities. An ultrasound of the abdomen demonstrates a normal gallbladder, biliary tree, liver, and pancreas. Liver and pancreatic enzyme levels are normal. A bile aspirate is obtained during upper endoscopy (see figure). Based on the findings, the following is recommended:

A. A trial of an anticholinergic agent
B. A trial of dissolution therapy with ursodeoxycholic acid
C. Cholecystectomy
D. ERCP with sphincter of Oddi manometry if there is no evidence of choledocholithiasis
E. Stimulated cholescintigraphy to calculate gallbladder ejection fraction

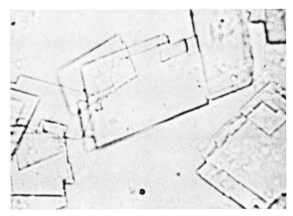

Figure for question **71**

72 Which of the following statements regarding very low-calorie diets is most accurate?

A. Very low-calorie diets do *not* result in long-term weight loss.
B. Very low-calorie diets cause more medical complications than do low-calorie diets.
C. Very low-calorie diets do *not* have a higher risk of gallstone formation.
D. Very low-calorie diets cause less rapid weight loss than standard low-calorie diets.

73 An 80-year-old man undergoes coronary artery bypass graft surgery and has a prolonged postoperative course in the intensive care unit (ICU) with respiratory failure. He receives nutrition by total parenteral nutrition. He experiences 2 days of fever and leukocytosis, and examination of the abdomen reveals diminished bowel sounds. A CT scan demonstrates a thickened gallbladder wall and pericholecystic fluid. The most likely etiology for this finding is:

A. Chemical and ischemic injury to the gallbladder
B. False-positive results
C. Gallstones
D. Ischemic hepatitis with secondary gallbladder involvement

74 A 55-year-old man undergoes ERCP with sphincterotomy for a retained common bile duct stone. After the procedure the patient experiences abdominal pain, prompting a CT scan of the abdomen. CT shows a small, contained retroduodenal perforation. The patient's lipase level is normal, there is no evidence of pancreatitis on CT, and the patient otherwise feels good and has no fever. Bowel sounds are normal and the abdomen is soft and nondistended with mild to moderate epigastric tenderness.

What is the best management strategy for this patient?

A. Admit him to the hospital and plan for elective surgery in the morning.
B. Admit him to the hospital for serial abdominal exams, nasogastric suction, and antibiotics.
C. Admit him to the hospital for observation, and if his condition improves, discharge him in the morning.
D. Perform surgery immediately.
E. Repeat ERCP in order to place a stent across the perforation.

75 A 42-year-old man is admitted to the hospital with his first episode of pancreatitis. He has no significant medical history and does not drink alcohol. Based on the results of his ultrasound (see figure) and assuming that no complications develop, what surgery would be recommended for this patient?

A. Cholecystectomy after the pancreatitis resolves, prior to discharge
B. Cholecystectomy 4 to 8 weeks after discharge
C. Immediate cholecystectomy
D. No surgery unless he has a repeat bout of pancreatitis

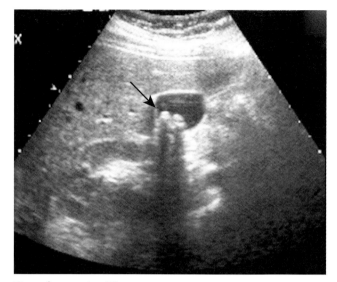

Figure for question **75**

76 Cholesterolosis of the gallbladder is:

A. Frequently present in individuals with cholesterol stones
B. Highly prevalent in certain ethnic groups
C. More common in women
D. Often symptomatic
E. Rare (<1% of autopsy specimens)

77 A 43-year-old man with ulcerative colitis is incidentally noted to have abnormal liver enzyme levels as follows (normal ranges): total bilirubin 1.0 mg/dL, direct bilirubin 0.8 mg/dL, alkaline phosphatase 244 IU/L (29 to 92 IU/L), AST 42 IU/L (7 to 42 IU/L), and ALT 45 IU/L (1 to 45 IU/L). An ultrasound and CT of the liver are both normal. The next step in his evaluation should be:

A. Antimitochondrial antibody testing
B. Antinuclear and smooth muscle antibody testing
C. Colonoscopy
D. ERCP
E. Hepatitis B and C testing

78 A 36-year-old man with a known history of Crohn's disease presents for evaluation of fatigue, decreased exercise tolerance, and dyspnea on exertion. He has predominantly distal ileal disease, which required surgical resection 2 years earlier. His disease has been relatively quiescent since his surgery, and his recent treatment consists of mesalamine. A CT scan and upper gastrointestinal (GI) series with small bowel follow-through confirms disease in the terminal ileum. He denies any bright red blood per rectum, melena, or change in bowel habits. On physical exam he is comfortable, temperature is 98.7°F, heart rate is 102 beats/minute, and blood pressure is 118/72 mmHg. A stool smear is heme negative, but serum hemoglobin is 9.2 mg/dL.

Which of the following deficiencies is the most likely cause of this patient's anemia?

A. Vitamin B_{12} deficiency
B. Folic acid deficiency
C. Iron deficiency
D. Zinc deficiency

79 Which of the following should be performed first when biliary colic is suspected?

A. CT
B. MRI
C. Endoscopic ultrasound (EUS)
D. ERCP
E. Transabdominal ultrasonography

80 Which of the following statements is most accurate regarding the natural history of primary sclerosing cholangitis (PSC)?

A. A clinically useful model of PSC progression is not available.
B. Asymptomatic PSC rarely becomes symptomatic.
C. "Small duct" PSC and "classic" PSC have the same prognosis.
D. Validated prognostic models for PSC are available.

81 Adenomyomatosis of the gallbladder:

A. Carries a high risk for malignancy
B. Is characterized by hyperplasia of the muscle layer
C. Is an indication for surgery when present as an isolated finding
D. Often causes symptoms of biliary colic or pancreatitis
E. Is typified by adenomas less than 0.25 mm in diameter

82 Which of the following agents has Food and Drug Administration (FDA) approval for use in patients with bulimia nervosa?

A. Desipramine
B. Trazodone
C. Naltrexone
D. Fluoxetine

83 A 41-year-old diabetic patient presents for outpatient evaluation of gallstones. Recently she had a CT of the chest to further evaluate a lung nodule. On the abdominal images, two small nonobstructing gallstones were seen. The patient has no history of abdominal pain, nausea, vomiting, or fever. What is the most appropriate therapy at this time?

A. Perform a hydroxy iminodiacetic acid (HIDA; nuclear medicine) scan of the gallbladder.
B. Observe; do not intervene at this time.
C. Obtain an ultrasound of the abdomen.
D. Schedule the patient for elective cholecystectomy.
E. Schedule the patient for urgent cholecystectomy.

84 Which of the following statements is most accurate regarding treatment of recurrent pyogenic cholangitis?

A. Cholangitis occurs in about one third of patients following hepaticojejunostomy.
B. Hepatectomy should not be performed because this disorder involves the entire biliary tree.
C. Liver transplant is contraindicated for this disorder due to the presence of chronic intrahepatic abscesses.
D. Surgery is a more effective treatment than ERCP for extrahepatic bile duct disease.

85 An 8-year-old boy who lives in Kenya has below-average height for age and weight for height. Marasmus is diagnosed. Which of the following clinical signs is associated with marasmus?

A. Protuberant abdomen
B. Intestinal distention and hepatomegaly
C. Peripheral edema is present
D. Weight loss and marked depletion of subcutaneous fat and muscle

86 Which of the following findings on ultrasound is most specific for cholecystitis?

A. Pericholecystic fluid
B. Gallbladder wall thickening
C. Focal tenderness under the transducer (Murphy sign)

87 A 27-year-old woman is pregnant and experiencing frequent bouts of RUQ pain associated with nausea and vomiting. Her symptoms have been increasing in severity and frequency during the last several weeks. She is unable to tolerate adequate oral intake secondary to abdominal pain and severe nausea. An ultrasound demonstrates several small gallstones but no evidence of acute cholecystitis. When is the ideal time to perform a cholecystectomy?

A. First trimester
B. Second trimester
C. Third trimester
D. Post partum

88 Which of the following is the best recommendation regarding management of gallbladder cancer?

A. Patients undergoing palliative surgery for advanced disease should not be offered radiation therapy.
B. Patients with Stage II, T2N0M0 (tumor has invaded perimuscular connective tissue) disease should undergo radical cholecystectomy.
C. Radical cholecystectomy should be avoided in patients with Stage III, T3 (tumor has perforated the serosa or directly invaded one adjacent organ) disease.
D. Simple cholecystectomy alone is insufficient for Stage I, T1N0M0 (tumor has invaded lamina propria or muscle layer) disease.

89 Which of the following studies is best at detecting choledocholithiasis?

A. Transabdominal ultrasound
B. MRCP
C. Endoscopic ultrasound (EUS)
D. CT

90 A 64-year-old man presents to the emergency department with a 2-hour history of RUQ pain without fever or chills. The pain resolves spontaneously. He has a past history of ischemic cardiomyopathy and implantation of a defibrillator. On initial evaluation he has a total bilirubin level of 4.2 mg/dL, alkaline phosphatase of 275 IU/L, AST of 175 IU/L, and ALT of 220 IU/L. Transabdominal ultrasound demonstrates intra- and extrahepatic ductal dilatation, a common bile duct (CBD) diameter of 1.2 cm, and an obstructing stone in the distal CBD. The patient is afebrile and has no tenderness on abdominal exam. Assuming all of the following are available, what is the best test for this patient?

A. Endoscopic retrograde cholangiopancreatography (ERCP)
B. Endoscopic ultrasound (EUS)
C. Laparoscopic cholecystectomy with intraoperative cholangiogram (IOC)
D. Magnetic resonance cholangiopancreatography (MRCP)
E. Percutaneous transhepatic cholangiography (THC)

91 A 40-year-old woman presents with a 2-year history of intermittent fever and chills. Physical exam reveals excoriations on her forearms and xanthomata. Laboratory tests show an alkaline phosphatase level of 340 IU/L, AST of 45 IU/L, ALT of 50 IU/L, albumin of 4.1, and prothrombin time of 13.4 seconds (INR = 1.03). Tests for ANA and smooth muscle antibody are both positive at a titer of 1:40, and the total immunoglobulin level is elevated. A liver biopsy is performed (see figure). What is the most likely diagnosis?

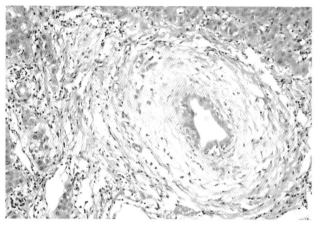

Figure for question **91**

A. Autoimmune cholangiopathy
B. Autoimmune hepatitis
C. Primary biliary cirrhosis
D. Primary sclerosing cholangitis
E. Wilson's disease

92 The essential amino acids are:

A. Alanine, tyrosine, and aspartic acid
B. Glycine, serine, and glutamine
C. Glutamine, cysteine, and asparagine
D. Histidine, phenylalanine, and lysine

93 Imaging is required of a 64-year-old woman's biliary system. ERCP has been attempted twice without success, and because the woman has a pacemaker, MRCP is not an option. Which statement regarding percutaneous transhepatic cholangiography (THC) is true?

A. The biliary tree can be visualized successfully in 99% of patients without dilated bile ducts.
B. The overall rate of serious complications is 8% to 10%.
C. The percutaneous puncture is through the 8th or 9th intercostal space in the right midclavicular line.
D. The risk of bile leak may be greater with a transcholecystic approach.

94 Several monogenic causes of obesity have been detected. Which one of the following is the most common monogenic cause of obesity?

A. Leptin gene mutation
B. Leptin receptor gene mutation
C. Pro-opiomelanocortin gene mutation
D. Melanocortin-4 receptor mutation

95 A 30-year-old Taiwanese man presents with abdominal pain, fever, and jaundice. An ultrasound shows dilation of the biliary tree, most prominent on the left, and numerous intrahepatic filling defects are present. A CT scan is obtained (see figure). Which of the following statements offers support for the leading theory explaining the etiology of this disease?

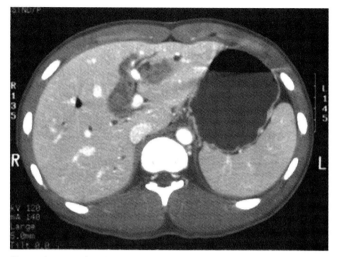

Figure for question **95**

A. A cholecystokinin (CCK)–stimulated HIDA scan demonstrates a markedly diminished gallbladder ejection fraction.
B. A history of total parenteral nutrition is common in these patients.
C. Numerous antibodies are present that cross-react with the colon and bile duct.
D. Ova have been detected in the bile and stool of these patients.
E. Patients have a genetic deficiency of bacterial glucuronidase.

96 Which of the following statements is true regarding fat-soluble vitamins?

A. The average daily dietary intake necessary to sustain normal physiologic operations is measured in milligrams or smaller quantities.
B. They are absorbed in the lipophilic phase of intestinal metabolism.
C. Bile acids are not necessary for intestinal absorption.
D. They serve as co-enzymes.

97 A 42-year-old man undergoes ERCP for evaluation of recurrent pancreatitis. ERCP performed for a similar indication 1 year earlier was complicated by post-ERCP pancreatitis. The ERCP findings on the current occasion include chronic pancreatitis and a duodenal diverticulum. No somatostatin or gabexate mesilate is given during the procedure. Which of the following places the patient at increased risk for pancreatitis after this second ERCP?

A. Age greater than 40
B. Duodenal diverticulum
C. Failure to use somatostatin or gabexate
D. Male gender
E. Previous history of post-ERCP pancreatitis

98 A 75-year-old woman is admitted to the hospital for treatment of dehydration secondary to intractable nausea and vomiting. She reports having nausea and vomiting and early satiety for the past 2 months. She is started on IV fluids and has a nasogastric tube placed, resulting in significant relief of her symptoms. During her hospitalization a gastric mass causing a gastric outlet obstruction is discovered, and she is started on TPN for nutritional support.
Three days later the patient goes into cardiac arrest. The results of analyzing serum samples drawn during the resuscitation attempt are as follows.

Sodium: 135 mEq/L
Potassium: 2.5 mEq/L
Chloride: 102 mmol/L
Carbon dioxide: 20 mmol/L
Blood urea nitrogen: 15 mg/dL
Creatinine: 0.9 mg/dL
Glucose: 124 mg/dL
Calcium: 8.4 mg/dL
Phosphate: 1.0 mg/dL
Magnesium: 0.8 mg/dL

What is the most likely cause of this patient's electrolyte abnormalities?

A. Dilutional effect secondary to volume repletion and TPN
B. Loss of gastrointestinal fluid via the nasogastric tube
C. Increased renal excretion of electrolytes
D. Intracellular electrolyte shifts
E. Miscalculation of the concentrations of electrolytes in the TPN solution

99 A healthy 50-year-old woman undergoes an ultrasound of the abdomen for evaluation of dyspepsia. A solitary 12-mm pedunculated polyp is seen in the gallbladder fundus. Which best explains the rationale for recommending surgery at this point?

A. This lesion frequently detaches and causes pancreatitis.
B. This lesion is likely to be an adenomyoma.
C. This lesion is too large to be an inflammatory polyp.
D. This lesion is the likely explanation for the patient's symptoms.
E. This lesion may be an adenoma.

100 A 45-year-old man known to have gallstones presents with painless jaundice. Which feature of this patient's presentation is most commonly associated with the CT findings shown in the figure?

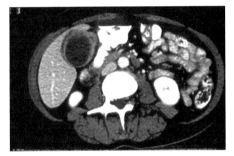

Figure for question **100**

A. Age of 45
B. Gallstones
C. Male gender
D. Painless jaundice

101 What organ systems are affected by protein energy malnutrition (PEM)?

A. Cardiovascular system and neurological system
B. Cardiovascular system and gastrointestinal system
C. Endocrine system and neurological system
D. Gastrointestinal system and neurological system

ANSWERS

1 B. (S&F, ch61)

Canalicular secretion is the rate-limiting step in the hepatic transport of bile acids from the blood into bile. Canalicular bile acid concentrations are more than 1000-fold higher than hepatocyte concentrations.

2 D. (S&F, ch19)

In 50% of individuals with ragweed-induced allergic rhinitis, melons (e.g., watermelon, cantaloupes, honeydew melons), and bananas will provoke symptoms. Those allergic to birch pollen may develop oral symptoms from ingesting raw potatoes, carrots, celery, apples, hazelnuts, and kiwi.

3 **C.** (S&F, ch66)

The surgical approach to cholangiocarcinoma is dependent on the location of the primary tumor. Cholangiocarcinoma occurring in the perihilar region or common hepatic duct bifurcation, the most common location for this tumor, requires a hepaticojejunostomy. Cholangiocarcinoma occurring in the distal common bile duct and head of the pancreas is resected by pancreaticoduodenectomy (Whipple procedure). Metastatic disease, such as liver metastasis or hepatic artery encasement, is not considered curable with surgery. Absence of lymph node involvement on MRI affirms the suitability of a candidate for surgical treatment, but does not influence the choice of surgical procedure.

4 **A.** (S&F, ch63)

The results of small, randomized trials suggest that there are no important differences in the efficacy and safety of precholecystectomy endoscopic sphincterotomy compared to open common bile duct exploration for treatment of choledocholithiasis. Equivalent efficacy and safety have also been shown for precholecystectomy endoscopic sphincterotomy and laparoscopic cholecystectomy with laparoscopic bile duct exploration.

5 **D.** (S&F, ch15)

Patients who have short gut syndrome are at risk for essential fatty acid deficiency due to moderate-to-severe fat malabsorption. Tube feeding formulas and parenteral lipids contain a mixture of essential fatty acids.

6 **B.** (S&F, ch67)

Strictures that develop after laparoscopic cholecystectomy tend to occur in the common hepatic duct. Symptoms this long (9 months) after surgery are usually due to thermal injury to the hilum from cautery and dissection probes.

7 **A.** (S&F, ch62)

The degree of cholesterol saturation is the most important determinant of crystal formation in the human gallbladder. Cholesterol is insoluble in water and therefore can only remain in solution through the detergent activity of bile salts and polar phospholipids. Supersaturation of bile leads to nucleation, crystallization, and, ultimately, stone formation.

8 **D.** (S&F, ch15)

Sugar-free candy contains sugar alcohols—sorbitol, mannitol, and xylitol—that can act as a laxative. Dairy foods, magnesium supplements, and a high-fiber diet can increase diarrhea.

9 **C.** (S&F, ch63)

The rate of gallstone recurrence after lithotripsy is 6% to 7% after the first year and 31% to 44% after 5 years.

10 **D.** (S&F, ch67)

Endoscopic sphincterotomy is the preferred treatment for retained common bile duct stones and is successful in more than 90% of cases. The sphincter muscle is cut at the ampulla with a monopolar blended current applied through a sphincterotome. The cut is performed with short bursts of current, so that the disruption is accomplished with minimal transmural burn, good coagulation, and minimal "unzipping."

11 **D.** (S&F, ch16)

"Vitamin E" is a group of eight compounds, known as tocols (saturated side chains) or tocotrienols (unsaturated side chains), that are found in plants. Alpha-tocopherol accounts for 75% of the total vitamin E found in man. The largest store of vitamin E is found in adipose tissue. The principal function of vitamin E is to protect cell membranes from the effects of oxidation. The major routes of vitamin E excretion are the feces and the skin. Deficiency of vitamin E is rare and generally occurs in individuals with a condition causing severe fat-soluble vitamin malabsorption such as short-bowel syndrome, cystic fibrosis, pancreatic insufficiency, or advanced liver disease. Vitamin E deficiency can lead to neuromuscular dysfunction.

12 **D.** (S&F, ch61)

Bile acid therapy, with ursodeoxycholic acid in particular, has been shown to slow the progression of liver fibrosis and lengthen survival in patients with PBC. Bile acid therapy also has favorable effects on other cholestatic conditions, such as cholestasis of pregnancy and cholestasis associated with total parenteral nutrition.

13 **C.** (S&F, ch66)

Thorium dioxide (Thorotrast) exposure, *Clonorchis sinensis* infection, and choledochal cyst are all important risk factors for cholangiocarcinoma. As many as 30% of patients with primary sclerosing cholangitis have cholangiocarcinoma documented at the time of autopsy.

14 **C.** (S&F, ch15)

Prealbumin, transferrin, and retinal binding protein (RBP) have shorter half lives than albumin and monitoring changes in the levels of these proteins is useful for assessing short-term changes in nutritional status.

15 **A.** (S&F, ch66)

Patients with familial adenomatous polyposis (FAP) have a markedly increased risk for ampullary carcinoma. Although these other neoplasms could present similarly, the likelihood of ampullary cancer is much higher given the history of FAP.

16 **A.** (S&F, ch16)

The preferred method of feeding this patient with severe gastroparesis is through an enteral feeding tube opening into the jejunum (DPJ).

Enteral feeding using the stomach would be contraindicated given the severity of this patient's gastroparesis, thus eliminating answer choices B and E.

Nasoenteric tube placement is the most common method of enteral access; however, these tubes may fail early because of either tube occlusion or tube dislodgment. Because tube failure interrupts tube feeding and medication regimens, these tubes should not be used in patients requiring tube feeding for more than one month, thus eliminating choice D.

A PEG/J allows for both gastric decompression and jejunal feeding and should be used in patients who will need jejunal feedings for more than one month; however, the jejunal feeding tube component of this system may fail because of tube occlusion or displacement if left in place for longer than 6 months. A retrospective study by Fan et al. compared the rate of physician re-interventions for J-tube complications in patients who had undergone PEG/J versus DPJ. The DPJ patients had significantly fewer re-interventions. Thus, DPJ should be performed in patients who will require jejunal feedings for longer than 6 months or in whom gastric access for decompression or medication instillation is not necessary.

17 **A.** (S&F, ch63)

This patient clearly has mild cholecystitis. Intravenous antibiotics are indicated because bile or gallbladder wall cultures are positive for bacteria in more than 40% of such patients. A cephalosporin, such as cefoxitin, is satisfactory for mildly ill patients. In cases of more severe illness, a combination of broad-spectrum antibiotics such as piperacillin-tazobactam or a third-generation cephalosporin and metronidazole are indicated. If gangrenous or emphysematous cholecystitis is suspected, an agent effective against anaerobic organisms should be included.

18 **E.** (S&F, ch67)

Sepsis can be prevented by not overdistending the gallbladder during percutaneous cholecystostomy (PC) catheter placement. PC has a success rate of between 95% and 100% and a complication rate of 8%. Bile peritonitis occurs only after a cholecystostomy catheter is inadvertently dislodged. Locking the pigtail catheter is advocated to prevent this complication. PC has gained popularity in the treatment of debilitated or severely ill patients with acalculous cholecystitis.

19 **D.** (S&F, ch65)

Primary sclerosing cholangitis (PSC) is associated with several complications. Bone mineral density is significantly lower in patients with PSC, independent of inflammatory bowel disease. These patients should be screened for osteoporosis. Cholangiocarcinoma is present in 7% to 36% of patients undergoing liver transplantation for PSC, but the sensitivity and specificity of CA 19-9 for diagnosing cholangiocarcinoma is variable. An optimal screening strategy for this malignancy has not yet been devised. PSC increases the already elevated risk for colon cancer in patients with ulcerative colitis. Screening with colonoscopy should begin immediately after PSC is diagnosed. Although bacterial cholangitis can complicate PSC and may hasten the need for liver transplant, long-term antibiotic prophylaxis is indicated in patients with recurring cholangitis. Finally, ursodeoxycholic acid at this dose is not effective for PSC, and the gallstones formed in PSC are primarily pigmented stones.

20 **B.** (S&F, ch17)

Anorexia nervosa and bulimia nervosa most commonly have their onset in adolescence. Binge eating disorder usually manifests in the third decade of life. Although eating disorders may develop at any time, they appear to be occurring more frequently in middle aged and older women. Eating disorders are much more common in female than in male patients.

21 **D.** (S&F, ch15)

Whole body glucose production decreases by more than half during the first few days of starvation (1 to 14 days of fasting) because of a marked reduction in hepatic glucose output.

The other answers are true regarding the metabolic response to long-term starvation (14 to 60 days).

22 **C.** (S&F, ch63)

This patient has a gallstone ileus with typical symptoms of mechanical intestinal obstruction, including abdominal pain and distention and vomiting. In most patients with this disorder, abdominal radiographs reveal an intestinal gas pattern compatible with intestinal obstruction. As the gallstone passes down the length of the gut, it obstructs the intestinal lumen intermittently. Characteristically, complete obstruction occurs in the ileum where the lumen is narrowest.

23 **A.** (S&F, ch17)

Because of lack of data, no pharmacologic agents currently can be recommended to promote weight gain in patients with anorexia nervosa. Risperidone has not been tested in randomized, controlled trials in this patient population. Cyproheptadine is associated with increased symptoms in patients with binge-purge anorexia nervosa. The safety and efficacy of zinc gluconate for long-term outpatient usage have not been established.

24 **B.** (S&F, ch67)

If an extrahepatic bile leak is detected, placing a stent across the disrupted duct will divert bile from the site of the injury and allow the injury to heal. Alternatively, bile leaks may be treated by diversion of bile via a percutaneous transhepatic drainage catheter. If the fistula does not resolve following simple biliary diversion, transcatheter occlusion techniques (e.g., sclerosis with tetracycline) may be used to close the leak.

25 **A.** (S&F, ch18)

Pancreatic cancer is associated with the greatest increase in obesity-related relative risk in men and women. Obese patients have an increased risk for the other cancers as well.

26 **C.** (S&F, ch61)

In patients with inherited disorders of bile acid conjugation, fat-soluble vitamin deficiency and steatorrhea develop. One would not expect vitamin B_{12} deficiency, fluid overload, or ascites.

27 **D.** (S&F, ch63)

This patient has a benign bile duct stricture from a surgical clip placed on the common bile duct.

Some such cases may be managed with ERCP and placement of a plastic biliary stent; however, of the options listed here, surgery is the best option. Several surgical approaches have been successful, but the best results occur with either resection of the stricture and an end-to-side Roux-en-Y choledochojejunostomy or hepaticojejunostomy.

28 **D.** (S&F, ch17)

Family therapy has emerged as the treatment of choice for patients with anorexia nervosa, especially those 19 or younger and those with a recent diagnosis. The other forms of psychotherapy are all legitimate and valuable as well.

29 **D.** (S&F, ch67)

This patient has cholangitis and requires immediate biliary decompression. Either PTBD or ERCP could be performed for nonsurgical biliary drainage. In this case, given the possible difficulty of reaching the choledochojejunostomy via ERCP, PTBD would be the treatment of choice.

30 **A.** (S&F, ch19)

Exclusive breast-feeding promotes the development of tolerance to oral antigens and may prevent the development of food allergy and atopic dermatitis. Breast milk contains S-IgA, which does provide protection. Evidence is accumulating that breast milk does affect infant immunity.

31 **C.** (S&F, ch60)

Patients with type III sphincter of Oddi dysfunction (SOD) have biliary-type pain without bile duct dilatation or abnormal liver enzymes. The response rate to sphincterotomy is less than 10% when the results of biliary manometry are normal and 55% to 60% when the results are abnormal. Therefore, biliary manometry should be performed prior to sphincterotomy in this case.

32 **D.** (S&F, ch67)

MRCP is a sensitive and specific noninvasive test for biliary obstruction. Were endoscopic ultrasound a choice, it would also be an excellent diagnostic option.

33 **D.** (S&F, ch19)

Of these choices, only dietary protein-induced enteropathy will resolve with elimination of milk. Dietary protein-induced enterocolitis syndrome manifests as vomiting and diarrhea without dehydration or fat malabsorption. Infants with dietary protein-induced enterocolitis proctocolitis appear healthy and have blood in their stool without diarrhea. Celiac disease may present in a similar manner, but it resolves only after gluten is withdrawn from the diet.

34 **D.** (S&F, ch59)

Biliary atresia is characterized by the complete obstruction of bile flow as a result of the destruction or absence of all or a portion of the extrahepatic bile ducts.

Laboratory studies initially reveal evidence of cholestasis, with a serum bilirubin level of 6 to 12 mg/dL, at least 50% of which is conjugated. Serum aminotransferase and alkaline phosphatase levels are moderately elevated. Serum gamma-glutamyl transpeptidase and 5′ nucleotidase levels also are elevated.

Histopathologic findings on initial liver biopsy specimens are of great importance in the management of patients with biliary atresia. Early in the course, hepatic architecture is generally preserved with a variable degree of bile duct

proliferation, canalicular and cellular bile stasis, and portal tract edema and fibrosis (see figure). The presence of bile plugs in portal triads is highly suggestive of large-duct obstruction. Bile duct epithelium shows varying degrees of injury, including swelling, vacuolization, and even sloughing of cells into the lumen. Portal tracts may be infiltrated with inflammatory cells, and in approximately 25% of patients, there may be giant cell transformation of hepatocytes to a degree more commonly observed in neonatal hepatitis. Bile ductules occasionally may assume a ductal plate configuration, suggesting that the disease process has interfered with the ductular remodeling that occurs during prenatal development. Biliary cirrhosis may be present initially or evolve rapidly over the first months of life, whether or not bile flow is successfully restored.

35 **D.** (S&F, ch19)

Celiac disease is strongly associated with HLA-DQ2, which is present in 90% of individuals with celiac disease. An extensive lymphocytic infiltrate is associated with sensitivity to gliadin, the alcohol-soluble portion of gluten, which is found in wheat, rye, barley, and perhaps oats. IgA

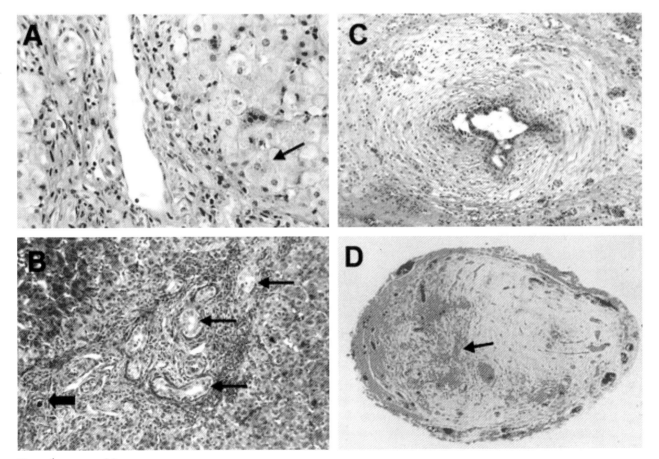

Figure for answer **34**

antibodies specific for celiac disease are present in more than 80% of adults and children with untreated celiac disease.

36 **D.** (S&F, ch67)

The image shows an anastamotic stricture that is 1.5 cm long and 2 mm in diameter. This is the result of technical complications or postoperative scarring. The differential diagnosis of post-transplant nonanastomotic strictures includes chronic graft rejection, ischemia, or cytomegalovirus (CMV) infection.

37 **D.** (S&F, ch16)

Energy requirements can be calculated using a variety of mathematical equations that incorporate measurements such as body surface area, body weight, body height, and the age of the patient. The most commonly used equation for calculating energy needs is the Harris-Benedict equation. The calculation for men or women is as follows:

Men:
Energy need in kilocalories/24 hours
$= 66 + (13.7 \times W) + (5 \times L) - (6.8 \times A)$

Women:
Energy need in kilocalories/24 hours
$= 655 + (9.6 \times W) + (1.7 \times L) - (4.7 \times A)$

where:
   W = weight in kilograms (kg),
   A = age in years, and
   L = height in centimeters (cm).

For patients, the calculated energy need is often increased by a "stress factor" of 10% for those with mild disease, 25% for those with moderate disease, and 50% for those with severe disease. In this case, the patient's baseline caloric need, calculated using the Harris-Benedict equation for a woman of her weight, age, and height, is 1858 kcal/day. Given the severity of this patient's condition, a stress factor of 0.5 (50%) should be used, adding 929 kcal/day to her energy need, for a total energy need of 2787 kcal/day.

38 **A.** (S&F, ch65)

Although this stricture could have been caused by cholangiocarcinoma, the more likely diagnosis is dominant stricture complicating primary sclerosing cholangitis. This complication should be suspected when patients develop worsening jaundice or pruritus, cholangitis, or abdominal pain. Dilation of strictures in these cases can improve clinical signs and symptoms, liver enzymes, and possibly slow the progression of disease and prolong survival.

39 **A.** (S&F, ch59)

Spontaneous perforation of the common bile duct is rare but can occur during infancy. The perforation usually occurs at the junction of the cystic and common ducts. The cause is unknown, but in some cases there is evidence of obstruction, secondary to stenosis or inspissated bile, at the distal end of the common bile duct. Congenital weakness and injury due to infection have also been implicated in some cases.

40 **D.** (S&F, ch19)

Gastrointestinal anaphylaxis is a relatively common form of IgE-mediated hypersensitivity. This generally occurs within minutes to 2 hours of an allergic reaction. Celiac disease, dietary protein–induced enterocolitis syndrome, and dietary protein–induced eosinophilic proctocolitis are examples of non–IgE-mediated food-induced gastrointestinal hypersensitivity disorders. Laboratory tests to detect IgE antibodies that are present in various foods are widely available, but such tests cannot identify the responsible food in non–IgE-mediated food-induced gastrointestinal hypersensitivity.

41 **C.** (S&F, ch65)

It is important to differentiate secondary sclerosing cholangitis from primary (idiopathic) sclerosing cholangitis (PSC). HIV cholangiopathy, cholangiocarcinoma, hepatic artery injury or occlusion, and choledocholithiasis can all cause secondary sclerosing cholangitis. Although it is a type of cholestatic liver disease, primary biliary cirrhosis does not cause the distinctive macroscopic changes to the biliary tree seen with PSC. Cirrhosis often causes attenuation or "pruning" of the biliary tree without the ductal irregularity or structuring seen in PSC.

42 **D.** (S&F, ch62)

TPN is associated with cholelithiasis, cholecystitis, and acalculous cholecystitis. Up to 45% of adults and 43% of children who receive TPN for 4 months will develop cholelithiasis. The incidence of gallbladder sludge among patients receiving TPN is even higher, and sludge may develop within 3 weeks of starting TPN. The primary problem seems to be gallbladder hypomotility and bile stasis from prolonged fasting. There may also be preferential flow of bile into the gallbladder due to failure of the sphincter of Oddi to relax.

43 **C.** (S&F, ch59)

The hallmark of Alagille's syndrome is a paucity of interlobular bile ducts. Paucity may be defined as a significantly decreased ratio (less than 0.4) of the numbers of interlobular portal bile ducts to portal tracts. The histologic features of liver biopsy specimens from patients with Alagille's syndrome presenting during the first months of life may overlap with those of neonatal hepatitis in that specimens in both cases may show evidence of ballooning of hepatocytes, variable cholestasis, portal inflammation, and giant cell transformation. Often, the number of interlobular bile ducts is not decreased in the initial liver biopsy specimen. However, there may be evidence of bile duct injury consisting of cellular infiltration of portal triads contiguous to interlobular bile ducts, lymphocytic infiltration and pyknosis of biliary epithelium, and periductal fibrosis. Serial biopsies of an individual patient may show bile duct proliferation initially, followed by a paucity of bile ducts, with a paucity of interlobular bile ducts usually becoming apparent by 3 months after diagnosis. There may also be mild periportal fibrosis, but progression to cirrhosis is uncommon. The extrahepatic bile ducts are patent but usually narrowed or hypoplastic.

44 **D.** (S&F, ch17)

Eating disorders carry the highest mortality risk of any psychiatric illness; the risk is equal to that of substance abuse.

45 **C.** (S&F, ch60)

Using the Modified Milwaukee Classification, the patient meets the criteria for Type I sphincter of Oddi dysfunction (SOD) in that she has biliary-type pain, AST elevation greater than 2 times normal on at least two occasions, and a bile duct dilated to more than 12 mm. Of patients with Type I SOD, 86% have an elevated basal sphincter of Oddi pressure. Because at least 90% of such patients have a favorable clinical response to endoscopic sphincterotomy, no further diagnostic studies or therapeutic trials are necessary. Furthermore, because the response rate is independent of the results of biliary manometry, this test poses more risk (pancreatitis) than benefit.

46 **C.** (S&F, ch59)

Acute noncalculous, noninflammatory distention of the gallbladder may occur in infants and children. The gallbladder is not acutely inflamed, and cultures of the bile are usually sterile. The absence of gallbladder inflammation is what distinguishes acute hydrops from acute cholecystitis. Acute hydrops has been associated with Kawasaki's disease and Henoch-Schönlein purpura. Patients present with acute onset of crampy abdominal pain and, often, nausea and vomiting. The right upper quadrant is usually tender and the gallbladder may be palpable. Ultrasonography reveals an enlarged, distended gallbladder without calculi.

Gallbladder hydrops often responds to nonsurgical treatment; with supportive care and management of the incurrent illness, the prognosis for return of normal gallbladder function is excellent.

47 **D.** (S&F, ch60)

Numerous medications have been studied with respect to their affect on the sphincter of Oddi (SO), and this has implications for the patient undergoing sphincter of Oddi manometry. Narcotics, such as morphine, stimulate the SO and raise the basal pressure. The exception is meperidine, which does not affect SO pressure when used at a moderate dose (1 mg/kg). Calcium channel blockers such as verapamil relax the SO. Diazepam does not affect SO pressure, but midazolam may lower basal pressure in hypertensive sphincters and should be avoided when performing biliary manometry.

48 **C.** (S&F, ch62)

Cholangitis due to purulent material under pressure in the biliary tree is the most rapidly fatal complication of gallstone disease. Infection can quickly spread to the bloodstream and cause septicemia. Early diagnosis and prompt treatment are essential.

49 **B.** (S&F, ch61)

The volume of bile secreted by the liver each day ranges from 500 mL to 600 mL. The predominant organic components are bile acids. Bile acids are almost completely re-absorbed by the terminal ileum and returned via the portal circulation to the liver.

50 **D.** (S&F, ch59)

The infantile form of choledochal cyst disease must be distinguished from other forms of hepatobiliary disease of the neonate, particularly biliary atresia. Disease often appears during the first months of life, and as many as 80% of patients have cholestatic jaundice and acholic stools. Vomiting, irritability, and failure to thrive may occur. Examination reveals hepatomegaly and, in approximately half of patients there is a palpable abdominal mass. In a series of 72 patients in whom a cyst was diagnosed postnatally, 50 (69%) were jaundiced; jaundice was associated with abdominal pain in 25 or a palpable mass in 3. Of the remaining 22, 13

(18% of the 72) had abdominal pain alone and 2 (3%) had an isolated palpable mass. Spontaneous perforation of a choledochal cyst may occur, particularly when bile flow is obstructed. Progressive hepatic injury can occur during the first months of life as a result of biliary obstruction (see figure).

The diagnosis of a choledochal cyst is best established by ultrasonography (see figure in which the arrow points to a type I choledochal cyst off the common bile duct of an infant).

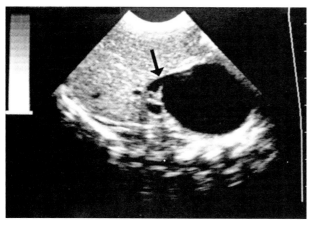

Figure for answer **50**

51 **B.** (S&F, ch61)

Cholecystectomy restores the normal rhythm of bile secretion. Bile acids are stored in the proximal small intestine and following a meal, intestinal contractions propel the stored bile acids to the distal small intestine where they are actively reabsorbed.

52 **B.** (S&F, ch16)

There has recently been an emphasis on evaluating a patient's weight and body habitus using the body mass index (BMI), defined as weight/height^2 in kg/m^2. The BMI is used to help categorize patients as underweight, ideal weight, overweight, obese, or super obese as follows:

BMI < 18	Underweight
BMI 18–26.5	Ideal weight
BMI 26.5–30	Overweight
BMI 30–40	Obese
BMI > 40	Super obese

53 **B.** (S&F, ch59)

Nonobstructive saccular or fusiform dilatation of the intrahepatic bile ducts is a rare, congenital disorder. In the pure form, known as Caroli's disease, dilatation is classically segmental and

saccular and associated with stone formation and recurrent bacterial cholangitis. A more common type, Caroli's syndrome, is associated with a portal tract lesion typical of congenital hepatic fibrosis. Dilatation of the extrahepatic bile ducts (choledochal cysts) also may be present. Renal disease occurs in both forms. Renal tubular ectasia occurs with the simple form, and both conditions can be associated with autosomal recessive polycystic renal disease or, rarely, autosomal dominant polycystic renal disease.

There may be mild to moderate elevations of serum bilirubin, alkaline phosphatase, and aminotransferase levels. Liver function may be normal initially, but repeated episodes of infection and biliary obstruction within the cystic bile ducts eventually may lead to hepatic failure. Inability to concentrate urine is the most frequent abnormality of renal function; variable elevations of blood urea nitrogen and serum creatinine levels reflect the severity of the underlying kidney disease.

Ultrasonography, MRI cholangiography, and computed tomography are of great value in demonstrating intrahepatic cystic dilatation. Renal cysts or hyperechogenicity of papillae may be detected. Cholangiography usually demonstrates a normal common duct with segmental, saccular dilatations of the intrahepatic bile ducts. Rarely, the process may be limited to one lobe of the liver.

54 **B.** (S&F, ch62)

Gallstone disease is the most common gastrointestinal disorder requiring hospitalization. The considerable cost of treating this disease justifies research into its pathophysiology and prevention.

55 **D.** (S&F, ch65)

The etiology and pathogenesis of PSC is poorly understood. Genetic factors have been studied and a variety of HLA haplotypes are found more often in patients with PSC compared to the general population. Similarly, at least one haplotype (DQ6) is associated with a reduced risk of disease progression. Infectious and toxic agents have been proposed to play an important role in the pathogenesis of PSC, but opportunistic infections such as *Cryptosporidium* and Cytomegalovirus have only been isolated from patients with AIDS cholangiopathy. Although hepatic artery injury can cause secondary sclerosing cholangitis, thromboses in patients with PSC have not been described. Finally, pANCA and numerous other antibodies have been identified in those with PSC. However, these antibodies are not specific for PSC and it is not clear whether they are involved in an immune-mediated mechanism or are an epiphenomenon.

56 **A.** (S&F, ch18)

Physical activity has many benefits including the prevention of obesity-related complications as well as successful management and maintenance of long-term weight loss. Unfortunately physical activity alone does not cause a significant increase in initial weight loss. Calorie restriction is required for this to occur.

57 **E.** (S&F, ch59)

Primary sclerosing cholangitis (PSC) is an uncommon, chronic, progressive disease of the biliary tract characterized by inflammation and fibrosis of the intrahepatic and extrahepatic biliary ductal systems leading to biliary cirrhosis. In adults, carcinoma of the bile ducts also must be excluded; however, this complication has not been reported in children. PSC is associated with inflammatory bowel disease (most often, ulcerative colitis) in 70% of adults and 50% to 80% of children with the disorder. A male preponderance has been reported in some, but not all, large series of children with PSC.

Inflammatory bowel disease–associated PSC most often occurs with ulcerative colitis, although cases have been reported in patients with Crohn's disease. The bowel symptoms can precede, occur simultaneously with, or appear years after the diagnosis of PSC. As in adults, treatment of the bowel disease in infants, including colectomy, does not influence the progression of PSC.

The prognosis of PSC in children is guarded. The clinical course of the disorder is variable but usually progressive. Analysis of survival factors at presentation indicates that older age, splenomegaly, and prolonged prothrombin time predict a poor outcome. The occurrence of jaundice after the neonatal period with a persistent serum bilirubin level of more than five times the upper limit of normal also was associated with a poor outcome. Hepato-cellular carcinoma also may occur, but cholangiocarcinoma, an important complication of adult PSC, has not been reported in children.

58 **A.** (S&F, ch62)

Octreotide, a somatostatin analog, increases the incidence of gallstones. Decreased gallbladder motility and bile stasis are the most likely

explanations. If anything, octreotide increases cholesterol secretion.

59 **C.** (S&F, ch17)

Patients with bulimia nervosa or binge eating disorder often have no abnormalities on physical examination and a normal or even high body weight. Patients with these disorders tend to avoid, not seek, medical care. Patients with anorexia nervosa frequently deny the seriousness of their medical condition and, by definition, are underweight.

60 **D.** (S&F, ch62)

This third-generation cephalosporin is largely excreted, unmetabolized, into the bile. When the drug's concentration in the bile exceeds saturation level, the drug complexes with calcium to form an insoluble salt. This "sludge" usually disappears after ceftriaxone treatment is stopped.

61 **A.** (S&F, ch59)

Black-pigmented gallstones are common in patients who have chronic hemolytic disorders. The stones are composed predominantly of calcium bilirubinate, with substantial amounts of crystalline calcium carbonate and phosphate. In those with sickle cell disease, the risk of gallstones increases with age; stones are diagnosed in at least 14% of children younger than 10 years of age and 36% of those between ages 10 and 20 years.

62 **E.** (S&F, ch16)

Zinc deficiency can result in a characteristic skin rash (acrodermatitis), poor wound healing, impaired or abnormal taste, glucose intolerance, alopecia, depression, and diarrhea.

63 **B.** (S&F, ch15)

Absorption of vitamin B_{12} tends to decrease with aging with concomitant increase in the prevalence of atrophic gastritis and consequent decrease of intrinsic factor.

64 **D.** (S&F, ch62)

A "porcelain" gallbladder (one that contains intramural calcifications that appear on imaging studies, including plain films of the abdomen and CT scans) is associated with a risk for gallbladder cancer approaching 20%. Prophylactic cholecystectomy is indicated in these cases to prevent the development of cancer.

65 **B.** (S&F, ch63)

Patient selection for oral dissolution therapy is a function of the stage of gallstone disease, gallbladder function, and the characteristics of the stone(s). Although oral dissolution therapy has been effective for stones up to 10 mm in diameter, results are superior for stones less than 5 mm in diameter.

66 **D.** (S&F, ch16)

Percutaneous endoscopic gastrostomy (PEG) was developed by Ponsky and Gauderer in the early 1980s. The procedure involves percutaneous placement of a gastrostomy tube, with the appropriate site for placement being chosen by endoscopic transillumination of the abdominal wall. The PEG tube may be placed by either the Sachs-Vine (push) or Ponsky (pull) technique. Prospective studies of PEG have found this procedure to be associated with few procedure-related complications.

The most common complication is peristomal wound infection, which is usually treated by oral administration for 7 days of an antibiotic, such as cephalexin, with activity against microorganisms that typically colonize the skin.

Other complications are rare. They include hematoma, peritonitis, gastric or colonic perforation, and fistula—hepatogastric, gastrocolic, or colocutaneous.

67 **B.** (S&F, ch63)

Acalculous cholecystitis usually occurs in patients hospitalized for serious illnesses such as trauma, burns, or major surgery. Outpatients at highest risk are elderly male patients with peripheral vascular disease. Sludge is generally present in the gallbladder and may obstruct the cystic duct. More often than with acute cholecystitis due to the presence of gallstones, acalculous cholecystitis may be complicated by gangrene and perforation.

68 **A.** (S&F, ch17)

Assessment of the appropriateness of weight for height is the most important initial assessment in a patient with a serious eating disorder, because the result helps determine the urgency of medical and psychiatric care. Patients who are dangerously underweight for their height may have normal serum chemistry profiles and electrocardiograms, and they cannot be relied upon to provide an accurate dietary history, nor can their friends and relatives provide an accurate history because patients may go to extreme lengths to deceive others into believing they are eating more than they do.

69 **A.** (S&F, ch59)

Ultrasonography can be used to assess the size and echogenicity of the liver. Even in neonates, high-frequency, real-time ultrasonography usually can outline the gallbladder so that its size and contours can be estimated. Ultrasound may also reveal stones and sludge in the bile ducts and gallbladder and cystic or obstructive dilatation of the biliary system. Extrahepatic anomalies also may be identified. The outline of a triangle 3 mm or greater in thickness, of a cone-shaped fibrotic mass cranial to the portal vein may be diagnostic of biliary atresia. The "ghost" triad of gallbladder length less than 1.9 cm, lack of a smooth (complete echogenic) mucosal lining, and an indistinct wall and irregular or lobular contour of the gallbladder on ultrasonography has also been proposed as diagnostic for biliary atresia.

70 **A.** (S&F, ch62)

Black-pigmented stones form in the gallbladder as a result of increased production of unconjugated bilirubin, which then precipitates and forms stones of calcium bilirubinate.

Chronic biliary infection is associated with formation of brown-pigmented stones. Brown stones may form anywhere in the biliary tree and are associated with bacterial colonization of bile and cholangitis.

71 **C.** (S&F, ch64)

This patient has acalculous biliary pain. Most patients with cholesterol crystals (cholesterol microlithiasis, as shown in the figure) will have evidence of cholecystitis at the time of surgery and will become symptom-free after cholecystectomy. If cholesterol crystals are seen in the bile aspirate, stimulated cholescintigraphy is unnecessary. Unless the patient is a poor surgical candidate, a trial of dissolution therapy is not warranted. ERCP with sphincter of Oddi manometry carries a risk of pancreatitis and is not indicated in this patient with an intact gallbladder and cholesterol crystals.

72 **B.** (S&F, ch18)

Very-low-calorie diets can result in long-term weight loss, and they can lead to more rapid weight loss than standard low-calorie diets. However, very-low-calorie diets pose significantly higher risk of medical complications, including gallstones.

73 **A.** (S&F, ch64)

Acalculous cholecystitis typically occurs in patients hospitalized in an intensive care unit with severe illness involving hemodynamic compromise and lack of oral nutrition. Fasting results in concentration of bile acids within the gallbladder due to the absence of cholecystokinin-stimulated gallbladder contraction (chemical injury), and splanchnic vasoconstriction occurs due to hemodynamic compromise (ischemic injury). Classic symptoms of cholecystitis, such as abdominal pain, may be absent initially in up to 75% of patients. Ultrasound, CT scan, and hepatobiliary scintigraphy have all been used to establish this diagnosis.

74 **B.** (S&F, ch67)

A small, contained retroduodenal perforation is best managed nonoperatively with nasogastric suctioning and antibiotics. If a "free" perforation is present, endoscopic stent placement or surgical repair should be considered.

75 **A.** (S&F, ch63)

The most likely cause of pancreatitis in this case is gallstones, which was confirmed by the ultrasound. For most patients with gallstone pancreatitis cholecystectomy may be performed safely during the initial hospitalization once the clinical signs of pancreatitis have resolved. Usually cholecystectomy can be performed laparoscopically. When surgery is delayed, up to half of patients have further episodes of pancreatitis.

76 **C.** (S&F, ch64)

Cholesterolosis is more common in women, although the gender difference is not as striking as it is for cholesterol stone disease. Cholesterolosis and cholesterol stones occur independently, although they can occur together. Cholesterolosis is present in 5% to 40% of autopsy specimens, typically as an incidental finding. No ethnic difference in prevalence has been demonstrated.

77 **D.** (S&F, ch65)

Primary sclerosing cholangitis (PSC) occurs as a complication of inflammatory bowel disease in 2.4% to 4.0% of patients with ulcerative colitis and 1.4% to 3.4% of patients with Crohn's disease. When patients with one of these disorders is found to have liver enzyme levels indicative of PSC, cholangiography should be performed. The biliary tree is often not dilated in patients with PSC, and the absence of dilatation

on ultrasound and computed tomography does not exclude the diagnosis. Cholangiography can be accomplished with ERCP or MRCP, the latter not being offered as an option in this question.

78 **A.** (S&F, ch16)

Vitamin B_{12} belongs to a group of compounds called corrinoids, which contain a cobalt atom in the center of four pyrrole rings with various side-chain attachments. Cyanocobalamin is the most common, commercially available form. Animal products are the only source of vitamin B_{12} for humans. Ingested cobalamin is liberated from proteins in the stomach by the action of pepsin and becomes bound to factors known as R-binders. In the small intestine, pancreatic enzymes cleave vitamin B_{12} from R-binders and facilitate the attachment of vitamin B_{12} to intrinsic factor (IF). In the distal ileum, the IF-B_{12} complex disassociates and the B_{12} molecule is absorbed and transported by specific proteins to the liver. Vitamin B_{12} is excreted in the bile. Although a vegan diet does not provide sufficient vitamin B_{12}, most cases of deficiency result from intrinsic factor deficiency, bacterial overgrowth, pancreatic insufficiency, distal ileal disease, or another disorder that impairs absorption of vitamin B_{12}. Deficiency usually manifests as megaloblastic anemia or peripheral neuropathy.

79 **E.** (S&F, ch62)

In patient's with suspected biliary colic, transabdominal ultrasonography should generally be the first imaging study performed. Transabdominal ultrasonography is a rapid, noninvasive, sensitive, and specific means of establishing the presence or absence of stones in the gallbladder. It is also relatively inexpensive and the equipment is portable, allowing examinations to be performed in a variety of outpatient settings.

80 **D.** (S&F, ch65)

Several validated prognostic models for PSC are available. Many are mathematically complex and some require invasive testing such as cholangiography or liver biopsy. The Mayo risk score, currently the most widely used, calculates the patient's prognosis based on age, serum bilirubin level, serum AST level, serum albumin level, and a history of variceal bleeding. When followed for a median of 6.25 years, 31% of asymptomatic patients with PSC developed liver failure and either died or underwent transplantation. A clinically useful model for PSC identifies 4 stages of disease: asymptomatic, biochemical, symptomatic, and decompensated cirrhosis. Small-duct PSC, although it progresses to classic PSC in a small percentage of cases, is associated with a better prognosis than classic PSC.

81 **B.** (S&F, ch64)

Adenomyomatosis is a hyperplastic condition of the gallbladder that is not associated with adenomas. Rarely, it causes biliary colic or pancreatitis, and the associated risk for gallbladder cancer appears to be very low. Surgery is a consideration for segmental adenomyomatosis (in which there may be a higher risk for cancer) and when biliary symptoms are present.

82 **D.** (S&F, ch17)

Of medications with established efficacy in treating bulimia nervosa, only fluoxetine has FDA approval for this indication. Desipramine may improve eating habits but is not well-tolerated in this population. Trazodone has not been adequately studied for its effects in patients with bulimia nervosa. Most of the studies of naltrexone for bulimia nervosa showed no benefit.

83 **B.** (S&F, ch63)

It has been thought that diabetic persons are more prone to develop gallstones, more likely to have complications from the stones, and more likely to have complications or die after emergency operations for complications of gallstone disease. These perceptions have not been borne out, however, when confounding variables, such as hyperlipidemia, obesity, cardiovascular disease, and chronic kidney disease are taken into account. Therefore, although prophylactic cholecystectomy does not appear warranted for an asymptomatic diabetic patient with gallstones, early intervention is indicated when symptoms develop, because such patients are at increased risk of developing gangrenous cholecystitis.

84 **A.** (S&F, ch65)

Hepaticojejunostomy and hepatectomy are both surgical options for management of recurrent pyogenic cholangitis (RPC). Surgery involving a biliary-enteric anastomosis carries a 31% risk for cholangitis. In patients presenting with focal, severe disease, hepatectomy is an option. Often, the left lobe is more involved than the right. Extrahepatic bile duct disease can be managed as effectively by ERCP as by surgery. Finally, liver transplantation is an option when RPC progresses to decompensated biliary cirrhosis.

85 **D.** (S&F, ch15)

Weight loss and marked depletion of subcutaneous fat and muscle are clinical signs associated with marasmus. Children with kwashiorkor have peripheral edema and a protuberant abdomen due to weakened abdominal muscles, intestinal distention, and hepatomegaly.

86 **C.** (S&F, ch62)

Although eliciting a Murphy sign during ultrasonography depends somewhat on the skill of the ultrasonographer, the sign has a positive predictive value of greater than 90% for acute cholecystitis if gallstones are present. The specificity of this sign is greater than a finding of gallbladder wall thickening and pericholecystic fluid, which are nonspecific for cholecystitis.

87 **B.** (S&F, ch63)

Indications for cholecystectomy during pregnancy include complicated gallstone disease, such as acute cholecystitis and pancreatitis, and inability of the mother to maintain adequate nutrition as a result of gallbladder disease. Surgery poses the lowest risk to fetus and mother during the second trimester.

88 **B.** (S&F, ch66)

Radical cholecystectomy for Stage II gallbladder cancer is associated with a 5-year survival rate of between 83% and 100%, compared to a rate of 35% to 40% for simple cholecystectomy. Radical cholecystectomy is also the surgical procedure of choice for many patients with T3 lesions. Simple cholecystectomy is adequate for resection of Stage I gallbladder cancer with a survival of rate of nearly 100%. Patients with advanced gallbladder cancer who have had palliative surgery or biopsy alone should be offered radiation therapy, as it is associated with longer survival.

89 **C.** (S&F, ch62)

Endoscopic ultrasound (EUS) allows visualization of the common bile duct (CBD) from inside the gastrointestinal lumen. This gives EUS a significant advantage over transabdominal ultrasonography in evaluating the CBD. EUS has been shown in several studies to be superior to MRCP.

90 **A.** (S&F, ch67)

The laboratory and imaging studies indicate that a stone is obstructing the CBD. Because it is the least invasive procedure for viewing and concurrently removing the stone, ERCP is preferred over a percutaneous approach or cholecystectomy. Endoscopic ultrasound and MRI cholangiography have no therapeutic benefit; furthermore, MRI is contraindicated in any patient with a pacemaker or defibrillator.

91 **D.** (S&F, ch65)

Although most histologic findings are not diagnostic for primary sclerosing cholangitis (PSC), the fibro-obliterative process leading to the "onion skin" appearance of the biopsy specimen (see figure) is characteristic of PSC. Also characteristic is the presentation with a history of intermittent fever and chills and physical findings of excoriations and xanthomata. The biochemical hallmark of PSC, chronic elevation of alkaline phosphatase, is present in at least 94% of patients. Nonspecific immunologic markers may also be present, such as IgM, anti-nuclear antibody, and anti-smooth muscle antibody, but these are not useful for diagnosis or prognosis.

92 **D.** (S&F, ch15)

Histidine, phenylalanine, and lysine are the essential amino acids because their carbon skeletons cannot be synthesized by the body. The other amino acids listed are nonessential because they can be synthesized from other proteins.

93 **D.** (S&F, ch67)

The risk of bile leak may be greater with a transcholecystic approach. The percutaneous puncture is through the 10th or 11th intercostal space to decrease the risk of pleural complications such as pneumothorax. The biliary tree can be successfully visualized in 99% of patients with dilated bile ducts and 40% to 90% of those with nondilated bile ducts. The overall rate of serious complications is 2% to 4%.

94 **D.** (S&F, ch18)

Melanocortin-4 receptor mutations are the most common of all monogenic causes of obesity and can be found in up to 5% of patients with obesity. The vast majority of obese persons, however, do not have a single gene mutation. Human obesity may involve multiple gene interactions.

95 **D.** (S&F, ch65)

This patient has recurrent pyogenic cholangitis (RPC). The leading theory links biliary infection with the parasites *Clonorchis sinenis*, *Opistorchis sp.*, and *Ascaris lumbricoides*. These infections are endemic in the regions with the highest incidence of this disorder, and ova have been cultured from biliary stones, bile, and stool. Patients with RPC may lack an inhibitor of bacterial glucuronidase, an enzyme that deconjugates bilirubin and thereby promotes formation of calcium bilirubinate stones. Cross-reactivity of antibodies between colon and biliary epithelium may be seen in primary sclerosing cholangitis, a much less likely diagnosis in this case. Gallbladder motility disorders can cause biliary colic and predispose to gallstone formation. Prolonged fasting increases the risk for gallstone formation and acalculous cholecystitis.

96 **B.** (S&F, ch15)

Fat-soluble vitamins are absorbed through the lipophilic phase of intestinal digestion.

97 **E.** (S&F, ch67)

The risk of post-ERCP pancreatitis is increased in women, patients with sphincter of Oddi dysfunction, those with previous ERCP-associated pancreatitis, patients in whom the pancreatic duct is filled excessively with contrast dye, and those in whom a pre-cut papillotomy is performed. Prophylactic use of somatostatin or gabexate mesilate may reduce the risk of pancreatitis; however, these agents are not used routinely because of controversy related to their efficacy, patient selection, ease of administration, and cost. In general, a duodenal diverticulum does not increase the risk of pancreatitis.

98 **D.** (S&F, ch16)

Refeeding syndrome is a common metabolic consequence of parenteral nutrition (PN). This syndrome results from sudden provision of a large amount of calories, especially carbohydrates, to a malnourished patient. When PN is started the metabolism of these patients rapidly becomes anabolic. As a result, insulin production is increased, which pushes potassium, phosphorus, and magnesium into intracellular compartments; this in turn leads to a decrease in serum levels of these electrolytes. Management of refeeding syndrome focuses on the close monitoring of electrolytes and adequate repletion as needed.

99 **E.** (S&F, ch64)

The ultrasound findings are consistent with an adenomatous polyp, although the findings may not be adequate for definitive diagnosis. Polyps within the gallbladder are an indication for cholecystectomy in a patient who is a good surgical candidate. Adenomas make up a small percentage of gallbladder polyps (~4%) but they do have malignant potential. Adenomyomatosis is far more common and very rarely leads to cancer. If an adenoma is less than 10 mm in diameter, the risk for malignancy is very low and surveillance is appropriate. However, when an adenoma is suspected or cannot be excluded, a cholecystectomy should be performed.

100 **B.** (S&F, ch66)

This CT scan shows a gallbladder cancer. The relationship between gallbladder cancer and gallstones is well established; at least 80% to 90% of patients with this malignancy have gallstones. Gallbladder cancer is 3 to 4 times more common in woman and occurs primarily in the elderly. Although up to 30% of patients with gallbladder cancer present with jaundice, abdominal pain is the most common symptom and occurs in more than 80% of patients with gallbladder cancer.

101 **B.** (S&F, ch15)

PEM affects every organ system except the brain, which is largely spared from any atrophy.

Topics Involving Multiple Organs

QUESTIONS

102 A 64-year-old white man is transferred from another hospital with severe diarrhea, abdominal pain, weight loss, electrolyte disorder, and malnutrition. On physical examination, he appears well developed and well nourished, and his vital signs are stable, but mucous membranes are dry. He states that he was fine prior to the onset of symptoms 6 weeks ago and has never noticed gross blood in the stool. The most notable findings on physical examination include alopecia, onycholysis, and shedding of some of the nails. His wife has noticed increased pigmentation on the patient's upper arms and thighs. The patient's brother had colon cancer at the age of 70 years. The patient's medical records from the previous hospital indicate that he had upper and lower endoscopies that showed multiple gastric and colonic polyps; analysis of the multiple biopsy specimens that were taken indicated that these were hyperplastic in nature. The most likely diagnosis is:

A. Cowden's syndrome
B. Gardner's syndrome
C. Muir-Torre syndrome
D. Peutz-Jeghers syndrome
E. Cronkhite-Canada syndrome

103 All of the following statements concerning nodular regenerative hyperplasia of the liver are correct *except*:

A. It can be associated with immune-mediated disease such as systemic lupus erythematosus (SLE), scleroderma, sarcoidosis, and Felty's syndrome.

B. It can be associated with hematologic disease such as polycythemia vera, agnogenic myeloid metaplasia, or sickle cell disease.
C. It can be associated with azathioprine use.
D. It can progress to end-stage cirrhosis.
E. It can be associated with portal hypertension and variceal bleeding.

104 A 46-year-old, obese African-American woman is referred to gastrointestinal (GI) clinic for evaluation of recurrent abdominal pain and intermittently elevated transaminase levels. She has mild hypertension and asthma but is otherwise healthy. Her past medical history is significant for two cesarean sections and cholecystectomy, performed 6 years ago.

On exam, she appears comfortable and her vital signs are stable. She is pain free at present, but states that she is tired of making recurrent visits to the emergency department and wants something done. She has heard about endoscopic retrograde cholangiopancreatography (ERCP), but is afraid to undergo this procedure because two of her sisters with complaints similar to hers had undergone ERCP and subsequently were hospitalized for a long time with more abdominal pain. Her medical record indicates that studies have been performed to rule out viral and other causes of hepatitis; an ultrasound (US) of her abdomen and magnetic resonance imaging (MRI) with magnetic resonance cholangiopancreatography (MRCP) show dilation of the common bile duct (CBD) lumen to 8 mm but no other abnormalities. Her levels of aspartate aminotransaminase (AST) and alanine aminotransaminase (ALT) are about 2 to 2.5 times normal. Sphincter of Oddi dysfunction (SOD) is suspected. The best way to decrease the likelihood of complications in this patient is to:

A. Place her on ursodiol (Actigall, Urso) for 3 months and follow clinically to see how she responds
B. Proceed with ERCP, but use only cutting current at the time of sphincterotomy to decrease the likelihood of pancreatitis
C. Prescribe anticholinergics and follow clinically
D. Refer her to a surgeon for bile duct exploration
E. Proceed with ERCP with placement of a temporary pancreatic stent to decrease the likelihood of post-ERCP pancreatitis

105 Which of the following techniques is contraindicated in endoscopic management of food impaction?

A. Forceful blinded pushing
B. Using forceps to disrupt and debulk the bolus
C. Insufflation and distention of the esophageal lumen
D. Use of an overtube
E. None of the above

106 A consult is requested on a hospitalized 24-year-old white man with anemia and stools positive for occult blood. He had been admitted to the hospital because of a nonhealing ulcer over the left medial malleolus that had not improved after surgery for varicose veins on the left leg 3 years ago. Medical history is significant for recurrent ulcer over the left medial malleolus, and the patient's parents report that he walks with a limp. On physical examination, there are multiple varicose veins over the left lower limb. There is predominant left lower limb hypertrophy, with the left limb being longer and larger. X-ray shows distinct soft tissue and osteohypertrophy of the left lower limb. Duplex scan of the left lower limb shows massive superficial venous varicosities and multiple anastomoses between the superficial and deep venous systems. An angiogram shows multiple arteriovenous fistulas. The most likely diagnosis is:

A. Klippel-Trénaunay syndrome
B. Blue rubber bleb nevus syndrome
C. Parkes Weber syndrome
D. Diffuse intestinal hemangiomatosis
E. None of the above

107 For each of the following circumstances, answer this statement true or false: Antibiotic prophylaxis should be given before this gastrointestinal procedure:

A. A 57-year-old white man who is about to undergo esophageal stricture dilatation had his left hip replaced 2 years ago
B. A 49-year-old man with a history of alcohol abuse, recurrent pancreatitis, and pancreatic pseudocyst about to undergo ERCP and possible pseudocyst drainage
C. A 90-year-old nursing home patient transferred for percutaneous endoscopic gastrostomy (PEG) tube placement
D. A 45-year-old white woman with mitral valve prolapse (MVP) and a 10-year history of ulcerative colitis who takes antibiotics prior to dental procedures and is about to undergo surveillance colonoscopy
E. A 50-year-old African-American man who had a defibrillator placed 6 months ago and is now admitted with painless obstructive jaundice and is about to undergo ERCP

108 The value of 18 positron emission tomography with fluorodeoxyglucose (FDG-PET) in evaluation of a gastrointestinal stromal tumor (GIST) includes:

A. It can illuminate even 1-cm implants on the omentum, which are difficult to see with computed tomography (CT).
B. It can demonstrate cystic/necrotic centers in tumors, which are indicative of malignancy.
C. It can demonstrate liver metastases, which are usually isodense with normal parenchyma and can be missed by CT.
D. All of the above.

109 Which of the following statements about congenital diaphragmatic hernias is correct?

A. Bochdalek hernias occur on the left side of the diaphragm in 80% of cases and are diagnosed in childhood; Morgagni hernias occur on the right side of the diaphragm in 80% of cases and are diagnosed in adults.
B. Bochdalek hernias occur on the right side of the diaphragm in 80% of cases and are diagnosed in childhood; Morgagni hernias occur on the right side of the diaphragm in 80% of cases and are diagnosed in adults.
C. Bochdalek hernias occur on the right side of the diaphragm in 80% of cases and are diagnosed in adults; Morgagni hernias occur on the left side of the diaphragm in 80% of cases and are diagnosed in childhood.
D. Bochdalek hernias occur on the left side of the diaphragm in 80% of cases and are diagnosed in adults; Morgagni hernias occur on the right side of the diaphragm in 80% of cases and are diagnosed in childhood.

110 All of the following statements about diabetic diarrhea are correct *except*:

A. May be aggravated by metformin or acarbose
B. Unaffected by diabetic control
C. Responds to clonidine
D. Can be associated with steatorrhea
E. Can respond to octreotide

111 A 19-year-old woman presents with right upper quadrant (RUQ) pain and a temperature of 101°F. On physical exam, she has RUQ tenderness with guarding and shifting dullness. Diagnostic paracentesis reveals a white blood cell (WBC) count of $525 \times 10^3/\mu L$ with 78% neutrophils and a protein concentration of 7.0 g/dL. Laparoscopy is performed (see figure). Which of the following drugs should be initiated as treatment?

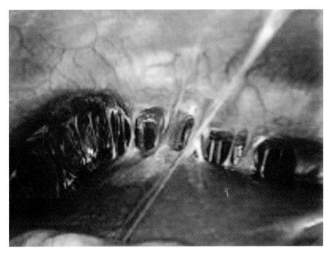

Figure for question **111**

A. Doxycycline
B. Rifampin
C. Vancomycin
D. Ganciclovir
E. Fluconazole

112 A 64-year-old woman with history of diverticulosis presents with left lower quadrant abdominal pain. A CT of the abdomen is performed and reveals a 1.2×2 cm abscess. The patient is admitted and started on intravenous (IV) antibiotics and her pain improves. A repeat CT is performed 4 days later, which reveals that the abscess is enlarging and now measures 4.0×4.2 cm. What is the next step in management of the patient?

A. Continue IV antibiotics and keep the patient on nothing by mouth.
B. Perform colonoscopy to evaluate the sigmoid colon.
C. Perform percutaneous drainage with catheter placement.
D. Perform surgical resection and debridement.
E. Perform percutaneous aspiration alone.

113 What is the most common hepatic abnormality in patients with sarcoid involvement of the liver?

A. Ultrasound showing heterogeneous echogenicity
B. Elevated bilirubin
C. Elevated alkaline phosphatase
D. Elevated AST and ALT

114 A 45-year-old African-American woman presents to the gastroenterologist's office with recurrent abdominal pain and intermittent elevation of liver enzymes. She underwent cholecystectomy 6 years ago, after the birth of her last child, because of gallstones. She describes the pain as being "similar to gallbladder pain." Results of a complete blood count (CBC) and prothrombin/partial thromboplastin (PT/PTT) are normal; AST is 70 U/L, ALT is 65 U/L, and alkaline phosphatase is 160 U/L. The results of MRI of the abdomen and MRCP show a CBD lumen diameter of 7 mm. The statement that describes the best course of action in this case is:

A. She probably has mild viral hepatitis, and blood samples should be sent to test for viral antigens.
B. She should be scheduled for a liver biopsy because she most likely has autoimmune hepatitis.
C. She has irritable bowel syndrome (IBS) and should be started on anticholinergics.
D. She should have a repeat imaging study to evaluate for cholangiocarcinoma.
E. If she undergoes ERCP, she has a high likelihood of developing post-ERCP pancreatitis.

115 Difficulty in establishing a specific food allergy as causative of eosinophilic gastroenteritis is due to all the following *except*:

A. Skin prick tests are sensitive, but food allergens used for testing must be fresh; otherwise false-negative results are likely.
B. Many of the allergens are not immunoglobulin E (IgE)–mediated.
C. The patient's subjective response to a food elimination diet makes its findings invalid.
D. Intradermal skin testing often yields false-positive results.

116 Ischemic bowel disease with bleeding or infarction can be found in which of the following systemic diseases:

A. Periarteritis nodosa
B. Mixed cryoglobulinemia
C. Systemic lupus erythematosus
D. Henoch-Schönlein purpura
E. **A** and **C**
F. **A**, **B**, **C**, and **D**

117 A 52-year-old Asian man presents to the emergency department with cramping lower abdominal pain and a low-grade fever 1 day after colonoscopy. He has passed flatus, but has not had any bowel movements after the colonoscopy; however, his main complaint is fever. His temperature is 100.6°F, but his other vital signs are normal. He has mild to moderate left lower quadrant (LLQ) abdominal tenderness. His WBC count is $12.6 \times 10^3/\mu L$ with a slight shift to the left. A plain film (scout film) of the abdomen obtained in the emergency department shows no free air. Review of the colonoscopy records show that he had left-sided diverticulosis and a 4-mm polyp in the sigmoid colon, which was snared using electrocautery. The patient wishes to go home. The next best step in his management is:

A. Because the scout film shows no perforation, discharge him home with a prescription for pain medication and instructions to return if fever recurs.
B. He has probably developed diverticulitis, so he should be discharged home with a prescription for a 2-week course of an antibiotic.
C. Obtain stool cultures and then begin antibiotic therapy.
D. Admit the patient, begin antibiotic therapy, and obtain CT scans of the abdomen and pelvis.

118 A 47-year-old white man is referred to the GI clinic with a history of recurrent heme-positive stools and normocytic anemia for 2 years. He has had two upper and lower endoscopies elsewhere, which showed no abnormality. He complains of yellow to orange redundant tissue on the side of his neck, which has been present for years. Recently, he has noticed similar yellow lesions in the axillary region. He is very upset because a week ago he was in the emergency department with chest pain and was told that he had a small "heart attack." He states, "I don't know what I'm doing wrong; I eat healthy and exercise regularly." True statements about this patient's condition include:

A. About 8% to 13% of patients with this condition develop GI bleeding.
B. This disorder occurs due to aberrant calcification of mature connective tissue.
C. The source of GI bleeding is often difficult to identify.
D. Biopsy of the skin will be diagnostic.
E. All of these statements are true.

119 For diagnosis of amyloidosis, it is advisable to biopsy all of the following sites *except*:

A. Stomach or duodenum
B. Liver

C. Colon
D. Subcutaneous abdominal fat pad

120 All of the following are true statements about the various purgatives used prior to colonoscopy *except*:

A. Polyethylene glycol (PEG) solutions are very well tolerated because they do not cause fluid shifts during preparation for colonoscopy.
B. Electrolyte abnormalities are common side effects of all purgatives currently given prior to colonoscopy.
C. Sodium phosphate should not be given to patients in renal failure.
D. Patients with severe diseases should be prepared for colonoscopy gradually over hours.

121 All of the following statements concerning clinical-pathologic correlation between site of eosinophilic infiltrate and presentation of disease are true *except*:

A. Infiltration of serosa can produce ascites with eosinophilic content.
B. Infiltration of bowel wall progresses to deep ulceration and can produce perforation.
C. Infiltration of muscularis propria more likely produces fibrosis and strictures.
D. Infiltration of mucosa can produce ulceration, bleeding, and protein-losing enteropathy.

122 A 35-year-old man with history of hepatitis B is being evaluated for hematopoietic cell transplant (HCT). The results of his liver function tests (LFTs) are normal, and imaging studies show some increase in echogenicity of the liver but no cirrhosis. The only abnormal results of serology are the presence of anti-HBc antibody. What should be recommended for this patient prior to HCT?

A. Weekly LFTs prior to transplant and then daily
B. Daily LFTs
C. Repeat blood testing
D. Initiation of lamivudine
E. None of the interventions listed

123 In a patient with a large unrepaired paraesophageal hernia, esophageal manometry and 2-hour pH measurements are useful for all of the following *except*:

A. To measure gastroesophageal reflux
B. To evaluate associated esophageal motor disorder
C. To determine the type and extent of fundoplication
D. To determine need for proton pump inhibitor (PPI) drug therapy postoperatively

124 The husband of a 30-year-old white woman brings her to the physician because of multiple GI complaints including postprandial abdominal pain, vomiting, and weight loss of 40 pounds in the last 2 months. The husband is extremely concerned that she may have an eating disorder. On exam, patient is pale, asthenic, weighs 96 lb., and is 5′6″ tall. She is tearful, very upset with her husband, and denies abuse of laxatives or any other symptoms of eating disorder. On further questioning, she says that her weight loss began in the hospital as the result of "bad hospital food" when she was admitted with spinal cord injury and had to be in a body cast, but the onset of vomiting is more recent. The physician should:

A. Obtain a gastric emptying scan
B. Initiate a nutrition consult with strict calorie counts
C. Obtain an upper GI series of x-rays with small bowel follow-through (SBFT)
D. Perform upper endoscopy
E. Start the patient on an antidepressant medication and obtain a psychiatry consult

125 A 35-year-old man who has had Crohn's disease for 8 years presents with voluminous diarrhea of 15 to 20 nonbloody bowel movements a day. His usual bowel habits are three to four soft bowel movements a day, but over the past week has had >1 L of output per day. There is no associated abdominal pain, nausea, or vomiting. However, he is complaining of lightheadedness and dizziness over the past 2 days. He is admitted to the hospital and started on fluid and electrolytes replacement therapy. What test is necessary for definitive diagnosis?

A. Colonoscopy
B. CT of the abdomen/pelvis
C. MRI of the abdomen
D. X-ray "obstruction" series
E. Upper GI x-rays with small bowel follow-through

126 A 60-year-old diabetic man has had chronic renal failure for 5 years and has been on hemodialysis for 3 years. Recurrent bouts of melena have required continuous oral iron supplementation plus Epogen every 2 weeks. Upper and lower endoscopy have not revealed a source for bleeding. The likely source of bleeding is:

A. Small bowel neoplasm
B. Angiodysplasia of small bowel
C. Meckel's diverticulum
D. Pyloric channel ulcer overlooked at endoscopy
E. Dieulafoy's lesion

127 A 55-year-old man presents with symptoms of dyspepsia, vomiting, and postprandial indigestion. He has a serum albumin level of 2.6 g/dL and creatinine of 0.8 mg/dL. He has noted increasing lower extremity edema. A CT scan of the abdomen reveals prominent and thick gastric folds. Which of the following medications should this patient be prescribed?

A. H₂ blockers
B. Omeprazole
C. Octreotide
D. Antacids
E. All of the above

128 In which of the following cases is gastric antral vascular ectasia (GAVE; also called watermelon stomach) least likely to be the diagnosis?

A. A 49-year-old white woman with iron deficiency anemia for 5 years and rheumatoid arthritis
B. A 50-year-old man with atrophic gastritis and heme-positive stools
C. A 47-year-old white man with cirrhosis secondary to hepatitis C, anemia, and possibly recurrent blood transfusions
D. A 65-year-old African-American man with a history of frequent nonsteroidal anti-inflammatory drug (NSAID) use who presents with hematemesis and anemia
E. A 27-year-old white woman with systemic sclerosis and anemia for 4 years

129 A 40-year-old woman is admitted with a 2-day history of nausea, vomiting, and abdominal distention. Obstructive series shows dilated loops of small bowel. On exam, the abdomen is soft, there is no local tenderness, and a rather indurated, tender nodule 2 to 3 cm in diameter is felt in the right groin. The most likely diagnosis is:

A. Neoplasm obstructing the small bowel and metastasis to the lymph nodes
B. Lymphoma presenting with inguinal adenopathy and perhaps small bowel involvement
C. Incarcerated femoral hernia
D. Small bowel obstruction with incidental inguinal adenopathy

130 A 50-year-old woman is confirmed to have a VIPoma. She continues to have approximately 3 L of stool per day and is requiring 200 mEq/day of potassium to maintain electrolyte balance. Which one of the following should be offered as a treatment?

A. Prednisone 60 mg/day
B. Clonidine
C. Indomethacin
D. Octreotide
E. Phenothiazine

131 A 39-year-old woman presents with acute onset of right lower quadrant (RLQ) abdominal pain. She denies any nausea, vomiting, or anorexia. She can locate the exact location of the pain in the RLQ with her index finger, and this spot is cephalad to McBurney's point. On the CT of the abdomen, she is found to have a hypoattenuating mass bordered by a hyperattenuating peripheral ring near the ascending colon. What is the diagnosis?

A. Acute appendicitis
B. Right-sided diverticulitis
C. Epiploic appendagitis
D. Localized abscess from perforated diverticulitis
E. Colon cancer

132 All of the following statements about traumatic hernias of the diaphragm are true *except*:

A. About 70% occur in the left side of the diaphragm.
B. The hernia may contain stomach, omentum, colon, spleen, or kidney.
C. They can be diagnosed by their immediate appearance after trauma.
D. Blunt trauma tends to produce a larger defect and hernia than penetrating injury.

133 A 63-year-old man presents with nausea, periumbilical pain, and a 10-lb. weight loss. A CT scan (see figure) shows a soft tissue mass in the retroperitoneum, encasing the aorta. Open biopsy of the mass showed inflammation and fibrosis with no evidence of tumor. What is the appropriate treatment for this patient?

A. Methysergide
B. Ergotamine
C. Colchicine
D. Glucocorticoid
E. Adriamycin

134 Regarding bleeding after polypectomy, all of the following statements are true *except*:

A. Patients taking warfarin are at increased risk of post-polypectomy bleeding.
B. Drugs such as aspirin, NSAIDs, ticlopidine, and clopidrogel have been clearly shown to increase the risk of postpolypectomy bleeding.
C. In patients with mechanical heart valves who are taking warfarin, low–molecular-weight heparin can be safely substituted for warfarin before and after the procedure.
D. This complication should always be discussed during the obtaining of informed consent.
E. The incidence of bleeding postpolypectomy is 1.5% to 3% of all cases.

135 A 24-year-old man is brought to the emergency department by the police because, after his arrest for suspected drug-dealing, he swallowed a few packets of white powder that was believed to be cocaine. The patient is completely asymptomatic and the results of his physical exam show no abnormalities. Abdominal radiographs show multiple sausage-shaped radiopaque areas in the small intestine. What is the next step in the management of this patient?

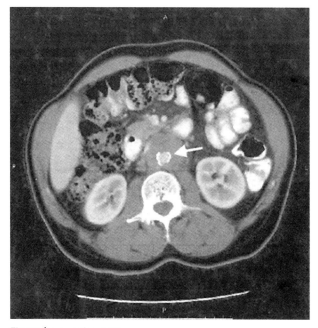

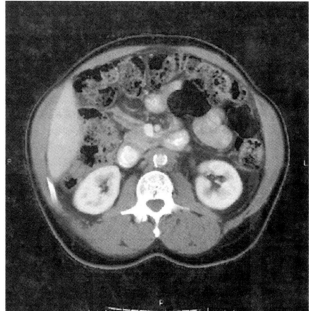

Figure for question **133**

A. Emergency surgery
B. Emergency endoscopic removal of the foreign bodies in the intestine
C. Inpatient observation with a clear liquid diet
D. None of the above
E. All of the above

136 A 61-year-old woman whose recovery from liver transplantation has been complicated by multiple bouts of rejection and has required high doses of immunosuppressant medications presents 14 months after the transplant with complaints of abdominal pain, intermittent fevers, night sweats, and some weight loss. She undergoes CT of the abdomen and pelvis (see figure). Which of the following is the likely diagnosis?

A. Intra-abdominal abscess
B. Post-transplant lymphoproliferative disease
C. Peritoneal tuberculosis
D. Nocardia
E. None of the above

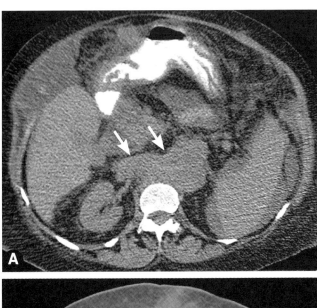
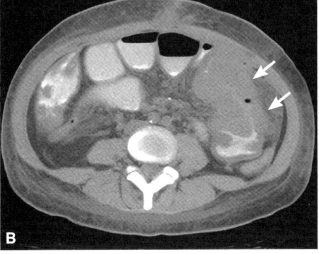

Figure for question **136**

137 A 70-year-old man presents with diffuse abdominal pain, nausea, and diarrhea for 4 weeks. His medical history includes rectal cancer treated with resection and radiation therapy 6 years ago. He had a recent colonoscopy, which he states was normal. On exam he is afebrile and has mild abdominal tenderness in both lower quadrants without rebound or guarding. His stool is brown and tests negative for hemoglobin, although he is anemic (hemoglobin level of 9.8 g/dL). A CT of the abdomen and pelvis is obtained and shows no evidence of obstruction or recurrence of tumor. Which of the following can be used to manage his symptoms?

A. High-fiber diet
B. Clonidine
C. Loperamide
D. Steroids
E. 5-Aminosalicylic acid (5-ASA) agents

138 A 40-year-old man presents to the emergency department with a 1-day history of abdominal pain, nausea, and vomiting. The symptoms began after he ate a large bag of popcorn at the movies the day prior to admission. His last bowel movement was more than 24 hours before the onset of his symptoms. A CT of the abdomen is obtained and reveals a ring-like soft tissue density in the lumen of the second portion of the duodenum. The density is outlined with contrast material and contains contrast material and a small amount of air (halo sign).

Which of the following is the most likely cause of the patient's small bowel obstruction?

A. Lymphoma
B. Crohn's disease
C. Duodenal diverticula
D. Adhesions
E. Strictures

139 A 39-year-old white man is referred by the dermatology clinic with a diagnosis of epidermolysis bullosa (EB). He has had dysphagia for several months, is unable to eat solid foods, and has lost a considerable amount of weight. However, his appetite is excellent, and he has no other GI complaints. He appears to be very nervous, but in no distress. On further discussion, it appears that his dermatologist had actually referred him to a thoracic surgeon for resection of a stricture in the esophagus and had advised him not to undergo esophageal dilatation. The patient is confused because his paternal uncle, who also suffers from EB, has a feeding tube and suggested that the patient request a GI evaluation. After a long discussion, the patient understands that all of the following are true *except*:

A. Esophageal stricture in EB is caused by repeated trauma from food and refluxed gastric acid.
B. The dermatologist is correct and the next best step in management is to see a surgeon for colonic interposition after esophageal stricture resection.
C. Recurrent esophageal stricture could be an ongoing problem.
D. The patient should undergo upper GI endoscopy with through-the-scope (TTS) balloon dilatation of the stricture.
E. The patient should have an upper GI imaging series.

140 All of the following statements about the relationship between somatostatin and carcinoid tumors are true *except*:

A. Somatostatin and its analogues inhibit synthesis and release of peptides produced by carcinoid tumors.
B. They do not block the effects of amines and peptides on target tissue.
C. Their role in carcinoid heart disease is unclear.
D. They have several side effects and are not very well tolerated by patients.
E. They are not effective in the treatment of abdominal pain due to carcinoid tumor.

141 Acrodermatitis enteropathica, a superficial scaling and blistering eruption of skin, is seen mainly in the perioral and groin area. It is a characteristic manifestation of:

A. Vitamin C deficiency
B. Zinc deficiency
C. Glucagon-secreting tumor of the pancreas
D. Whipple's disease
E. Tropical sprue

142 A 28-year-old woman who is 28 weeks pregnant presents to the emergency department with a 1-day history of RLQ pain. She also complains of nausea and anorexia over the past 2 days. She denies any changes in her bowel movements or blood in her stool. She does state that she has had low-grade fevers over the past 2 days. Her lab work reveals a mildly elevated leukocyte count (12,000 cells/mL). Which of the following is the diagnostic test of choice in this patient?

A. CT of the abdomen/pelvis
B. Exploratory laparoscopy
C. Graded-compression ultrasound of the abdomen
D. MRI of the abdomen/pelvis

143 The following are all feature of the pathology of mucosa-associated lymphoid tissue (MALT) gastric lymphoma *except*:

A. Destruction of gastric glands by proliferating lymphocytes
B. Predominance of large, atypical B lymphocytes in the tumor
C. Presence of periodic acid–Schiff (PAS)–positive Dutcher bodies in plasma cells
D. Diffuse infiltration of the lamina propria and follicular colonization (invasion of germinal centers of follicles)

144 A 40-year-old man presenting with diarrhea and weight loss is found to have a duodenal lesion, which on histopathologic evaluation is found to contain psammoma bodies. Which one of the following hormones will be produced by this lesion?

A. Somatostatin
B. Insulin
C. Glucagon
D. Vasoactive intestinal polypeptide (VIP)
E. None, because this lesion is a carcinoid

145 All of the following increase the risk of recurrence after inguinal hernia repair *except*:

A. Smoking
B. Overlooked hernia on initial repair
C. Steroid therapy
D. Alcoholism

146 All of the following are true about Parkes Weber syndrome *except*:

A. Several genetic defects in the regulation of angiogenic factor VG5Q occur in patients with this syndrome.
B. Bony elongation of the affected limb is the result of increased blood supply to that limb.
C. This condition is often associated with protein-losing enteropathy.
D. The syndrome can be diagnosed on the basis of physical examination findings alone.
E. Endoscopic therapy is often useful in controlling GI bleeding in patients with this syndrome.

147 All of the following are required in the evaluation of a patient with suspected foreign body ingestion *except*:

A. Careful history and physical exam
B. Anteroposterior and lateral radiographs of the chest
C. Barium esophagram
D. Radiographs of the abdomen

148 Bouts of jaundice and upper abdominal pain with elevated liver enzymes in patients with sickle cell disease can be attributable to all of the following *except*:

A. Ischemic liver injury
B. Hepatitis B infection
C. Hepatitis C infection
D. Zinc deficiency
E. Cholecystitis

149 All of the following statements about Kaposi's sarcoma (KS) are true *except*:

A. It is thought to be associated with infection with herpesvirus type 8.
B. Lesions are red to purple oval macules that develop into papules, plaques, and nodules that almost always ulcerate.
C. It can involve any viscera.
D. Treatment is usually palliative.
E. Recently, there has been a significant decline in the incidence of KS.

150 A 25-year-old woman with a 6-year history of Crohn's disease comes to see her physician. She is recently married and is considering becoming pregnant. Her Crohn's disease has been well controlled on mesalamine (Pentasa) and her last flare, which was 3 years ago, was treated with a course of oral glucocorticoids. Which of the following is true regarding inflammatory bowel disease (IBD) and pregnancy?

A. Female fertility in patients with IBD is significantly reduced even while in remission after medical or surgical therapy.
B. Initial presentation of IBD during pregnancy is common.
C. Pregnancy increases the severity of preexisting IBD.
D. Glucocorticoid therapy during pregnancy has been shown to be unsafe.
E. Immunosuppressive therapy with mercaptopurine (6-MP) seems to be safe in pregnant women.

151 Which of the following patient populations are at risk for foreign body ingestion?

A. Patients with psychiatric disorders
B. Prisoners
C. Patients with dentures and dental bridgework
D. Intoxicated patients
E. All of the above

152 A 29-year-old woman experiences a gradual increase in serum bilirubin, alkaline phosphatase, and aminotransferase enzyme levels 1 month after HCT. Her liver biopsy results are shown in the figure. What is the diagnosis?

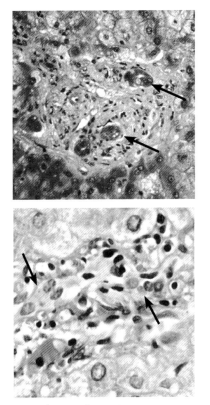

Figure for question **152**

A. Varicella zoster virus (VZV) infection
B. Adenovirus infection
C. Cytomegalovirus (CMV) infection
D. Graft-versus-host disease (GVHD)
E. Herpes simplex virus (HSV) infection

153 A 65-year-old man presents to his primary care physician complaining of nocturnal regurgitation of food for several months. Symptoms have recently become worse, waking him up at night. He denies any dysphagia or odynophagia. His wife has also noticed that his voice has been changing and has complained to him often that he has severe halitosis. He states that he has no other medical problems but his current symptoms have affected his quality of life. What is the most useful diagnostic study?

A. Endoscopy
B. Barium swallow
C. 24-Hour pH monitoring
D. Esophageal manometry
E. CT scan of the chest

154 A 24-year-old woman in her 34th week of pregnancy presents with new onset of jaundice. Her husband noted 2 days ago that her eyes appeared yellow and brought her in after she became lethargic and confused. On exam she is oriented only to person and place. Physical examination is notable for asterixis as well as the gravid uterus. Her white blood cell count is elevated ($13 \times 10^3/\mu L$), AST is 800 U/L, ALT is 780 U/L, total bilirubin is 4.9 mg/dL, international normalized ratio (INR) is 2.0, and PTT is 66 seconds. Which of the following is the likely diagnosis?

A. Acute fatty liver of pregnancy
B. Cholestasis of pregnancy
C. Pre-eclampsia
D. Hemolysis, elevated liver enzymes, and low platelets (HELLP) syndrome
E. Viral hepatitis

155 A Bochdalek hernia may be associated with which of the following?

A. Trisomy of chromosomes 13, 18, and 21
B. Bilateral pulmonary hypoplasia
C. Pulmonary hypertension
D. All of the above

156 A 49-year-old woman presents with painless abdominal distention and anorexia. She denies any history of liver disease and any risk factors for chronic liver diseases. On physical exam, she has a "doughy" abdomen. This is most likely secondary to which of the following?

A. Mucinous cyst adenocarcinoma of the appendix
B. Hepatocellular carcinoma
C. Retroperitoneal fibrosis
D. All of the above

157 All of the following are true regarding percutaneous endoscopic gastrostomy (PEG) tube placement *except*:

A. Starting antibiotic medications before the procedure has been shown to reduce the risk of local wound infection.
B. The most frequent complication of PEG tube placement is infection at the PEG tube entry site.
C. "Buried bumper" syndrome is a known complication.
D. The commonest cause of aspiration pneumonia in patients fed via PEG tube is reflux of their enteral feedings.

158 Internal abdominal hernias have been reported after all of the following operations *except*:

A. Gastric bypass
B. Aortofemoral bypass
C. Appendectomy
D. Billroth II gastric resection
E. Colostomy

159 All of the following statements about oral hairy leukoplakia are true *except*:

A. It presents as dark, black, lesions along the lateral border of the tongue; hence the name.
B. It is usually asymptomatic.
C. Development of hairy leukoplakia in a person with human immunodeficiency virus (HIV) infection usually presages the development of acquired immunodeficiency syndrome (AIDS) in about 24 months.
D. This condition can occur in solid organ transplant recipients.
E. The epithelium of patients with this condition contains Epstein-Barr virus.

160 Match the following disorders of the mouth and oral cavity to the disease they are associated with:

Condition	Associated Disease
1. Glossodynia	A. Chronic smoking
2. Glossitis	B. Sjögren's syndrome
3. Xerostomia	C. Psychiatric disease
4. Black hairy tongue	D. Magnesium deficiency
5. Dysgeusia	E. Pernicious anemia

161 Which of the following tumors is a nonfunctional pancreatic endocrine tumor?

A. Pancreatic polypeptide (PP)–secreting tumor
B. Insulinoma
C. VIPoma
D. Gastrinoma
E. GFR-secreting tumor

162 A 55-year-old man has received a liver transplant for hepatitis C–related liver disease. Approximately 3 months after the transplant, he is admitted with cholangitis. ERCP reveals left hepatic duct stricture and multiple biliary casts, which are treated during the ERCP. Which of the following should now be performed?

A. Nothing
B. Surgical revision
C. Long-term antibiotic therapy
D. Repeat ERCP in 2 weeks
E. Ultrasound to assess for hepatic artery patency

163 A 60-year-old obese woman who underwent surgical repair of a large incisional hernia a few hours ago is noted to be tachypneic and in respiratory distress. Ventilation-perfusion (V/Q) scan of the lungs and electrocardiography (ECG) are nondiagnostic. A likely mechanism for these symptoms would be:

A. Decreased venous return to the heart
B. Undetected pulmonary embolism
C. Compression of lungs due to postoperative increase in the size of the abdomen or pressure on the lungs
D. Early myocardial infarction
E. **A** and **C**

164 All of the following have been used in the treatment of recurrent aphthous ulcers in the oral cavity *except*:

A. Multivitamin supplementation
B. Metronidazole, 500 mg PO twice a day for 14 days
C. Oral colchicine at a dose of 0.6 mg three times a day
D. Topical or systemic prednisone
E. 2% viscous lidocaine with sucralfate

165 A 29-year-old man with AIDS whose last known CD4 count was 58 presents to the emergency department with a history of diarrhea for several days. He has not been taking his highly active antiretroviral therapy (HAART) medications. The diarrhea is large volume, nonbloody, and associated with nausea but not with abdominal pain. What is the most likely cause of the patient's diarrhea?

A. *Campylobacter* species
B. *Microsporidium*
C. *E. coli*
D. *Salmonella*
E. *Shigella*

166 Which of the following is an infectious complication seen during the first month following a liver transplant?

A. Biliary sepsis
B. HSV infection
C. CMV infection
D. EBV infection
E. Fungal infection

167 A 70-year-old man with a history of hypertension, diabetes mellitus, and coronary artery disease presents to the emergency department with two episodes of melena in the last 24 hours. He thinks he may have had dark, black stool 2 to 3 days ago but is not sure. He had dizziness earlier in the day but never lost consciousness. He feels fine now. He is accompanied by his wife who has his list of the medications he is taking, which include oral hypoglycemic agents, an angiotensin-converting enzyme (ACE) inhibitor, a beta-adrenergic blocker, and NSAIDs for arthritis. His medical history includes appendectomy several years ago, abdominal aortic aneurysm repair 20 years ago, and a cardiac catheterization a year ago. He appears pale but is alert and oriented. His vital signs are: pulse, 90 beats/minute; blood pressure, 105/80 mmHg; respiratory rate, 22 to 24 breaths/minute; and temperature, 100.2°F. He does not have orthostatic hypotension, abdominal pain, nausea, vomiting, or hematemesis. During evaluation in the

emergency department, he has another episode of melena. An IV infusion is started, and a blood sample obtained preparatory to upper endoscopy His hemoglobin is 9.6 gm% with normal mean corpuscular volume (MCV); however, his bicarbonate level is 16 mEq/L. Esophagogastroduodenoscopy (EGD) performed in the emergency department shows a single, small, white-based ulcer in the duodenal bulb. There is no blood in the stomach or visualized portions of the duodenum. The patient now feels much better. The best approach at this point is:

A. Stop NSAIDs, admit the patient, continue administration of IV fluids, and begin IV PPI.
B. Stop NSAIDs and discharge the patient with a prescription for an oral PPI medication twice daily.
C. Admit the patient, continue administration of IV fluids, start IV administration of a PPI medication, and repeat EGD with a pediatric endoscope the next day.
D. Admit the patient, continue IV fluid administration, start IV administration of a PPI medication, and obtain a CT scan of abdomen stat.
E. None of the above.

168 A 22-year-old man comes to the emergency department after ingesting an alkaline substance He has no symptoms. Upper GI endoscopy reveals grade IIA injury. What should be done next?

A. Keep NPO and start total parenteral nutrition.
B. Keep NPO and insert a nasoenteral feeding tube.
C. Start him on a liquid diet and advance to a regular diet in 24 to 48 hours.
D. Perform a barium swallow before allowing oral intake.
E. None of the above.

169 All of the following are true about the association between dermatitis herpetiformis (DH) and celiac sprue *except*:

A. More than 80% of patients with celiac sprue will have dermatitis herpetiformis.
B. DH presents as papulovesicular lesions that are symmetrical and involve the extensor surfaces of extremities, trunk, buttock, scalp, and neck.
C. Withdrawal of gluten reverses the condition in 6 to 12 months.
D. Although the exact pathogenesis of DH remains unclear, it is thought that antibodies to gluten that are formed in the small intestine are deposited at the dermoepidermal junction.
E. DH is rarely diagnosed in childhood.

170 A 45-year-old man who has received a cadaveric kidney transplant for polycystic kidney disease presents to the emergency department with crampy left lower quadrant abdominal pain that awoke him from sleep at 3 o'clock in the morning. He also had one episode of a bloody bowel movement and feels he has a low-grade fever. Which of the following is the most likely diagnosis?

A. Diverticular bleeding
B. Infectious colitis
C. Ulcerative colitis
D. Ischemic colitis
E. None of the above

171 A 33-year-old woman a with history of endometriosis who is currently receiving hormone therapy presents with abdominal pain. A CT scan shows nodules on the peritoneum, and during laparoscopy, multiple small, rubbery nodules are seen along the peritoneum. What is the diagnosis?

A. Mesenteric cysts
B. Pelvic lipomatosis
C. Leiomyomatosis peritonealis
D. Sarcoma
E. None of the above

172 A 41-year-old woman with history of chronic renal failure due to polycystic kidney disease was evaluated by her physician for symptoms of gastroesophageal reflux disease (GERD). Her fasting serum gastrin level was found to be 800 pg/mL, and *H. pylori* antibodies are found in a serum sample obtained after treatment for GERD was stopped. Which of the following should be performed next?

A. Tests for secretin and basal acid output
B. Computed tomography of abdomen and pelvis
C. Endoscopic ultrasound
D. Exploratory laparotomy
E. None of the above

173 True statements about the cutaneous manifestations of inflammatory bowel disease include all of the following *except*:

A. Cutaneous lesions are more common in people with Crohn's disease than in people with ulcerative colitis.
B. Erythema nodosum can occur in those with Crohn's disease or ulcerative colitis.
C. Treatment of the underlying disease usually improves the skin lesions.
D. Pyoderma gangrenosum presents as painless ulcers in 5% of patients with ulcerative colitis and 1% of patients with Crohn's disease.

E. Pyostomatitis vegetans may appear years before the onset of GI symptoms in those with IBD.

174 A 32-year-old man with acute myelogenous leukemia (AML) underwent hematopoietic cell transplant 20 days ago and still remains neutropenic. He is now complaining of severe pain near the anal canal, and this pain is worse with defecation. External examination shows no abnormalities. What should be done next?

A. Start acyclovir.
B. Start ganciclovir.
C. Obtain a CT scan of the pelvis.
D. Perform flexible sigmoidoscopy.
E. None of the above.

175 A 68-year-old woman presents with painless rectal bleeding that has lasted 1 day. She denies having any abdominal pain and has no fever. Over the past 24 hours, she has had five episodes of passing bright red blood per rectum. She denies any shortness of breath, dizziness, or chest pain. Her medical history includes hypertension, and 8 years ago she was diagnosed with cervical cancer and treated with chemotherapy and radiation therapy. The patient undergoes colonoscopy, which reveals friable mucosa with multiple telangiectasias.

What is the best treatment for this lesion?

A. Argon plasma coagulation
B. Mesalamine enemas
C. Metronidazole
D. Steroids
E. Surgery

176 In a patient suspected of having somatostatinoma, which of the following tests should be conducted?

A. CT of the abdomen and pelvis
B. Measurement of plasma somatostatin-like immunoreactivity (SLI) level
C. Secretin stimulation test
D. Surgical exploration
E. Endoscopic ultrasound

177 Which of the following best describes protein-losing enteropathy?

A. Malabsorption of digested amino acids
B. Lack of pancreatic digestion of dietary proteins
C. Excessive leakage of plasma proteins into the lumen of the GI tract
D. Excessive protein catabolism
E. An inborn error of protein biosynthesis

178 Which of the following lists the correct sequence of damage to intestinal epithelium after ingestion of a caustic substance?

A. Necrosis, ulceration, fibrosis, stricture, carcinoma
B. Ulceration, necrosis, fibrosis, stricture, carcinoma
C. Necrosis, fibrosis, ulceration, stricture, carcinoma
D. Ulceration, fibrosis, necrosis, stricture, carcinoma
E. None of the above

179 All of the following are true statements about CMV infection in adults *except*:

A. Symptomatic CMV infections usually occur in immunocompromised individuals.
B. CMV affects 40% to 80% of adults.
C. CMV infection is often associated with retinitis.
D. Skin ulcers are common and appear as punched-out, deep ulcers of varying sizes.
E. Histologic examination of a biopsy specimen from an ulcer due to CMV infection will show intracytoplasmic and intranuclear inclusions.

180 A 47-year-old man who has undergone heart and lung transplant (HLT) presents with complaints of early satiety, some abdominal bloating, and some pyrosis. Which one of the following should be performed next?

A. Upper GI series
B. CT of abdomen
C. Gastric emptying scan
D. Upper endoscopy
E. None of the above

181 A boy undergoes successful endoscopic removal of a disc battery from his esophagus. What follow-up care should he receive?

A. No follow-up care is needed.
B. He should undergo yearly upper endoscopy examinations to screen for esophageal cancer.
C. A barium esophagram should be performed in 2 weeks to evaluate for stricture.
D. A bronchoscopy should be performed in 2 weeks to evaluate for tracheoesophageal fistula.
E. His blood and urine mercury levels should be measured.

182 All of the following conditions/states may mask the pain of peritonitis *except*:

A. Administration of analgesics
B. Chronic glucocorticoid therapy
C. Diabetes with advanced neuropathy

D. Cirrhosis and ascites
E. All of those above

183 All of the following types of small bowel lymphoma are considered to be nonimmunoproliferative small intestine diseases (non-IPSIDs) *except*:

A. Diffuse large B-cell lymphoma
B. Heavy chain/Mediterranean lymphoma
C. Mantle cell lymphoma
D. Burkett's lymphoma
E. Follicular lymphoma

184 A 55-year-old woman with chronic heartburn is found to have a 5-cm sliding hiatal hernia on upper GI barium-contrast x-rays. Her hemoglobin is 7.5 g/dL and MCV is 75/μm^3. Evaluation 3 years ago for anemia included normal EGD, colonoscopy, and small bowel barium study. Of the following statements, all are true *except*:

A. There is a 5% chance of finding Cameron ulcers on repeat EGD.
B. Further evaluation of small bowel by video capsule could be important in her evaluation.
C. If the results of repeat upper and lower endoscopy are normal, a site for blood loss must be postulated in the small bowel.
D. Such hiatal hernias pose a threefold increased risk of iron deficiency anemia.

185 Abnormal liver function and hepatomegaly in cases of multiple myeloma are due to:

A. Malignant plasma cell infiltration
B. Amyloidosis
C. Extramedullary hematopoiesis from myelophthesis
D. Both **A** and **B**
E. **A**, **B**, and **C**

186 Compared to laparotomy, laparoscopy is associated with:

A. Peritoneal macrophage response
B. Less cortisol release
C. Less reduction in natural killer (NK) cell subsets
D. Less of a systemic inflammatory response
E. All of the above

187 All of the following statements concerning Spigelian hernias are true *except*:

A. They are readily diagnosed as a bulge in the abdominal wall lateral to the rectus sheath and below the umbilicus.
B. They do not traverse the entire abdominal wall.
C. The pain can be mistaken for acute appendicitis or diverticulitis.
D. About 25% are not diagnosed before surgery.

188 A 32-year-old woman of Ashkenazi Jewish descent who is 15 weeks pregnant was just admitted by the high-risk obstetrics group because of multiple skin lesions and odynophagia. She denies abdominal pain, but has had nausea for 2 weeks. She has some constipation but has not noticed any blood in the stool. She states that she "was doing fine till 3 weeks ago when the skin lesions started." Her medical history is significant for appendectomy. She is otherwise healthy and takes prenatal vitamins. On physical examination, she is afebrile. There are multiple erosions and pustules over the skin on the arms, chest, abdomen, and thighs. Similar lesions are seen in the oral cavity and gingiva. All of the following statements about this illness are true *except*:

A. A definitive diagnosis of this condition is made by biopsy and demonstration of antibody and complement in the basement membrane zone by immunofluorescence.
B. IV immunoglobulin G (IgG) has been used in the treatment of this disorder.
C. Patients with serum IgG and IgA antibodies are less likely to respond to medications.
D. Oral ulcerations are present in 100% of patients with this condition.
E. Glucocorticoid medications, both topical and systemic, have been used to treat this condition.

189 Which of the following neurologic diseases is/are associated with involvement of the pharynx and/or esophagus and dysphagia?

A. Amyotrophic lateral sclerosis
B. Parkinsonism
C. Multiple sclerosis
D. Myotonic dystrophy
E. **A**, **B**, and **D**

190 A 58-year-old woman presents with chest pain and difficulty swallowing solid foods for the past week. She was recently diagnosed with lung cancer and is undergoing chemotherapy and completed radiation therapy 2 weeks ago. The chest pain is unrelated to eating but she does have odynophagia at times. What is the most likely finding on barium swallow?

A. Esophageal stricture
B. Esophageal stenosis
C. Esophageal dysmotility
D. Esophageal ulceration

191 A 55-year-old patient presents with crampy abdominal pain and profuse diarrhea. Stool studies reveal mild to moderate elevation in the WBC count. Colonoscopy reveals mild erythema of the sigmoid and descending colon and biopsies show an eosinophilic colonic infiltrate. Which of the following could be responsible for the findings in this patient?

A. Mycophenolate mofetil (MMF)
B. Cyclosporine
C. Rapamune
D. Prednisone
E. **A** and **B**

192 What proportion of patients with MALT lymphomas test negative for *H. pylori*?

A. 5%
B. 15%
C. 25%
D. 35%

193 A 25-year-old man is hospitalized for evaluation of multiple episodes of documented hypoglycemia. He is found lying on the floor, and a blood test shows a blood glucose concentration of 17 mg/dL. Which of the following additional blood test results would suggest factitious hypoglycemia?

A. Elevated insulin, proinsulin, and C peptide levels
B. Elevated insulin and proinsulin levels but no detectable level of C peptide
C. Elevated insulin but normal proinsulin and C peptide levels
D. Elevated insulin, slightly decreased proinsulin, and very low C peptide levels
E. Elevated insulin, decreased proinsulin, and elevated C peptide levels

194 Foreign body ingestion should be suspected in infants and children with which of the following symptoms?

A. Choking
B. Respiratory distress
C. Failure to thrive
D. Refusal to eat
E. All of the above

195 Match each of the following skin disorders with its associated GI pathology:

Skin Disorder	GI Pathology
1. Dermatitis herpetiformis	A. Pancreatic tumor
2. Porphyria cutanea tarda	B. Crohn's disease
3. Necrolytic migratory erythema	C. Celiac sprue
4. Erythema nodosum	D. Hepatitis C infection
5. Sister Mary Joseph nodule	E. Gastric cancer

196 A 52-year-old African-American woman is referred for evaluation of postprandial abdominal discomfort, mainly above the periumbilical region, without any radiation. She has a history of poorly differentiated adenocarcinoma of the lung (right upper lobe) that was treated by lobectomy 3 years previously, followed by radiation therapy. She lost 35 lb. during treatment and has been unable to regain the weight. She denies hematemesis, melena, dysphagia, diarrhea, and any bright red blood per rectum. She says she feels weak and tired and is concerned about the weight loss. An upper endoscopy performed by another gastroenterologist 2 weeks ago shows only a small hiatal hernia. The most likely etiology of her symptoms is:

A. Linitus plastica
B. Recurrence of lung cancer in the other lung
C. Superior mesenteric artery syndrome
D. Esophageal stricture from radiation esophagitis
E. None of the above

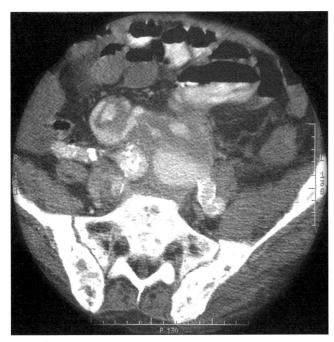

Figure for question **196**

197 True statements about perforation during upper endoscopy include:

A. Patients with large cervical osteophytes are at an increased risk.
B. The incidence of perforation in upper endoscopy is 2 to 3 per 10,000 procedures.
C. Most perforations in the neck can be managed conservatively.
D. Perforation is more likely to occur if the stricture is in the proximal esophagus.
E. All of the above are true.

198 Which of the following is a characteristic of glucagonoma?

A. Hypoaminoacidemia
B. Essential fatty acid deficiencies
C. Anorexia and weight loss
D. Normochromic anemia
E. All of the above

199 A 32-year-old woman who has undergone a successful liver transplant for primary biliary cirrhosis develops anorexia, nausea, and intermittent vomiting 1 month after the transplant. Her immunosuppressant regimen includes tacrolimus and prednisone. The next step should be:

A. Endoscopy
B. Reduce tacrolimus dose
C. Add a proton pump inhibitor medication
D. Stop tacrolimus and add mycophenolate mofetil
E. Start metoclopramide

200 A 39-year-old woman complains of progressive swelling in her hands and feet, numbness in her hands and other symptoms of carpal tunnel syndrome, and intermittent galactorrhea. MRI of the head fails to reveal any pituitary abnormality, but there is a mass in the abdomen. What is the appropriate treatment for this patient?

A. Streptozocin
B. Doxarubicin
C. Octreotide
D. Surgical exploration
E. Bromocriptine

201 Which of the following alterations in GI physiology is seen during normal gestation?

A. Resting lower esophageal sphincter pressures progressively decrease during gestation.
B. Transit time of intestinal contents is prolonged during gestation.
C. There is an increase in weight of the small intestine and in villus height, in conjunction with mucosal hypertrophy.
D. There is an increase in pooling of bile acids associated with greater residual gallbladder volumes in both the fasting and fed states.
E. All of the above.

202 A 34-year-old man presents with a several months' history of gnawing midepigastric abdominal pain and reflux. His symptoms were initially controlled with a once-daily dose of a proton pump inhibitor medication, but now he is experiencing symptoms while taking the medication twice a day. He has history of nephrolithiasis that was managed without surgery. His family history is significant for hyperparathyroidism. On physical exam, he complains of tenderness in the midepigastric region. What is the most likely diagnosis?

A. Sporadic Zollinger-Ellison syndrome (ZES)
B. ZES with multiple endocrine neoplasia type I (MEN-I)
C. Glucagonoma
D. Multiple endocrine neoplasia type IIa (MEN2a)
E. Multiple endocrine neoplasia type IIb (MEN2b)

203 Which of the following statements is *not* true about Dieulafoy's lesion (DL):

A. The most common site of bleeding from this lesion is 6 cm from the cardioesophageal junction.
B. These lesions are more common in men than in women.
C. The diagnosis is best made by early endoscopy.
D. These lesions were thought to represent the early stage of gastric ulcers.
E. These lesions cannot occur outside the GI tract.

204 The most common complication following colonoscopy with polypectomy is:

A. Perforation of hollow viscus
B. Infection
C. Immediate postoperative bleeding
D. Cardiorespiratory complications
E. Delayed postoperative bleeding

205 Eosinophilic esophagitis may be difficult to distinguish from GERD for all the following reasons *except*:

A. Both are associated with esophageal strictures.
B. Both can present with food bolus impaction.
C. Both are associated with similar numbers of eosinophils in the mucosa.
D. Both are associated with the symptom of heartburn.

206 A 42-year-old man presents 1 month after attempting suicide by drinking a caustic agent. He has been experiencing early satiety and progressive emesis that have resulted in a 5-pound weight loss. Upper endoscopy of the stomach is performed (see figure). What is the appropriate next step in treatment of this patient?

A. Endoscopic dilation
B. Refer to a surgeon for antrectomy
C. Refer to a surgeon for vagotomy and antrectomy
D. Refer to a surgeon for pyloroplasty and gastroenterostomy
E. Refer to a surgeon for subtotal gastrectomy

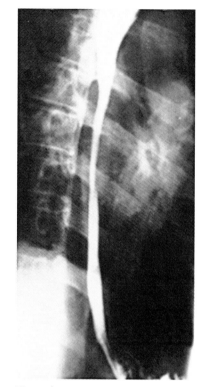

Figure for question **206**

207 Which one of the following types of multiple endocrine neoplasia (MEN) is characterized by pancreatic endocrine tumor?

A. MEN1
B. MEN2a
C. MEN2b
D. B and C
E. All of the above

208 A 40-year-old woman with history of pruritic hyperpigmented skin rash, migraine, and asthma has developed persistent diarrhea. The results of an upper GI series and small bowel x-ray show thickened folds in the stomach and jejunum with a "bull's eye" lesion in the jejunum. Of the following statements about this patient's condition, all are correct *except*:

A. Endoscopic biopsy would be expected to show diffuse mast cell infiltration throughout the mucosa and submucosa.
B. D-Xylose and vitamin B_{12} malabsorption will be present.
C. Duodenal ulcer disease might complicate her course.
D. Her symptoms are likely to show a dramatic response to administration of imatinib (Gleevac).
E. The disease is associated with activating mutations in the *C-kit* gene.

209 A 32-year-old man is admitted with perforated gastric ulcer. In addition to broad-spectrum beta-lactamase–producing antibiotics, which medications should be considered in the treatment of peritonitis?

A. Vancomycin
B. Ganciclovir
C. Acyclovir
D. Fluconazole
E. None of the above

210 Regarding newly diagnosed metastatic carcinoid, all of the following statements are true *except*:

A. The patient should undergo cross-sectional imaging at the level of the tumor and liver.
B. Positron emission tomography (PET) is advantageous in these cases because it can identify disease throughout the body.
C. Identification of metastatic disease is more difficult than identification of primary tumor.
D. Somatostatin scintigraphy is very helpful in these cases.

211 A 17-year-old girl is brought to the emergency room by her parents for symptoms of persistent salivation and vomiting. She admits to drinking bleach in an attempt to commit suicide. She develops hoarseness and stridor during the history and physical examination. Which of the following is the appropriate *next* step?

A. Portable chest radiography
B. Urgent endoscopy
C. Urgent intubation
D. Abdominal radiography
E. CT of the esophagus

212 A 50-year-old man presents with acute onset of subxiphoid pain associated with repeated retching, but no material is vomited. The results of ECG and his levels of cardiac enzymes, liver function enzymes, amylase, and lipase are all normal. An attempt is made to pass a nasogastric tube, but resistance is encountered at the gastroesophageal junction. On physical exam the epigastrium is tender, but the abdomen is soft with peristalsis. The most likely diagnosis is:

A. Ruptured abdominal aneurysm
B. Perforated peptic ulcer
C. Gastric volvulus
D. Esophageal carcinoma

213 In the patient described in question 212, the simplest test for confirmation of the diagnosis would be:

A. EGD
B. Barium swallow
C. CT of the abdomen
D. Chest X-ray

214 Match the following disorders of the oral cavity to the treatment:

Oral Cavity Condition
1. Xerostomia
2. Black hairy tongue
3. Oral thrush
4. Oral hairy leukoplakia
5. Geographic tongue

Treatment
A. Topical tretinoin gel
B. Topical anesthetics
C. Oral acyclovir
D. Oral mycostatin
E. Oral cevimeline

215 A 54-year-old white man presents for a screening colonoscopy. He has not noticed any change in his bowel habit or any blood in the stool. He does not have any gastrointestinal symptoms. Family history is significant for father developing colon cancer at 75 years of age. His laboratory test results show no abnormality in CBC, metabolic panel, thyroid-stimulating hormone (TSH) level, or prothrombin time/partial thromboplastin time (PT/PTT). He reports taking aspirin 81 mg/day for cardioprotective reasons and enalapril (Vasotec) for control of mild hypertension. Colonoscopy is performed to the cecal tip without difficulty and shows scattered diverticula in the left and transverse colon and a lesion in the cecum (see figure). Which of the following is a true statement about this lesion?

A. It should be treated with a heater probe to prevent occurrence of lower GI bleeding.
B. It indicates that the patient should have an angiogram after the colonoscopy to ensure he does not have other similar lesions.
C. It indicates that the patient should be offered hormonal therapy.

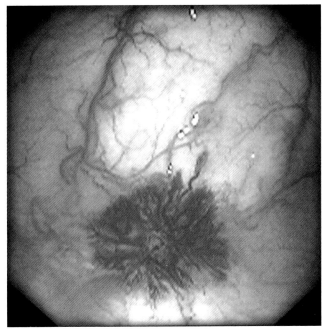

Figure for question **215**

D. It should be treated with argon plasma coagulation (APC) because this kind of lesion is a common cause of recurrent lower GI bleeding.

E. It does not require any treatment because the risk of bleeding from this lesion is very small.

216 A woman is referred by a dermatologist because of pruritus. She is 30 weeks' pregnant and has had an uncomplicated pregnancy thus far. She states that 1 week ago she began to have severe itching of her palms and soles, most intensely at night. She denies any abdominal pain, nausea, or vomiting. Lab tests show elevated levels of bilirubin (total, 5.6 mg/dL; direct, 4.3 mg/dL), AST (500 U/L), ALT (660 U/L), and alkaline phosphatase (400 U/L). Her hemoglobin level of 9.6 g/dL is consistent with levels measured on prenatal visits. Which of the following is the most likely diagnosis?

A. Acute fatty liver of pregnancy
B. Acute viral hepatitis
C. Choledocholithiasis
D. Cholecystitis
E. Cholestasis of pregnancy

217 A 54-year-old woman presents with a 4-cm lesion in the tail of the pancreas that is diagnosed as a glucagonoma. There is no evidence of metastatic disease. What is the best treatment for this patient?

A. Octreotide
B. Chemotherapy
C. Further evaluation, including a PET scan
D. Surgical resection

218 The following statements concerning the *KIT* gene and its role in the generation of gastrointestinal stromal tumor (GIST) are true *except*:

A. Normal *KIT* activation produces signal transduction, resulting in a controlled proliferation of cells and their survival.
B. Mutation in the *KIT* gene results in a gain of function in the signal for cell proliferation.
C. Interstitial cells of Cajal and mast cells normally stain for CD-117.
D. CD-117 is a marker for *KIT* receptor tyrosine kinase, which enables the signal from the gene.
E. About 5% of patients with GISTs test negative for CD-117 and a mutation in the *PDGFRA* gene is found to account for the hyperactivated kinase responsible for the tumor.
F. All of the above statements are false.

219 A 45-year-old woman who has just undergone HCT for multiple myeloma develops abrupt onset of severe retrosternal pain, odynophagia, and hematemesis. What should be the diagnostic test of choice?

A. Urgent endoscopy
B. Barium esophagram
C. CT of the chest with water-soluble contrast
D. CT of the chest without contrast
E. Radiography of the chest

220 The GI manifestations and associations of Sjögren's syndrome include:

A. GAVE (watermelon stomach)
B. Duodenal ulcer disease
C. Dysphagia
D. Primary biliary cirrhosis
E. **A**, **C**, and **D**

221 A 40-year-old alcoholic man is hospitalized with typical physical and x-ray findings of right lower lobe pneumonia. He has been started on an antibiotic medication. Gram-positive cocci are seen on Gram stain. On the 2nd hospital day, he appears slightly jaundiced, and jaundice is worse the following day. Liver function test results are as follows: alkaline phosphatase, twice normal; AST, 55 U/L; ALT, 70 U/L; bilirubin, 5 mg% (direct, 3.5 mg%); and gamma glutamyl transferase (GGT), twice normal. An ultrasound of the liver is unremarkable. The best next step in managing this patient's condition is:

A. Test for hepatitis A and B, cytomegalovirus (CMV), Epstein-Barr (EB) virus, and herpes simplex virus.
B. Perform urgent ERCP.
C. Observe and re-evaluate liver function daily.
D. Perform magnetic resonance imaging (MRI) and MRI with cholangiopancreatography (MRI-MRCP).
E. Immediately change to another antibiotic medication.

222 Emergency laparotomy or laparoscopy is not indicated in cases of peritonitis *except*:

A. When it is due to a perforated gastric ulcer
B. In patients with diverticulitis
C. When there is a contained perforation of the appendix with abscess (appendicitis)
D. When it is due to acute pancreatitis
E. None of the above; they all require surgical intervention

223 A 70-year-old white man is referred to the GI clinic for recent change in bowel habits and rectal bleeding. Change of bowel habits is characterized by a 5- to 6-month history of watery, nonmucousy, nonbloody diarrhea three to five times a day. In addition, he has noticed intermittent, lower abdominal crampy pain accompanied by a small amount of bright red blood on the toilet paper after a bowel movement for the past 3 months. He has no history of fever, recent travel outside the country, unusual environmental exposures, or contact with ill individuals. On physical examination he has mild, lower abdominal tenderness without rebound and normal rectal sphincter tone with no palpable rectal masses. A stool sample is brown but tests heme positive. Lab test results are normal. A colonoscopy is performed to the terminal ileum without difficulty. Findings include pandiverticulosis, a normal-appearing terminal ileum, and a 3.5-cm yellow nodule in the rectum, which is biopsied. The histopathology report is carcinoid tumor. All of the following statements about this patient's condition are true *except*:

A. Rectal carcinoids >2 cm in diameter pose a 60% to 80% risk of metastasis.
B. The incidence of rectal carcinoids is three times higher in whites than in African Americans.
C. Carcinoid syndrome is an uncommon feature of rectal carcinoids.
D. Invasion of the muscularis propria at diagnosis is a poor prognostic sign.
E. The overall survival rate for patients with rectal carcinoids is 87%.

224 A 45-year-old woman with a history of systemic lupus erythematosus presents with a 2-day history of diffuse abdominal pain and severe watery diarrhea. Her serum albumin level is 2.9 g/dL, and her creatinine level is 0.6 mg/dL. Examinations of a stool specimen are negative for pathogens. A CT scan of the abdomen reveals diffuse thickening of the wall of the small bowel.

Which of the following is the best treatment for this patient?

A. IV metronidazole
B. A 5-aminosalicylic acid (5-ASA) medication
C. Nothing by mouth and IV fluids for hydration alone
D. IV solumedrol
E. Exploratory laparotomy

225 Which of the following treatments may be used to manage bezoars?

A. Prokinetic agent such as metoclopramide
B. Nasogastric lavage
C. Cellulase
D. Mechanical disruption during endoscopy
E. All of the above

226 How is the liver affected in Hodgkin's disease?

A. Diffuse lobular hepatitis
B. Interface hepatitis

C. Sclerosing cholangitis
D. Idiopathic cholestatic hepatitis

227 A 35-year-old white woman presents to the emergency department with RLQ abdominal pain, anorexia, nausea, and vomiting. She has a temperature of 101°F. Based on her symptoms, physical examination findings, and abdominal CT scan findings, a diagnosis of acute appendicitis is made. The patient undergoes emergency appendectomy and is discharged home. Histopathologic examination of the appendix results in discovery of a 2.5-cm carcinoid tumor, and she is referred to a gastroenterologist. Which of the following statements regarding this patient is true?

A. She had carcinoid of the appendix that has been cured by appendectomy.
B. She may have metastatic disease and needs to undergo CT of the abdomen and pelvis every 3 months.
C. She is likely to have recurrence of the tumor.
D. Her prognosis is poor; the 5-year survival rate for patients with carcinoid is 10%.
E. She should undergo right hemicolectomy.

228 A 43-year-old man comes to the emergency department because of severe abdominal pain. On physical exam, percussible hepatic dullness is absent. Which of the following is the likely diagnosis?

A. Spontaneous bacterial peritonitis
B. Peritoneal carcinomatosis
C. Hepatocellular carcinoma
D. Perforated gastric ulcer
E. None of the above

229 Which of the following tumors may cause hypergastrinemia?

A. Ovarian cancer
B. Bronchogenic carcinoma
C. Acoustic neuroma
D. All of the above
E. None of the above

230 Flushing is a symptom commonly associated with carcinoid syndrome. Other conditions in which flushing can occur include all of the following *except*:

A. Pheochromocytoma
B. VIPoma
C. Amyloidosis
D. Medullary carcinoma of the thyroid
E. Anaphylaxis

231 The preferred treatment for diffuse, large, B-cell lymphoma is:

A. Rituximab alone
B. Radiation therapy alone
C. Surgery only
D. Chemotherapy (cycles of CHOP) alone
E. **A**, **B**, and **D**

232 Incidental infiltration of the GI tract with eosinophils, focal or diffuse, may be found in all the following diseases *except:*

A. Following solid organ transplant
B. Inflammatory bowel disease
C. Peptic ulcer disease
D. Celiac sprue
E. Juvenile polyps

233 A 56-year-old man with a recent diagnosis of glucagonoma presents with complaints of diarrhea, weight loss, and new onset of shortness of breath. Which of the following conditions should be ruled out?

A. Steatorrhea
B. Metastatic disease
C. Pulmonary emboli
D. Anemia
E. Hypoaminoacidemia

234 The following statements concerning enteropathy-associated T-cell lymphomas are true *except:*

A. Sprue is discovered at the time lymphoma is diagnosed in half of patients.
B. Following a gluten-free diet for 5 years or more can decrease the risk of lymphoma developing.
C. Anemia and perforation are rare presentations.
D. Celiac sprue is present an average of 3 to 5 years prior to diagnosis of lymphoma.

235 A 40-year-old man infected with HIV and a CD4 count of 59 presents with RUQ pain, nausea, and vomiting. He reports intermittent RUQ pain over the past year. On exam he is febrile (temperature 101.0°F) and has significant tenderness in the RUQ but without rebound or guarding. His lab results are as follows: WBC count of $13.6 \times 10^3 \mu L/$, alkaline phosphatase of 400 U/L, total bilirubin of 2.2 mg/dL, direct bilirubin of 1.3 mg/dL, AST of 60 U/L, and ALT of 80 U/L.

A CT of the abdomen is obtained and reveals intra- and extrahepatic ductal dilatation. The patient undergoes ERCP, which reveals papillary stenosis and focal strictures and dilatation of the intrahepatic and extrahepatic bile ducts. Which of the following could cause these findings?

A. CMV
B. *Cryptosporidium*
C. *Mycobacterium avium-intracellulare* (MAI) infection

D. *Microsporidium*
E. All of the above

236 The treatment of most proven benefit for familial Mediterranean fever is:

A. Glucocorticoids
B. Immunosuppressants (cyclophosphamide [Cytoxan], azathioprine [Imuran])
C. Colchicine
D. NSAIDs

237 The first step in treatment of a lymphoma in a patient who is immunosuppressed owing to organ transplant is:

A. Exploratory laparotomy for staging
B. Stopping immunosuppressive drugs
C. Chemotherapy with CHOP (cyclophosphamide, hydroxydaunomycin, Oncovin [vincristine], prednisone)
D. Radiation of the tumor if there is no indication of disseminated disease

238 False-positive elevations of 5-hydroxyindole acetic acid (5-HIAA) levels in urine can result from ingestion of all of the following *except:*

A. Melatonin
B. Methyldopa
C. Walnuts
D. Rifampin
E. Isoniazid (INH)

239 A 44-year-old woman presents with a 2-month history of worsening diarrhea and cramps in the lower extremities. She describes passing large amounts of watery stool that is the color of dilute tea. Stool studies fail to reveal any WBCs or infection, but the stool osmolar gap is less than 50. A VIPoma is suspected. What other laboratory abnormalities would be expected if this diagnosis is correct?

A. Hyperglycemia
B. Hypochlorhydria
C. Hypokalemia
D. Hypercalcemia
E. All of the above

240 The molecular marker(s) found in more than 95% of gastrointestinal stromal tumors (GISTs) is (are):

A. CD-34
B. CD-117
C. Smooth muscle actin
D. S-100
E. All of the above

241 Which of the following statements is true regarding hepatitis B infection in pregnancy?

A. Most women of childbearing age with chronic hepatitis B have a high risk of developing complications of their disease during gestation.

B. Maternal–fetal transmission is responsible for most cases of hepatitis B worldwide.

C. Mothers who test negative for the hepatitis B e-antigen cannot transmit the virus to their fetuses.

D. Women with hepatitis B can be treated with interferon during pregnancy.

E. Women with hepatitis B should not be treated with lamivudine during pregnancy.

242 A 22-year-old man with AIDS presents with abdominal pain and chronic diarrhea. On colonoscopy he is found to have mucosal ulceration and subepithelial hemorrhage. Biopsies reveal viral inclusions. Which of the following is true regarding the viral infection in the colon?

A. This infection usually occurs early in the course of HIV infection, when the CD4 count is >100/L.

B. This infection is rarely found in the colon; it usually affects the esophagus and small bowel.

C. It can be treated with ganciclovir.

D. Recurrences are very uncommon following withdrawal of therapy.

E. Long-term antiviral therapy is needed, even for patients being treated with HAART.

243 All of the following statements are correct *except*:

A. At least half of patients with Felty's syndrome (splenomegaly, leukopenia) have liver enzyme abnormality.

B. The degree of enzyme abnormality is unrelated to histopathology in Felty's syndrome.

C. Portal hypertension and variceal bleeding rarely occur with Felty's syndrome.

D. Adult-onset Still's disease can present with hepatosplenomegaly and abnormal LFT results.

E. Acute liver failure is not a feature of Still's disease.

244 In patients with which of the following tumors would hormone release be increased after calcium infusion?

A. Neurotensinoma

B. Gastrinoma

C. Adrenocorticotropic hormone (ACTH) tumor

D. VIPoma

E. All of the above

245 Which of the following statements regarding management of carcinoid syndrome is most accurate?

A. Serotonin antagonists such as methysergide, ondansetron, and cyproheptadine provide excellent control of flushing episodes.

B. Hypertension is best treated with angiotensin-converting enzyme (ACE) inhibitors.

C. Bronchospasm is best treated with beta-adrenergic receptor agonists.

D. Ondansetron is very effective in controlling diarrhea due to carcinoid syndrome.

E. Glucocorticoids should not be given to a patient with carcinoid syndrome who develops hypotension.

246 All of the following statements are true about the course of imatinib therapy for GISTs *except*:

A. About 20% of GISTs are refractory to therapy with an initial trial of imatinib.

B. Doubling the dose from 400 mg to 800 mg daily will usually decrease the nonresponse rate by 50%.

C. Lack of efficacy after an initial favorable response to imatinib has been attributed to additional mutation of a clone of the tumor.

D. If the tumor grows, partial surgical resection along with continuation of imatinib therapy to control the bulk of the tumor may be advisable.

E. Imatinib cannot provide enough benefit to allow resection in a patient with an initially nonresectable tumor.

247 The following statements about pathology of diffuse, large, cell B-lymphoma of the stomach are true *except*.

A. Some areas of a low-grade MALT lymphoma can be recognized intermixed with the predominant large cell population of the tumor.

B. P53 and P16 mutations can be found.

C. Large cell lymphomas discovered early may occasionally respond to *H. pylori* eradication, suggesting a role for this bacteria in their origin.

D. Initially these tumors can be confined to the mucosa.

248 Which of the following aerobic bacteria are most often found in intra-abdominal abscesses?

A. *Escherichia coli*

B. *Streptococcus pneumoniae*

C. *Klebsiella*

D. *Pseudomonas*

E. *Staphylococcus epidermidis*

249 A 49-year-old woman with a somatostatinoma that is being treated with octreotide presents with severe right upper quadrant and midepigastric pain along with fevers and chills. Which of the following could be causing her symptoms?

A. Diabetic ketoacidosis
B. Perforated ulcer
C. Pancreatitis
D. Cholecystitis
E. All of the above

250 A 55-year-old kidney transplant patient with fever and diffuse adenopathy 4 months after transplant is found to have Epstein-Barr virus DNA in the bloodstream. Which one of the following is the best treatment for this patient?

A. Increase doses of immunosuppressant medications
B. Start acyclovir
C. Start rituxan
D. Start ganciclovir
E. Start systemic chemotherapy

251 Which of the following protozoa most often cause diarrheal illness in HIV-infected patients?

A. *Blastocystis hominis*
B. *Cryptosporidium*
C. *Entamoeba histolytica*
D. *Giardia lamblia*
E. *Microsporidia*

252 A 40-year-old man with acute myeloid leukemia has just completed induction chemotherapy and has severe neutropenia (absolute neutrophil count [ANC] <500) and thrombocytopenia. He presents with fever, RLQ abdominal pain, and blood-tinged diarrhea. An abdominal CT shows marked thickening of the cecal wall without prominence of the appendix. The most likely cause of symptoms is:

A. Acute appendicitis; proceed with surgery directly
B. Bowel perforation with early collection in the right paracolic gutter
C. Leukemic infiltration of the bowel wall; this should subside with chemotherapy
D. Typhlitis (cecitis) associated with leukemia; treat with IV fluid therapy, administration of blood products to correct cytopenias, and a broad-spectrum antibiotic

253 A 41-year-old woman experienced palpitations, tremors, and sweating when she started skipping breakfast as part of a new diet. Which one of the following would help establish the diagnosis of insulinoma?

A. Surgical exploration
B. Overnight fasting blood sugar measure
C. Overnight fasting blood sugar measure with simultaneous plasma insulin level
D. Plasma insulin:glucose ratio measure
E. All of the above

254 Concerning MALT lymphoma, which of the following statements is *incorrect*:

A. Gastric tissue does not normally contain MALT unless chronically exposed to an infectious agent such as *H. pylori*.
B. The incidence of MALT lymphoma is proportional to the prevalence of *H. pylori* infection in that population.
C. Treatment of *H. pylori* occasionally leads to resolution of a MALT lymphoma.
D. T-cells in MALT lymphomas that are specifically reactive to *H. pylori* can drive the proliferation of malignant B-cells.

255 Flushing is a distinctive feature of carcinoid syndrome and is present in 30% to 94% of patients with carcinoid syndrome at some time during the course of their illness. All of the following are incorrect statements about the proposed etiology of flushing *except*:

A. Flushing occurs due to release of a number of polypeptide hormones.
B. Many studies have found a direct correlation between serotonin levels and degree of flushing.
C. Norepinephrine levels are not correlated with flushing episodes.
D. Flushing in carcinoid syndrome is not worsened by emotional or physical stress.

256 A patient who has undergone HCT presents with nausea and a history of two episodes of hematemesis. Upper endoscopy is performed (see figure). What is the best treatment for this patient?

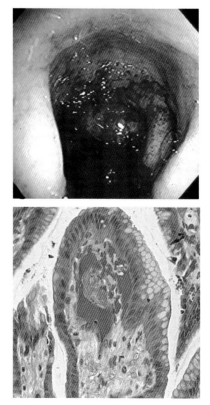

Figure for question **256**

A. Endoscopic laser therapy
B. Angiography with embolization
C. Proton pump inhibitor drip
D. Surgery
E. None of the above

257 All of the following diseases can be associated with diarrhea *except*:

A. Addison's disease
B. Hyperthyroidism
C. Hyperparathyroidism
D. Medullary thyroid carcinoma
E. Pheochromocytoma

258 A 41-year-old man with a history of MEN1 with hyperparathyroidism and ZES has been requiring higher doses of antisecretory drugs to control his symptoms. What else can be recommended at this time?

A. Surgical exploration to look for gastrinoma
B. Parathyroidectomy
C. Nissen fundoplication
D. *H. pylori* testing
E. All of the above

259 Which of the following statements about alpha heavy chain disease (Mediterranean lymphoma) is *incorrect*:

A. It is most prevalent in North Africa, Israel, the Middle East, and other Mediterranean countries.
B. It is associated with lack of sanitation and poor socioeconomic status.
C. It has been reported to be associated with *C. jejuni* infection.
D. The tumor secretes a polyclonal immunoglobulin.
E. It is associated with giardiasis.

260 All of the following are true statements about the adverse effects of imatinib *except*:

A. It has not been reported to cause myelotoxicity.
B. Diarrhea, myalgias, and skin rash reportedly occur in 30% to 45% of patients receiving the drug.
C. Its adverse effects tend to ameliorate with continued treatment.
D. GI hemorrhage from shrinking tumor masses has been noted in 5% of patients receiving this medication.

261 Which of the following statements about rectal carcinoid tumors are true:

A. The rectum is a very rare site of carcinoid tumors.

B. Rectal carcinoid is more common in female than in male patients.
C. Carcinoid syndrome is a common feature of rectal carcinoid.
D. Radical resection via a low anterior or abdominoperineal approach is the treatment of choice in cases of rectal carcinoid.
E. The primary determinant of the prognosis for patients with rectal carcinoid is the underlying tumor biology.

262 The following characteristics of a GIST predict greater likelihood of malignancy:

A. More mitoses in biopsy specimen
B. Smooth edges on endoscopic ultrasound
C. Tumor diameter >4 cm
D. None of the above
E. All of the above

263 A patient with abrupt onset of retrosternal pain, hematemesis, and painful swallowing undergoes imaging (see figure). What is the most likely diagnosis?

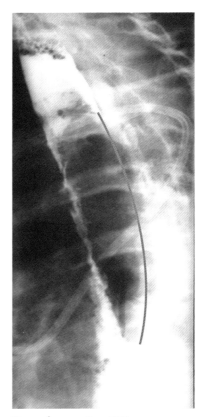

Figure for question **263**

A. Esophageal rupture
B. Mallory-Weiss syndrome (esophageal tear)
C. Esophageal wall hematoma
D. HSV esophagitis
E. CMV esophagitis

264 Which of the following can result from foreign body ingestion?

A. Pericarditis
B. Esophagoaortic fistula
C. Lung abscess
D. Mediastinitis
E. All of the above

265 GISTs can present in all of the following ways *except*:

A. Asymptomatic abdominal mass
B. Enlarged left supraclavicular (Virchow's) node
C. Gastric outlet obstruction
D. GI bleeding (intraluminal)
E. Intraperitoneal bleeding

266 A 55-year-old man with new diagnoses of diabetes mellitus and a pancreatic mass is brought to the emergency department with tachycardia, hypotension, and flushing. On physical exam, he has cyanosis. Which of the following levels should be checked?

A. Pancreatic peptide level
B. Insulin level
C. Glucagon level
D. Neurotensin level
E. ACTH level

267 The prognosis for survival of a patient who has had a stage I MALT lymphoma for 5 years is:

A. 20% to 25%
B. 40% to 50%
C. 60% to 76%
D. 80% to 95%

268 True statements regarding the relation between carcinoid tumor of the gut and urine levels of 5-HIAA include all of the following *except*:

A. Urine excretion rates of 5-HIAA of more than 25 mg/24 hours is diagnostic.
B. The excretion rate of 5-HIAA in the urine corresponds well with carcinoid tumor mass.
C. Midgut carcinoid tumors are associated with increased excretion rate of 5-HIAA in urine.
D. Foregut carcinoids may be associated with normal urinary levels of 5-HIAA.
E. All of these are true.

269 Which one of the following is elevated in patients with pancreatic polypeptide (PP) tumors?

A. Chromogranin A
B. Chromogranin B
C. Neuron-specific enolase

D. α-Human chorionic gonadotropin (α-HCG)
E. All of the above

270 Which one of the following is invariably elevated in patients with carcinoid?

A. Chromogranin C
B. Alpha subunit of human chorionic gonadotropin
C. Neuron-specific enolase
D. Chromogranin A
E. Synaptophysin

271 A 64-year-old woman who underwent liver transplant for cryptogenic cirrhosis 32 days ago arrives in the emergency department with right upper quadrant pain and jaundice. She has temperature of 100.9°F. Her bilirubin level is 9.2 mg/dL, and alkaline phosphatase is 482 IU/L. ERCP is performed (see figure). Based on these findings, what is the best treatment option?

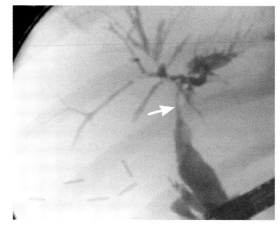

Figure for question **271**

A. Percutaneous biliary drainage
B. Surgical correction
C. Sphincterotomy
D. Balloon dilation and stent placement
E. Any of the above

272 A 30-year-old woman taking glucocorticoids for systemic lupus erythematosus (SLE) develops subacute periumbilical abdominal pain. The pain is most likely due to:

A. Peritonitis
B. Budd-Chiari syndrome
C. Mesenteric ischemia
D. Pancreatitis
E. Any of the above

273 A patient is suspected of having metastatic glucagonoma. What is the best test to identify metastatic disease?

A. Somatostatin receptor scintigraphy (SRS)
B. Endoscopic ultrasound (EUS)
C. CT of the abdomen and pelvis
D. Selective abdominal angiography
E. Surgical exploration

274 All of the following statements are correct concerning positive immunohistologic staining for CD-117 *except*:

A. Ewing sarcoma, angiosarcoma, small-cell lung cancer, and ovarian cancer can stain positive.
B. A positive stain implies a mutation in the *KIT* gene.
C. Positive staining can be found in acute myeloid leukemia and rarely in lymphoma.
D. Positive staining can be absent in 5% of GISTs.

275 A 25-year-old man with no significant medical history presents with pitting edema in the lower extremities and diarrhea that has lasted 2 weeks. Stool studies are negative for pathogens. He reports a 20-pound weight loss over the past month. His albumin level is 2.6 g/dL, and his creatinine level is 0.6 mg/dL. A urine sample tests negative for protein. His hemoglobin is 10.5 gm/dL, and coagulation values are mildly elevated. Which if the following tests would be most useful for diagnosis?

A. 24-hour urine protein excretion
B. 72-hour fecal fat concentration
C. 24-hour stool alpha-1 antitrypsin content
D. Stool phenophthalein test
E. Stool magnesium level

276 A 52-year-old woman with newly diagnosed type 2 diabetes mellitus presents with a rash (see figure) and a 7-pound weight loss in the last month. As the rash heals, hyperpigmentation develops. Which of the following is a possible diagnosis?

A. Insulinoma
B. Gastrinoma
C. Glucagonoma
D. Necrobiosis lipoidica diabeticorum
E. None of the above

277 A 37-year-old woman with AIDS who is receiving antiretroviral therapy presents with increasing abdominal girth and fullness. She has a temperature of 100.8°F and ascites. Diagnostic paracentesis is performed, and straw-colored fluid is withdrawn. The patient's serum-to-ascites albumin gradient is 0.9, she has a low glucose level of 18 gm/dL, and her WBC is 540 thousand with 68% lymphocytes. Which of

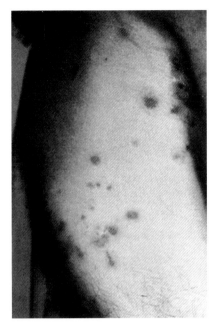

Figure for question **276**

the following tests may help arrive at a diagnosis in this case?

A. CA-125
B. Cytology of ascites fluid
C. Laparoscopy
D. **B** and **C**
E. **A** and **B**

278 A 28-year-old man with a history of Crohn's disease for 10 years presents with right lower quadrant abdominal pain, fever, and leukocytosis. His last colonoscopy (2 years ago) revealed ileal disease, which has been well controlled with 5-ASA. He has a temperature of 101°F and fullness in the right lower quadrant. Which imaging study should be performed?

A. Abdominal ultrasound
B. CT of the abdomen/pelvis
C. MRI of the abdomen
D. Small bowel x-ray
E. None of the above

279 A 65-year-old man with a 30-pack-year history of tobacco use presents with increasing obstipation for the past year. His abdomen is distended, and few peristaltic sounds are heard. An x-ray to evaluate for obstruction shows diffuse dilation (up to 8 cm) of the small bowel and colon, which is visible as far as the rectosigmoid. A 2-cm mass visible in the left lung is suspected to be a carcinoma. In addition to direct biopsy of the lung lesion, which of the following chemistry lab studies would help to clarify the cause of the symptoms in this case?

A. Serum gastrin level measurement
B. 24-hour urine collection for measurement of 5-HIAA
C. Serum calcium measurement
D. Serum antineuronal nuclear antibody (ANNA-1) test

280 Which of the following is the most important prognostic factor for a pancreatic endocrine tumor?

A. Liver metastases
B. Location of the tumor
C. Size of the tumor
D. Type of hormone secreted by the tumor
E. All of the above

281 A 13-year-old boy is brought in to the emergency department by his parents after he accidentally ingested a button battery. The child appears well and is interacting appropriately. What should be done next?

A. No further treatment is required; the patient can be safely discharged.
B. Obtain posteroanterior and lateral radiographs from mouth to anus.
C. Perform blind passage of a Foley catheter balloon.
D. Perform blind passage of a magnetic retrieval device.
E. None of the above.

282 A 47-year-old man develops dysphagia and the sense of esophageal obstruction along with chest pain while eating a steak. What treatment is indicated for this patient?

A. Trial of sips of water
B. Esophagraphy using a water-soluble contrast
C. IV glucagon administration
D. Urgent endoscopy using a rigid endoscope and intravenous sedation
E. Urgent endoscopy using a rigid endoscope and general anesthesia.

283 A patient with marfanoid habitus, puffy lips, and mucosal neuromas is now found to have bilateral pheochromocytomas. Which of the following is responsible for this patient's condition?

A. Neurofibromatosis with MEN1
B. MEN1
C. MEN1b
D. MEN2a
E. MEN2b

284 A 29-year-old woman who has undergone HCT for acute myelogenous leukemia (AML), subtype 3 has developed intractable anorexia, nausea, and intermittent vomiting on day 25 after the

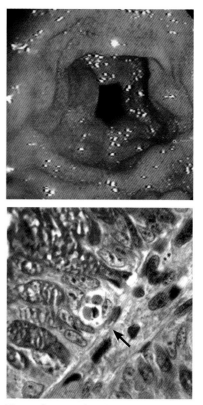

Figure for question **284**

transplant. Upper endoscopy of the duodenum is performed (see figure). Based on the findings, which of the following would be the best treatment at this time?

A. Start acyclovir
B. Start ganciclovir
C. Start 1 mg/kg of prednisone by mouth daily
D. Start fluconazole
E. None of the above

285 A 46-year-old woman with type 2 diabetes, hypertension, and gastroparesis was recently started on nifedipine by her physician. She now presents with a vague feeling of epigastric distress and worsening early satiety. Her physical exam findings are unremarkable. An endoscopy performed 2 months ago for dyspepsia showed no abnormalities, but an upper GI series with barium contrast shows a gastric-filling defect. What is the most likely diagnosis?

A. Gastric ulcer
B. Gastric cancer
C. Lymphoma
D. Pharmacobezoar
E. None of the above

286 A 49-year-old man undergoing chemotherapy for chronic myelogenous leukemia (CML) has pancytopenia, fever, right lower quadrant pain, nausea, and diarrhea that tests positive for heme. What antibiotics, if any, should be started?

A. None
B. Ciprofloxacin and metronidazole
C. Fluconazole
D. Oral vancomycin
E. Imipenem, oral vancomycin, and an antifungal agent

287 Which of the following statements is true regarding treatment of Zenker's diverticulum?

A. All patients with Zenker's diverticula should be offered surgery regardless of the size of the diverticulum and symptoms.
B. An open surgical approach is recommended for patients with large diverticula that extend into the thorax.
C. Compared to endoscopic techniques, open surgical procedures have a higher recurrence rate.
D. Compared to endoscopic techniques, open surgical procedures have a lower complication rate.

288 Pellagra may occur as a result of any of the following conditions *except*:

A. Inadequate intake of niacin
B. VIPoma
C. Carcinoid syndrome
D. Prolonged treatment with INH
E. Inflammatory bowel disease

289 A 33-year-old woman undergoes high-dose chemotherapy for HCT, and soon thereafter progressive lethargy, confusion, vomiting, gait loss of coordination, and hyperventilation are noted. Her medical history is remarkable only for AML, subtype 5. Which one of the following tests/studies should be performed to establish the diagnosis?

A. Liver function tests
B. Ammonia levels
C. Immediate CT of the head
D. Electroencephalography (EEG)
E. Blood cultures to rule out infection

290 Risk factors for diabetic autonomic neuropathy include all of the following *except*:

A. Older age
B. Poor control of diabetes mellitus
C. Use of oral hypoglycemic agents
D. Peripheral neuropathy

291 Which of the following cells gives rise to pancreatic endocrine tumors?

A. Neuron-specific enolase
B. Amine precursor uptake and decarboxylation

C. Chromogranin A
D. Chromogranin C
E. Synaptophysin

292 The best treatment for IPSID (also called alpha-heavy chain disease) is:

A. Surgery followed by radiation
B. Chemotherapy
C. Antibiotics followed by chemotherapy
D. Combined radiation and chemotherapy

293 Which is the most common cause of liver function test abnormalities in HIV-infected patients?

A. Acute hepatitis
B. CMV infection
C. HAART-induced injury
D. MAI infection

294 A patient who has undergone bilateral lung transplant (LT) is brought to the emergency department with severe midepigastric pain and reflux. His stool is positive for heme, and his serum hemoglobin level is 8.2 g/dL. Upper GI endoscopy reveals a clean-based ulcer that is 4 cm in diameter. Which of the patient's medications may have contributed to this ulcer?

A. Cyclosporine
B. MMF
C. Tacrolimus
D. Bactrim
E. All of the above

295 Paresthesias of the medial thigh and increased pain in the hip or medial thigh with extension and medial rotation of the hip are typical signs of:

A. Sciatic hernia
B. Spigelian hernia
C. Obturator hernia
D. Perineal hernia

296 Sarcoidosis with liver involvement may present:

A. Asymptomatically in a patient with normal liver function
B. Asymptomatically in a patient with elevated alkaline phosphatase level
C. As cirrhosis of the liver with portal hypertension
D. As cholestatic liver disease with jaundice, pruritus, and biopsy findings indistinguishable from those of primary biliary cirrhosis
E. As any of the above

297 Which of the following statements about post-ERCP pancreatitis is *not* true?

A. Pancreatitis is the most common complication of ERCP.
B. Risk factors for post ERCP pancreatitis have been well defined and include both patient and procedural factors.
C. The only definitive way to minimize the complication rate is to avoid performing ERCP for diagnostic purposes.
D. Treatment of post-ERCP pancreatitis is supportive.
E. Using pure cutting current for sphincterotomy will decrease the risk of pancreatitis.

298 A 20-year-old white woman who was diagnosed with hematochezia when she was 5 days old is seeking a second opinion. She has multiple cutaneous vascular lesions that have been present since 5 days of age. She has received blood transfusions on three occasions following hematochezia episodes. An emergent exploratory laparotomy showed a large pelvic vascular malformation, which was not treated. On physical examination, she is asthenic and appears pale but in no distress. She has multiple, bluish, nodular, soft, compressible, nontender lesions on her face, soft palate, arms, legs, hands, and trunk. No abdominal or rectal abnormalities are found on exam, and she is not orthostatic. All of the following statements about this young woman's diagnosis are true *except*:

A. GI bleeding is a rare feature of this condition.
B. Intussusception may be a presenting feature.
C. This can be transmitted in an autosomal dominant fashion.
D. The cutaneous nodules are venous malformations, for which no treatment is needed.

299 Cirrhosis of the liver in patients with sickle cell disease can be attributed to:

A. Hepatitis C
B. Ischemic liver injury
C. Hepatic siderosis
D. Hepatitis B
E. All of the above

300 A 25-year-old woman in the 30th week of her first pregnancy presents with nausea, vomiting, and headaches. She had been feeling well until 1 week ago when she began to have headaches accompanied by some blurring in vision. Her blood pressure has increased to 150/95 mmHg and some of her lab values are abnormal: WBC count, $4.5 \times 10^3/\mu L$; hemoglobin, 8.0 mg/dL; platelets, $57 \times 10^3/\mu L$, AST, 280 U/L; ALT, 180 U/L; and total bilirubin, 2.0 mg/dL. Which of the following is the correct diagnosis?

A. Acute fatty liver of pregnancy
B. Cholestasis of pregnancy

C. Pre-eclampsia
D. HELLP syndrome
E. Viral hepatitis

301 Which of the following is/are associated with increased occurrence of pancreatic endocrine tumor?

A. von Hippel-Lindau disease
B. von Reckinghausen's disease
C. Tuberous sclerosis
D. MEN1
E. All of the above

302 The following statements concerning elevated alkaline phosphatase in a case of uncomplicated rheumatoid arthritis are correct *except*:

A. It is usually associated with progressive hepatic disease.
B. It can be found in 18% of patients.
C. It can be associated with fatty liver.
D. Fluctuations correlate with disease activity.

303 A 52-year-old man with end-stage renal disease underwent continuous ambulatory peritoneal dialysis (CAPD) and now presents with diffuse abdominal pain and low-grade fever. On physical exam, the abdomen is diffusely tender. The catheter site appears normal, without erythema. Which of the following treatments should be initiated?

A. Imipenem
B. Piperacillin–tazobactam
C. Piperacillin–tazobactam and an aminoglycoside
D. Vancomycin and ceftriaxone
E. Hospitalization followed by removal of catheter

304 A 70-year-old man was diagnosed 2 weeks ago with diverticulitis and a diverticular abscess. A percutaneous drain was placed in the abscess, and the patient was discharged on antibiotics and scheduled for surgical resection as an outpatient. He now returns with increasing abdominal pain and increased output from the drain. What is the most likely cause of these symptoms?

A. Catheter dislodgement from the abscess cavity
B. Undrained loculation
C. New abscess
D. Perforation
E. Fistula tract

305 Match the stage of MALT gastric lymphoma with the preferred treatment (more than one treatment may be used per stage).

Stage	Treatment
1. Stage I	**A.** Surgery
2. Stage II	**B.** Antibiotics
3. Stage IV	**C.** Chemotherapy
	D. Radiation

306 A 23-year-old medical student complains of "very embarrassing loud noises in the stomach" that are worse after eating. He has no abdominal pain, his appetite is good, and he feels well without any other complaints. On questioning, he admits that he has lost about 12 pounds in the last 6 months, which he attributes that to skipping meals due to a very busy schedule. He also complains of an intermittent, sudden feeling of "warmth" and is concerned about his thyroid gland, especially because his mother had Grave's disease. Physical examination reveals mild periumbilical tenderness and hyperactive bowel sounds. Rectal exam is normal, but he is heme occult positive. Lab testing that he done elsewhere reported all levels including TSH as normal, but the patient wonders if there was lab error. The next indicated test is:

A. Mesenteric angiography
B. PET scan
C. Upper GI radiographic examination with small bowel follow-through
D. Enteroclysis
E. None of the above

307 A 33-year-old man who has undergone HCT following chemotherapy that included cyclophosphamide presents with progressive weight gain and edema 30 days after the transplant. His bilirubin, AST, and ALT values are also rising. Which one of the following is the best treatment option?

A. Intravenous defibrotide (25 mg/kg/day)
B. Prednisone 1 mg/kg/day
C. Intravenous heparin
D. **A** and **C**
E. **B** and **C**

308 A 29-year-old white woman who is 24 weeks pregnant presents with dysphagia and odynophagia that started about a week ago and have progressed in severity. She has pruritus and severe oral pain, for which she has started taking pain medication. She has no significant medical history and, prior to this, her only routine medication is a prenatal vitamin. On physical exam, she is alert and oriented, but appears uncomfortable and has a temperature of 99.6°F. She has multiple, lace-like lesions in her oral cavity with overlying ulcerations and small-to-medium, flat-topped pruritic and violaceous papules all over her skin. All of the following are true statements about her condition *except*:

A. Upper GI endoscopy will likely show erythema, ulcers, and webs in the proximal esophagus.
B. The condition should be treated with topical and systemic glucocorticoids.
C. The condition is associated with increased prevalence of chronic liver disease.
D. Treatment of this condition will decrease the risk of development of esophageal cancer.

309 Which of the following is true regarding radiation-induced enteritis?

A. Symptoms of radiation-induced enteritis may appear within a week of radiation therapy.
B. Younger patients are affected more than older patients.
C. Concurrent chemotherapy has not been shown to intensify the effects of radiation therapy.
D. Colonoscopy is the diagnostic test of choice for radiation enteritis.
E. Symptoms such as abdominal pain and diarrhea will not subside after discontinuation of radiation.

310 Which of the following is the drug of choice in treatment of insulinoma?

A. Diazoxide
B. Trichlormethiazide
C. Verapamil
D. Glucocorticoids
E. Propranolol

311 All of the following associations between viral hepatitis and rheumatoid arthritis have been described *except*:

A. A majority of patients with hepatitis C have serum positive for rheumatoid factor.
B. Treatment of rheumatoid arthritis with anti-TNF drugs can cause a flare of concomitant hepatitis B.
C. New-onset rheumatoid arthritis does not occur when chronic hepatitis C is present.
D. Cryoglobulinemia associated with hepatitis C presenting with arthralgia can be mislabeled as rheumatoid arthritis.

312 Which of the following are indications for surgical interventions in management of foreign body ingestions?

A. Perforation
B. Fistula formation
C. Failed endoscopic retrieval
D. Colonic obstruction
E. All of the above

313 All of the following studies should be performed to stage a gastric MALT lymphoma *except*:

A. EGD with biopsy of areas of involvement as well as normal-appearing areas of the stomach
B. Endoscopic ultrasound
C. Polymerase chain reaction amplification of specific mutations in the B-lymphocyte population of the gastric mucosa
D. CT of the chest and abdomen
E. Bone marrow biopsy

314 Which of the following is the most common predisposing factor in patients with food bolus impaction?

A. Benign esophageal stenoses
B. Surgical anastomosis
C. Esophageal cancer
D. Esophageal motility disorder
E. All of the above

315 Which of the following factors predict fibrosis and progression to cirrhosis in patients with hepatitis C who are also infected with HIV?

A. Higher ALT levels
B. Older age at infection
C. Higher inflammatory activity
D. Alcohol consumption of more than 50 g/day
E. All of the above

316 Which of the following studies is useful in detecting a coin in the hypopharynx or cervical esophagus?

A. Anteroposterior and lateral radiographs of the chest
B. A careful history and physical exam
C. CT scan
D. X-ray "obstruction" series
E. None of the above

317 Disorders that occur more often in diabetics include all of the following *except*:

A. Pancreatitis
B. Abdominal pain due to lower thoracic radiculopathy
C. Pancreatic cancer
D. Crohn's disease
E. Cholecystitis

318 All of the following are true statements about esophageal dilatation during upper endoscopy *except*:

A. Patients with eosinophilic esophagitis should not undergo dilation because they are at very high risk of perforation.
B. The esophageal stricture should always be dilated to the size of an uninvolved lumen for symptom relief.
C. The greatest risk of esophageal dilatation is perforation.
D. The type of dilator used during the procedure is a very important determinant of the risk of perforation.
E. Proximal esophageal strictures are more likely to perforate than mid or distal strictures.

319 Which of the following determines how severely ingestion of a caustic agent injures the gastrointestinal tract?

A. Concentration of the agent
B. Quantity of the agent ingested
C. Physical state of the agent (solid or liquid)
D. Duration of the exposure
E. All of the above

320 All of the following are areas of physiologic narrowing in the esophagus where foreign bodies are apt to become impacted *except*:

A. Upper esophageal sphincter
B. Aortic arch
C. Crossing of the mainstem bronchus
D. Gastroesophageal junction
E. Distal one third of esophagus

321 A 23-year-old woman presents with fatigue and a one-year history of intermittent diarrhea. She reports a 10-pound weight loss over the past year. She is found to have iron deficiency anemia. What is the best test for diagnosis of the underlying condition?

A. CT of the abdomen/pelvis
B. MRI of the abdomen
C. Ultrasound examination of the RUQ of the abdomen
D. Colonoscopy with random biopsies
E. Upper GI endoscopy with small bowel biopsies

322 Which of the following is needed to make the diagnosis of ZES?

A. Acid hypersecretion
B. Hypergastrinemia
C. Hypergastrinemia in a patient who is not being treated with a proton-pump inhibitor (PPI)
D. Acid hypersecretion in a patient with hypergastrinemia
E. A tissue sample showing characteristic changes

323 A 30-year-old man presents with profuse watery diarrhea and pitting edema of the lower extremities. No pathogens are found in stool samples. His albumin level is 2.6 g/dL, creatinine is 0.8 mg/dL, and low levels of IgG, IgM, and IgA are present. Which of the following treatments is the most important in management of the patient's hypoproteinemia and edema?

A. A high-fat diet
B. A high-protein diet
C. Administration of a glucocorticoid agent
D. Metronidazole 500 mg by mouth three times a day
E. A 5-aminosalicylic acid agent

324 Which of the following is the recommended treatment for peritonitis?

A. Glucocorticoids
B. Fluid resuscitation and antibiotic therapy followed by urgent laparotomy or laparoscopy
C. Fluid resuscitation and antibiotic therapy
D. Vasopressors such as dopamine
E. None of the above

325 A 40-year-old white man comes to the emergency department because of melena of 2 days' duration and dizziness. He has been taking over-the-counter NSAIDs for 3 days for a sports-related injury. He has multiple cherry-red spots on his lips and tongue. All of the following statements are true about this patient's condition *except*:

A. It is inherited.
B. It is characterized by telangiectasias that occur more commonly in the stomach and small intestines than in the colon.
C. The diagnosis is usually made by endoscopy.
D. Vascular involvement of the liver can present as a giant hemangioma.

326 The 5-year survival rate for enteropathy-associated T-cell lymphoma is:

A. 11% to 20%
B. 31% to 40%
C. 51% to 60%
D. 71% to 80%

327 Which one of the following has been recommended to treat caustic esophageal strictures?

A. Intralesional steroid injections
B. Repeat dilation
C. Esophageal resection
D. All of the above

328 Which of the following statements regarding *Mycobacterium avium* complex (MAC) in the GI tract is true?

A. MAC is the most commonly identified organism in patients with chronic diarrhea and low CD4 counts.
B. Many patients with MAC infection will have asymptomatic infection of the gut.
C. Duodenal involvement is common.
D. The diagnosis of MAC infection is best made by endoscopic biopsy.
E. All statements are true.

329 Which of the following liver diseases may recur after orthotopic liver transplantation?

A. Hepatitis C
B. Hepatitis B
C. Autoimmune hepatitis
D. Primary sclerosing cholangitis (PSC)
E. All of the above

330 All of the following statements regarding the incidence of carcinoid tumors in the gut are true *except*:

A. Carcinoid tumors of the esophagus are rare.
B. The stomach is the most common foregut location for carcinoid tumors.
C. The appendix is the most common site in the gut for carcinoid tumors.
D. In the colon, carcinoids are more likely to occur on the right side.
E. The incidence of rectal carcinoids is on the rise.

331 The incidence of liver involvement with acute myeloid or lymphoid leukemia is approximately:

A. 20% to 25%
B. 30% to 40%
C. 50% to 60%
D. 75% to 95%

332 Match the following cutaneous markers to the gastrointestinal malignancy with which each has been historically associated:

Cutaneous Marker	Gastrointestinal Malignancy
1. Tylosis	A. Gastric cancer
2. Sweet's syndrome	B. Pancreatic cancer
3. Trousseau's syndrome	C. Lymphoma
4. Dermatomyositis	D. Esophageal cancer
5. Subcutaneous fat necrosis	E. Colorectal cancer

333 A 32-year-old man is brought to the emergency department from a psychiatric ward where he was observed to have swallowed a round plastic chip. The patient has no complaints, and the results of the physical exam are within normal limits. On radiographs of the gut, a round object 2.3 cm in diameter can be seen within the stomach. What is the next step in the management of this patient?

A. Emergent surgery
B. Endoscopic retrieval
C. Observation for 5 to 7 days, and if the foreign object is not passed, endoscopic or surgical retrieval
D. No intervention; the foreign object will pass spontaneously

334 A patient who has undergone kidney transplantation complains of left lower quadrant abdominal pain. Abdominal imaging shows pneumatosis intestinalis. The patient is taking high doses of glucocorticoids and cyclosporine. What, other than infection, may be contributing to the findings in this case?

A. Glucocorticoid therapy
B. Cyclosporine therapy
C. Ischemia
D. **A** and **C**
E. **B** and **C**

335 All of the following statements about mycotic aneurysms are correct *except*:

A. The main risk factor for development of mycotic aneurysm is IV drug use.
B. The celiac artery is the commonest site.
C. They are most commonly caused by fungal infection and hence the name.
D. Early presenting symptoms are nonspecific and include abdominal pain.
E. They usually need to be treated by surgery.

336 Which of the following locations in the esophagus is more susceptible to stricture formation with alkali ingestion?

A. Level of the cricopharyngeus
B. Level of the aortic arch
C. Near the tracheal bifurcation
D. Lower esophageal sphincter
E. All of the above

337 Which of the following is *not* indicated in the follow-up care of a patient who underwent successful endoscopic removal of a food impaction?

A. Education on methods of reducing further impactions
B. Repeat endoscopy within 48 hours
C. 24-hour pH study and/or manometry study
D. Proton-pump inhibitors
E. All of the above

338 A 30-year-old man with AIDS presents with a 1-week history of progressive dysphagia and odynophagia that has resulted in a 5-pound weight loss. On exam he is afebrile and there is no evidence of thrush or ulcers in the oropharynx, but his mucous membranes are dry. Which of the following is the most likely finding on endoscopy?

A. Extensive, deep ulcerations throughout the esophagus
B. Diffuse, shallow ulcerations with areas of vesicles
C. Friability and ulceration of the distal esophagus
D. Focal or diffuse white plaques in association with mucosal hyperemia and friability

339 Malabsorption syndromes can be associate with all of the following diseases *except*:

A. Abetalipoproteinemia
B. Hypoparathyroidism
C. Addison's disease
D. Hyperthyroidism

340 A 55-year-old woman with scleroderma is referred for recurrent abdominal pain, bloating, and diarrhea. She says she hears loud rumbling sounds in her belly, particularly after each meal, and has intermittent diarrhea. Her lab studies reveal a macrocytic anemia. Stool studies are negative for blood, fecal leukocytes, ova, and parasites. Colonoscopy shows no abnormalities.

Which of the following is the best explanation for the patient's symptoms?

A. Collagenous colitis
B. Jejunal diverticulosis with bacterial overgrowth
C. Irritable bowel syndrome
D. *Clostridium difficile* enterocolitis
E. Inflammatory bowel disease

341 All of the following are true statements regarding carcinoid syndrome *except*:

A. Atypical carcinoid syndrome is caused by foregut carcinoids.
B. Flushing and diarrhea are the first symptoms of carcinoid syndrome.
C. Typical carcinoid syndrome is caused by midgut carcinoids.
D. Patients with atypical carcinoid syndrome have normal serotonin levels.
E. Patients with typical carcinoid syndrome have elevated rates of urine 5-HIAA excretion.

342 A 29-year-old man infected with the HIV (CD4 count of 100) presents with a 1-week history of bloody diarrhea (five to six bowel movements a day with bright red blood mixed with the stool). He denies any fevers, nausea, vomiting, contact with persons who are ill, or recent travel. He does complain of tenesmus associated with the diarrhea. Stool studies reveal fecal leukocytes but are negative for *Salmonella, Shigella, Campylobacter,* and *Clostridium difficile*. An antibiotic medication is selected empirically, but the patient's condition fails to improve. What is the next step in treatment of this patient?

A. CT scan of the abdomen
B. EGD with small bowel biopsies
C. Flexible sigmoidoscopy with biopsies
D. MRI of the abdomen

343 The most common site for non-Hodgkin's lymphoma of non–lymph node origin (primary GI lymphoma) is:

A. Stomach
B. Small intestine
C. Pancreas
D. Colon

344 Which of the following statements is most correct concerning surgical repair of inguinal hernias?

A. Recurrence is lower after mesh graft repair than after tissue-to-tissue repair.
B. Laparoscopic repair is associated with greater risk of recurrences than open repair.
C. Laparoscopic repair is associated with a greater complication rate than open repair.
D. A, B, and C.

345 A 37-year-old woman presents with episodic arthralgias, pleuritic chest pain, and vague abdominal pain. Her parents had suffered from similar complaints and one of her cousins also has had similar complaints. Which of the following treatments should be initiated?

A. Diagnostic laparoscopy
B. Prednisone
C. Colchicine
D. Malphalan
E. No treatment

346 Which grade of esophageal injury is more likely to lead to stricture formation?

A. Grade I
B. Grade IIB
C. Grade III
D. Grade IIB and grade III
E. Grade IIA

347 The following statements about GISTs occurring in a family are true *except*:

A. They can be associated with hyperpigmented areas of the skin.

B. The inheritance pattern is autosomal dominant.
C. They occur as part of Carney's triad, with pulmonary chondromas and extra-adrenal paragangliomas.
D. The association with neurofibromatosis is related to a common mutation in the *KIT* gene.
E. They tend to be multifocal.

348 The following are true statements about familial adenomatosis polyposis (FAP) and its variant, Gardner's syndrome, *except*:

A. There are multiple osteomas within the oral cavity of these patients.
B. It is an autosomal dominant condition.
C. Multiple sebaceous cysts appear on the face, scalp, and extremities of these patients before puberty.
D. The APC gene located on chromosome 5q21 is mutated in these patients.

349 Eosinophils are found in many sites in the normal GI tract; these include all of the following *except*:

A. Esophagus
B. Stomach
C. Cecum and appendix
D. Colon

350 A 55-year-old man presents 7 weeks after liver transplantation with complaints of fever of 101.1°F, malaise, myalgias, and odynophagia. His immunosuppression therapy includes mycophenolate mofetil and prednisone. Liver function tests reveal mild elevation of serum ALT. Upper endoscopy is performed (see figure). Which of the following should he have received post-transplant to reduce the risk of this complication?

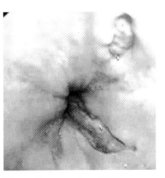

Figure for question **350**

A. Fluconazole
B. Cyclosporine
C. Ganciclovir
D. Acyclovir
E. Trimethoprim–sulfamethoxazole

351 In a patient with a history of food bolus impaction, symptoms of retrosternal chest pain can localize the level of impaction to the middle of the esophagus.

  A. True
  B. False

352 Which of the following techniques reduces the likelihood of radiation enteritis?

  A. Use only anterior and posterior fields for pelvic radiation.
  B. Administer radiotherapy in a supine position.
  C. Maintain an empty bladder during radiation therapy.
  D. Use misoprostol suppositories in patients undergoing radiation.

353 A patient who has undergone a liver transplantation for primary sclerosing cholangitis (PSC) would be at risk for which of the following malignancies?

  A. Colon cancer
  B. Lymphomas
  C. Skin cancers
  D. Kaposi's sarcoma
  E. All of the above

354 What is the frequency with which granulomas are found on liver biopsy of patients with sarcoidosis?

  A. 10% to 20%
  B. 30% to 40%
  C. 50% to 60%
  D. 80% to 90%

355 Which of the following products are involved in most cases of caustic ingestion in the United States?

  A. Nonhousehold acid/alkali products
  B. Drain cleaners and openers
  C. Rust removers
  D. Bleaches

356 What is the main cause of mortality in patients with GI fistulas?

  A. Arrhythmias due to electrolyte imbalance
  B. Underlying disease such as cancer
  C. Sepsis with multiorgan failure
  D. Complications of parenteral feeding

ANSWERS

102 **E.** (S&F, ch20)

Cronkhite-Canada syndrome is a rare, sporadic syndrome of GI polyposis, mucocutaneous hyperpigmentation, alopecia, malabsorption, and nail dystrophy. Diarrhea, nail changes, abdominal pain, and weight loss are the most common symptoms. Alopecia occurs in more than 95% of patients and involves loss of both scalp and body hair. Hyperpigmentation occurs in 85% of patients and more commonly involves the upper extremities. Death can occur in about 50% of the patients as a result of malnutrition from the diarrhea. Aggressive nutritional support by total parenteral nutrition can lead to complete resolution of symptoms.

103 **D.** (S&F, ch34)

Nodular regenerative hyperplasia is a subtle lesion occasionally picked up as hypodense areas on CT or abnormal echogenicity on ultrasound. However, these macro nodules have the same function as normal liver parenchyma when the diagnosis is clarified by MRI. Cirrhosis does not develop, and liver biopsy usually reveals tissue similar to normal parenchyma. They are associated with autoimmune and hematologic

diseases and with the drug azathioprine (and 6-thioguanine).

104 **E.** (S&F, ch39)

Acute pancreatitis is the commonest and most feared complication of ERCP. The risk factors for ERCP include both patient and procedural factors. Young age, female gender, and suspected SOD; all of which are present in this patient, put her at an increased risk for post-ERCP pancreatitis. Prescribing Actigall or an anticholinergic agent is not going to affect her symptoms significantly. Use of cutting current for ERCP has not been shown definitely to reduce the risk of post-ERCP pancreatitis. Placing a temporary pancreatic duct stent at the time of ERCP has been shown to significantly reduce the risk of post-ERCP pancreatitis in high-risk patients such as this one. Sending her to a surgeon at this point for bile duct exploration would be inappropriate.

105 **A.** (S&F, ch23)

The high association of underlying esophageal pathology accompanying food bolus impactions makes the practice of forceful blind pushing with the endoscope unacceptable. Esophageal muscular relaxation induced by sedation and expansion of the lumen with air insufflation may help food boluses pass with a gentle nudge forward with the tip of the endoscope, termed the push technique.

106 **C.** (S&F, ch35)

This patient most likely has Parkes Weber syndrome, which is a variant of Klippel-Trénaunay syndrome, differentiated from the latter by the fact that arteriovenous fistulae are common in the former. This syndrome consists of (a) vascular nevus of the lower limb, (b) varicose veins of the affected limb, (c) hypertrophy of all tissues including bone of the affected limb, and (d) arteriovenous fistulae. It usually manifests at birth; the results of the physical examination are almost always diagnostic.

107 **A**, false; **B**, true; **C**, true; **D**, false; **E**, true (S&F, ch39)

108 **D.** (S&F, ch29)

PET scan is of great value in staging GISTs for all the reasons listed. Almost all GISTs readily pick up fluorodeoxyglucose, making PET with FDG a preferred method to evaluate metastatic tumor.

109 **A.** (S&F, ch22)

Bochdalek hernias are large, present in the posterior left hemithorax, can be a neonatal emergency due to respiratory compromise, and require urgent surgery. Morgagni hernias occur through a smaller defect in the right anterior chest and present later in life.

110 **B.** (S&F, ch34)

Strict control of blood sugar levels may improve the condition and should be attempted first. Metformin and acarbose both have adverse effects, which include diarrhea. Steatorrhea is commonly found with this entity in patients without pancreatic or other small bowel disease. Clonidine and octreotide have both been used successfully.

111 **A.** (S&F, ch36)

This is a classic presentation of Fitz-Hugh-Curtis syndrome, or perihepatitis. Laparoscopy is very helpful in confirming the diagnosis, revealing "violin strings" and "bridal veil" adhesions from the abdominal wall to the liver. These signs were formerly most commonly associated with

Gonococcus infection. However, in recent years, *Chlamydia* infection is increasingly implicated in the development of perihepatitis. Doxycycline is usually curative.

112 **C.** (S&F, ch25)

The patient has diverticulitis with a diverticular abscess. The abscess did not resolve with antibiotics alone and therefore, it needs to be drained. Percutaneous drainage with catheter placement is preferred for collections greater than 3 cm in diameter, and systemic antibiotic therapy should be administered after drainage.

113 **C.** (S&F, ch34)

114 **E.** (S&F, ch39)

In this young woman with intermittent abdominal pain and abnormal liver enzyme values, the most likely diagnosis is sphincter of Oddi dysfunction (SOD). Patients suspected of having SOD have a high likelihood of developing post-ERCP pancreatitis.

115 **C.** (S&F, ch26)

Food elimination diets may be the only way to test for allergy if the allergen is not IgE mediated. These tests need to be performed in a double-blinded placebo-controlled fashion to be valid. Radioallergosorbent tests (RASTs) only help to identify IgE-mediated responses, which are not invoked by most of the allergens responsible for these diseases. Recently extracted allergens (less then 1 year old) must be used for skin-prick testing; older allergens are likely to cause false-negative responses.

116 **F.** (S&F, ch34)

These systemic vasculitides can all affect mesenteric circulation, causing ulceration and bleeding from the small bowel, and infarction with or without perforation. Of note, periarteritis nodosa is frequently accompanied by acute, acalculous cholecystitis that is ischemic in origin.

117 **D.** (S&F, ch39)

This patient most likely has postpolypectomy coagulation syndrome, which is characterized by full-thickness electrocautery burn following polypectomy. Patients with this condition usually present, as in this case, with localized abdominal pain, fever, and leukocytosis without any evidence of free air on a scout film. In mild cases, the patient can be discharged home on antibiotics but this patient needs to be observed in the hospital. It would only be by coincidence that diverticulitis would develop a day after a patient underwent colonoscopy, so this diagnosis is not likely.

118 **E.** (S&F, ch20)

This patient has pseudoxanthoma elasticum, which is a rare disorder characterized by aberrant calcification of mature elastic tissue. Skin lesions are usually the initial manifestation, appearing in the second decade as yellow to orange papules in the lateral neck ("plucked chicken skin"). Major complications of this condition such as retinal bleeding, intermittent claudication, premature onset of coronary artery disease (CAD), and GI bleeding are the result of calcification of the elastic tissue of the arteries. GI bleeding occurs in 8% to 13% of the patients, and the younger patients are more likely to be affected. GI bleeding is usually from the stomach, and often no specific bleeding site is found. Skin lesions may not be visible at the time of a GI bleed, and therefore, a blind skin biopsy may be needed to make the diagnosis.

119 **B.** (S&F, ch34)

Increased risk of bleeding (up to 4% in one report) after biopsy of a liver affected by amyloidosis has been reported. It is better to obtain tissue from other sites where bleeding can be controlled if it occurs.

120 **A.** (S&F, ch39)

PEG solutions, although they are considered safe for preparation for colonoscopy, can cause fluid shifts in patients. All of the other statements are true.

121 **B.** (S&F, ch26)

More extensive infiltrate of the bowel wall tends to produce fibrosis and stricture rather than deep ulceration. Perforation is not a reported complication. **A** and **D** have both been reported.

122 **D.** (S&F, ch33)

In the absence of antiviral prophylaxis, fatal fulminant hepatitis develops in approximately 15% of HCT recipients who are infected with hepatitis B virus (HBV). There is a 35% risk of post-HCT reactivation of HBV in patients with isolated anti-HBc antibodies, usually during treatment for acute graft-versus-host disease (GVHD). Severe hepatitis B infection has been seen in anti-HBc+/anti-HBs+ patients and in a patient with occult hepatitis B infection. Therefore, patients receiving an HCT should be immunized against HBV.

123 **D.** (S&F, ch22)

Determining the extent of gastroesophageal reflux and motor disorder of the esophagus allows the clinician to decrease the risk of postoperative complications by adjusting the tightness of the fundoplication used with these repairs.

124 **C.** (S&F, ch35)

This patient has superior mesenteric artery (SMA) syndrome, which is a condition in which the third part of the duodenum is compressed by the root of the SMA, leading to symptoms of intestinal obstruction. Typical symptoms include episodic epigastric distress, vomiting, and, in severe cases, weight loss. Diagnosis is by barium study, which typically shows an abrupt cutoff in the third part of the duodenum, with proximal dilatation (particularly when the patient is supine). The syndrome has been associated with immobilization in a body cast, rapid growth in children, and marked rapid weight loss in adults. Treatment includes small feedings or a liquid diet; symptoms generally improve after body weight is gained. Surgery is rarely needed. Duodenojejunostomy has been performed laparoscopically.

125 **E.** (S&F, ch25)

This patient has large-volume diarrhea suggestive of a fistula originating in the small bowel. Early management is directed to fluid and electrolyte replacement. Historically, conservative management of fistulas associated with Crohn's disease has been unrewarding, because most abdominal and perianal fistulas require surgical correction. However, infliximab, an anti-TNF alpha antibody, has shown efficacy in the closure of fistulas secondary to Crohn's disease and should therefore be first-line treatment for fistulous disease in patients with Crohn's disease.

126 **B.** (S&F, ch34)

Angiodysplasias are the most frequent cause of recurrent GI bleeding in patients on dialysis, especially when disease is long-standing. The first three conditions are not detectable by routine endoscopy and the last two are not infrequently missed at endoscopy.

127 **E.** (S&F, ch27)

This patient has giant hypertrophic gastropathy (Ménétrier's disease), which is the most common gastric lesion causing severe protein loss. Patients usually have dyspepsia, postprandial nausea, emesis, edema, and weight loss. Prominent and thick gastric folds with protein-rich exudates are seen. In this disorder, tight junctions between cells are wider than those found in healthy subjects, and it is believed that proteins traverse the gastric mucosa through these widened spaces. Histamine receptor antagonists, anticholinergic agents, proton pump inhibitors (PPIs), and octreotide may be used to improve symptoms; however, most patients with persistent abdominal pain or severe protein loss require subtotal or total gastrectomy.

128 **D.** (S&F, ch35)

GAVE or watermelon stomach is a vascular lesion of the gastric antrum that consists of tortuous dilated vessels radiating outwards from the pylorus like the spokes on a wheel and resembling the stripes on a watermelon. This lesion can cause both occult bleeding and acute hemorrhage. This condition is seen particularly in middle-aged or older women with achlorhydria, atrophic gastritis, or cirrhosis; with calcinosis cutis, Raynaud's phenomenon, esophageal dysfunction, sclerodactyly, and telangiectasia (CREST syndrome); or after bone marrow transplantation. This 65-year-old man presenting with hematemesis and a history of NSAID does not fit the classic picture of a patient with GAVE.

129 **C.** (S&F, ch22)

While all of the conditions listed could be present, the most likely diagnosis is incarcerated hernia, which can be completely corrected by relatively simple surgery.

130 **D.** (S&F, ch31)

The following drugs have been reported to control diarrhea, to varying degrees, in a few patients with vipoma: prednisone (60 to 100 mg/day), clonidine, indomethacin, phenothiazines, lithium, propranolol, metoclopramide, loperamide, lidamidine, angiotensin II, and norepinephrine. It is proposed that these agents primarily enhance sodium absorption in the proximal small intestine or inhibit secretion. Currently, long-acting somatostatin analogues such as octreotide or lanreotide are the agents of choice.

131 **C.** (S&F, ch36)

Epiploic appendagitis is often confused with appendicitis. It typically presents with RLQ abdominal pain. However, constitutional symptoms such as nausea, vomiting, and anorexia are less frequent, and the pain tends to have a more sudden onset. The patient can typically point to the exact location of the pain with one finger, and this point tends to be more

localized and slightly more cephalad than in appendicitis. Epiploic appendagitis can be diagnosed by CT, on it appears as a mass with negative attenuation values, indicating the presence of fat. This hypoattenuating mass may be bordered by a hyperattenuating peripheral ring corresponding to the edematous serosa.

132 **C.** (S&F, ch22)

The right side of the diaphragm is protected by liver; therefore, more traumatic hernias occur on the left side of the diaphragm. Many organs can be contained in hernia. Blunt trauma is more likely to produce hernia. Hernias may not be apparent immediately post-trauma but enlarge over time with the cessation of positive intrathoracic pressure from a ventilator or the traction of normal negative intrathoracic pressure.

133 **D.** (S&F, ch36)

This patient's history is compatible with retroperitoneal fibrosis. Treatment is usually with an immunosuppressant drugs such as azathioprine and steroids.

134 **B.** (S&F, ch39)

Although it is a common practice to stop aspirin and NSAIDs 7 days prior to an elective endoscopic procedure, these drugs have never been shown clearly to increase the risk of bleeding during an endoscopic procedure. On the other hand, patients receiving an anticoagulant are at an increased risk of bleeding during procedures; to decrease the risk, warfarin, a long-acting anticoagulant, needs to be temporarily stopped and short-acting low–molecular-weight heparin should be substituted before endoscopy.

135 **C.** (S&F, ch23)

Endoscopic removal of narcotic packets is absolutely contraindicated to avoid inadvertent rupture of the packages and release of the toxic contents. If the patient is asymptomatic, inpatient observation with a clear liquid diet is recommended. Whole-gut lavage and gentle purgatives have been reported to hasten the decontamination of the gut but remain controversial because of the potential to promote package rupture. Surgery is the definitive therapy for signs of intestinal obstruction, failure of packets to progress, and suspected rupture.

136 **B.** (S&F, ch33)

Post-transplant lymphoproliferative disease continues to be a problem for recipients of a liver transplant because they require continued high doses of immunosuppressant drugs. Both B- and T-cell lymphomas can develop in these patients.

137 **C.** (S&F, ch38)

In this patient, chronic radiation enteritis has caused intestinal dysmotility and mucosal dysfunction. Faster intestinal transit time and reduced bile acid and lactose absorption are observed in patients with chronic radiation enteritis. These effects are improved after the administration of loperamide. Antibiotics are indicated if there is evidence of small bowel bacterial overgrowth.

138 **C.** (S&F, ch21)

The most common symptoms of an intraluminal duodenal diverticulum are those of duodenal obstruction. Obstruction may be precipitated by retention of vegetable material or foreign bodies. Typical radiologic appearance on CT has been reported as a ring-like soft tissue density outlined with oral contrast and containing oral contrast and air, referred to as the "halo sign."

139 **B.** (S&F, ch20)

Epidermolysis bullosa (EB) is a heterogeneous group of rare inherited disorders of skin fragility. They are characterized by the formation of blisters with minimal trauma and are of different forms. Esophageal strictures are the most common complication of dystrophic EB and most commonly occur in the upper third of the esophagus. The esophageal strictures are probably induced by repeated trauma due to the passage of food or refluxed gastric contents. Balloon dilatation remains the mainstay of treatment for esophageal strictures. Although surgical excision of the esophageal stricture followed by colonic interposition is a possible treatment for this condition, it is not the next best step.

140 **B.** (S&F, ch30)

Somatostatin and its analogues do block the effects of amines and peptides on target tissue. This results in decreased gut motility, blood flow, and both exocrine and endocrine function. They are most effective in the treatment of diarrhea and to some degree in the treatment of flushing, but they are not effective in the treatment of abdominal pain due to carcinoid tumor.

141 **B.** (S&F, ch20)

Acrodermatitis enteropathica is a superficial scaling and blistering condition of the skin seen mainly in the groin area and periorally. It is often associated with alopecia. Replacement with zinc leads to rapid resolution of both alopecia and skin lesions. It is usually seen in patients with Crohn's disease, those on hyperalimentation, in children with congenital metabolic disorders, and in alcoholics with cirrhosis.

142 **C.** (S&F, ch37)

Graded-compression ultrasonography is the diagnostic test of choice for pregnant patients suspected of having appendicitis. Right lower quadrant pain is the most common presenting symptom of appendicitis. Pregnant patients during any trimester may undergo laparoscopic appendectomy, although potential interference by the gravid uterus may be a relative contraindication to this procedure during the third trimester.

143 **B.** (S&F, ch28)

Large, atypical cells are abundant in large, follicular B-cell lymphomas of the stomach. The predominant cell of MALT lymphoma is a small to medium lymphocyte with cellular atypia. Dutcher bodies are periodic acid–Schiff (PAS) positive inclusions in the nuclei of lymphomatous plasma cells. Destruction of gastric glands and germinal centers of lymphoid follicles is part of the neoplastic invasive process.

144 **A.** (S&F, ch31)

Somatostatinomas are neuroendocrine tumors that usually originate in the pancreas or intestine and release large amounts of somatostatin, which causes a distinct clinical syndrome characterized by diabetes mellitus, gallbladder disease, diarrhea, and weight loss. Histologically, a specific feature of duodenal somatostatinoma is the presence of psammoma bodies that are rarely found in pancreatic somatostatinomas or other types of duodenal carcinoid tumors.

145 **D.** (S&F, ch22)

Alcoholism is not listed as a risk for recurrence. Generally diseases that cause tissue deterioration, such as malignancy and chronic renal or liver disease or glucocorticoid therapy allow hernias to occur and recur.

146 **B.** (S&F, ch35)

The etiology of bony elongation of the affected limb in Parkes Weber syndrome is unclear but it is thought to occur due to in utero venous hypertension and stasis. Endoscopic control of GI bleeds is especially effective when the lesions are localized.

147 **C.** (S&F, ch23)

A careful history is important in eliciting risk factors for foreign body impaction. the results of physical examination tendsto be unremarkable or nonspecific but the exam must be carefully performed to recognize complications of foreign body ingestions such as perforation. Plain radiographs of the chest and abdomen can help determine the presence, type, and location of the foreign body. Radiographic contrast studies are relatively contraindicated in the evaluation of foreign body ingestions. Barium esophagrams should not be performed becausethey may make the performance of subsequent therapeutic endoscopy more difficult.

148 **D.** (S&F, ch34)

Although zinc deficiency is more common in patients with sickle cell disease due to renal loss of zinc, it is not a cause of acute liver damage, whereas the other diagnoses listed do cause damage. Zinc supplementation has been recommended for patients in sickle crisis in the past. Liver ischemia due to intrasinusoidal sickling can add to the toxicity of **B**, **C**, and **E**.

149 **B.** (S&F, ch20)

Kaposi's sarcoma (KS) is a common consequence of HIV infection and is associated with human herpes virus type 8 infection. The lesions appear as asymptomatic, red to purple oval macules that develop into papules, plaques, or nodules. These lesions rarely ulcerate. Treatment is usually palliative. It is true that recently there has been a decline in the number of KS cases.

150 **E.** (S&F, ch37)

Female fertility does not seem to be affected significantly by IBD. An exception may be among women who have undergone proctocolectomy for ulcerative colitis with ileoanal J-pouch anastomosis. These women reportedly have more difficulty becoming pregnant than do women without IBD, probably because women with IBD have pelvic adhesions and scarring of the fallopian tubes. Initial presentation of IBD during pregnancy is unusual. When IBD does develop in a pregnant woman, it most often does so during the first trimester. Pregnancy does not appear to increase the severity of pre-existing IBD. Most of the drugs routinely prescribed to manage IBD are safe during pregnancy.

151 **E.** (S&F, ch23)

Several groups are at above-average risk for intentional or accidental foreign body ingestion. Eighty percent of cases occur in the pediatric population, with a peak incidence between the ages of 6 months and 3 years. Intentional foreign body ingestion by an adult is most apt to occur among patients with psychiatric disorders, malingerers, and the incarcerated. Those at risk for accidental ingestion include the very elderly, those who are demented, those who wear dentures or have dental bridgework, and the intoxicated.

152 **D.** (S&F, ch33)

Hepatic GVHD usually follows cutaneous and/or intestinal GVHD and is heralded by a gradual rise in serum bilirubin, alkaline phosphatase, and aminotransferase enzyme levels. Characteristic liver biopsy findings in those with GVHD include lymphocytic infiltration of small bile ducts with nuclear pleomorphism and epithelial cell dropout. Because these patients are frequently pancytopenic, inflammatory infiltrates may be minimal.

153 **B.** (S&F, ch21)

This patient has a Zenker's diverticulum. Presenting symptoms in patients with Zenker's diverticulum include dysphagia, regurgitation, halitosis, aspiration, voice changes, and weight loss. A barium swallow is the most useful diagnostic study. At endoscopy it may be difficult to distinguish the lumen of the diverticula from the true lumen of the esophagus.

154 **A.** (S&F, ch37)

Acute fatty liver of pregnancy (AFLP) is a form of microvesicular fatty liver disease unique to human gestation that presents late in pregnancy, often as fulminant hepatic failure with sudden onset of coagulopathy and encephalopathy in a woman without a prior history of liver disease. In the majority of cases, symptoms develop between 34 and 37 weeks of gestation, although cases beginning as early as 19 to 20 weeks of gestation have been reported. Patients with AFLP frequently are confused and have pregnancy-related complications such as premature labor, vaginal bleeding, and decreased fetal movement. On laboratory evaluation, women with AFLP often have prolonged prothrombin times and decreased serum fibrinogen levels as well as leukocytosis. Their serum aminotransferase levels usually are moderately elevated (750 U/L), but rarely may be very high or even normal. Jaundice is common but not invariably present. The diagnosis of AFLP almost always is based on the appearance of typical clinical and laboratory features of the disorder in a woman in the later stages of pregnancy. Patients with AFLP should be managed in an intensive-care setting, preferably by obstetricians with special qualifications in the practice of maternal-fetal medicine, in cooperation with other specialists as appropriate. Early diagnosis and prompt delivery of the infant are imperative to minimize maternal and fetal morbidity and mortality.

155 **D.** (S&F, ch22)

All three congenital abnormalities have been described in neonatal Bochdalek hernias. Emergency surgical repair can require cardiopulmonary bypass because of poor lung function.

156 **A.** (S&F, ch36)

Pseudomyxoma peritonei represents a rare and special case in peritoneal tumors. Three-quarters of patients are women between 45 and 75 years of age. The sites of origin of the tumor are the ovary and the appendix. The diagnosis is made by finding jelly-like material in one of these locations at laparotomy or laparoscopy.

157 **D.** (S&F, ch39)

Although aspiration pneumonia can occur in patients receiving enteral feedings from aspiration of either oropharyngeal contents or an enteral feeding, the former is more usual. "Buried bumper syndrome" is a condition in which the external bolster of the PEG tube is so tight that the internal bolster migrates into the gastric wall. The commonest complication of PEG tube placement is local infection at the site of entry of the tube into the skin. The risk of this occurring can be reduced by preprocedure administration of an antibiotic medication.

158 **C.** (S&F, ch22)

All of the operations listed except appendectomy can create a new space through which bowel can herniate.

159 **A.** (S&F, ch20)

Oral hairy leukoplakia (HL) presents as corrugated white lesions on the lateral border of the tongue. Therefore, **A** is wrong. It is usually asymptomatic and may be an early sign of HIV infection. Although the severity of HL does not correlate with the severity of HIV, the presence of HL in an HIV-infected person has prognostic implications. It usually indicates that the time to development of AIDS is 24 months. It

can also occur in kidney and other solid-organ transplant recipients. Biopsy may be needed to confirm the diagnosis. Treatment is with oral acyclovir, topical retinoic acid and podophyllum. HL recurs with the discontinuation of treatment.

160 1-**D**, 2-**E**, 3-**B**, 4-**A**, 5-**C** (S&F, ch20)

Glossodynia (burning sensation or pain in the tongue) may occur as a result of a deficiency of magnesium, vitamin B_{12}, or folate. In addition, it may also be found with anxiety or depression. Glossitis or inflammation of the tongue occurs in a heterogeneous group of disorders including ingestion of chemical irritants, nutritional deficiencies, iron deficiency, and pernicious anemia. Xerostomia or dry mouth is often seen in patients with Sjögren's syndrome. Black hairy tongue is often seen in chronic smokers and occurs due to exogenous pigment trapped within the elongated keratin strands of the filiform papillae. Although dysgeusia may occur in association with glossitis, it is also seen in a variety of psychiatric disorders.

161 **A.** (S&F, ch31)

PETs are classified as nonfunctional if they are not associated with a clinical syndrome due to hormone release. Nonfunctional PETs have the histological characteristics of a PET but no associated elevation in plasma hormones or a clinical syndrome. Examples of such include PETs that release pancreatic polypeptide (PPomas), ghrelin, neurotensin (neurotensinomas), or other peptides that do not cause a distinct clinical syndrome.

162 **E.** (S&F, ch33)

The incidence of biliary cast syndrome has recently decreased to 5% to 20%, and most cases occur within the first year after orthotopic liver transplantation. Clinical factors associated with development of biliary casts include hepatic ischemia and biliary strictures. Hepatic artery patency should be assessed by ultrasound. Endoscopic and percutaneous therapy is successful in up to 70% of cases, but surgical intervention may be required, and mortality is reported at 10% to 30%.

163 **E.** (S&F, ch22)

This patient has so called "eventration syndrome," which occurs when a large-volume incisional hernia is repaired; with reduction of abdominal contents of the hernia, a major increase in intra-abdominal pressure occurs. Decreased venous return to the heart as well as compression of the lungs is the mechanism for dyspnea.

164 **B.** (S&F, ch20)

Aphthous ulcers, also called canker sores, are painful shallow ulcers that appear almost exclusively on unkeratinized oral mucosa. They are covered by yellowish-white or grayish-white exudate and surrounded by an erythematous margin. Rarely, they may occur in the esophagus, upper or lower GI tract, or in the anorectal mucosa. Management includes palliative and curative measures. All of the treatments listed have been used except B.

165 **B.** (S&F, ch32)

Microsporidium has emerged as one of the most common intestinal infections in patients with AIDS. Intestinal and hepatobiliary disease may be caused by two species: *Enterocytozoon bienusi* and *Encephalitozoon intestinalis*. Typical symptoms include watery, nonbloody diarrhea of mild to moderate severity, usually without associated crampy abdominal pain. Weight loss is common. Infection is associated with severe immunodeficiency with median CD4 counts less than 100/L.

166 **A.** (S&F, ch33)

During the first month following a solid organ transplant, infections include those present prior to transplant (e.g., urinary tract infection, UTI), those related to technical complications of the procedure itself (e.g., biliary sepsis), or those transmitted with the allograft. Opportunistic viral, fungal, and parasitic infections are more likely to develop after the first month.

167 **D.** (S&F, ch35)

It must absolutely confirm that this patient does not have an aortoenteric fistula, which usually is seen between the third and fourth portions of the duodenum. Although a clean-based duodenal bulb ulcer was found on the upper endoscopy, the likelihood of this patient bleeding from that is small. That, together with the fact that he had a similar episode of melena 2 to 3 days ago (which could have been a herald bleed from the aortoenteric fistula), CT of the abdomen is indicated and the patient needs to be hospitalized. No test is diagnostic for AE fistula; therefore, if the CT of the abdomen fails to show any abnormality and he continues to have melena, surgical intervention is needed. Repeating EGD with a pediatric colonoscope to visualize the third part of the duodenum is acceptable practice but only when it is performed the same day.

168 **C.** (S&F, ch24)

The majority of patients with caustic ingestions can be safely started on oral liquids after 24 to 48 hours. Grade I or IIA injury is noncircumferential, and these patients can be safely fed a liquid diet after the endoscopy. In patients with grade IIB or III injuries, oral feedings may not be tolerated right away and if this is the case after 48 hours, a nasoenteric tube can be inserted.

169 **A.** (S&F, ch20)

DH is an extremely pruritic skin disorder seen in early adulthood. All of the statements about DH are true except **A**. Fewer than 5% of patients with celiac sprue will have DH. However, more than 80% of patients with DH have celiac sprue. Gluten has been shown to be a dietary trigger of DH. Introduction of gluten to the diet of a patient with celiac disease who has been on a gluten-free diet will lead to reappearance of DH. Dapsone has been used to treat this condition.

170 **D.** (S&F, ch33)

Kidney transplant recipients are at higher risk for the development of intestinal ischemia compared to other organ transplant recipients; however, the incidence of ischemia is low (less than 5%), and the etiology is multifactorial. Recipients with polycystic kidney disease more often develop intestinal ischemia and obstruction. Intestinal ischemia in these patients carries a high mortality. Ischemia should be considered in kidney transplant recipients with abdominal pain, particularly older patients (older than 40 years) who have received a cadaveric kidney.

171 **C.** (S&F, ch36)

Multifocal leiomyomas, also called leiomyomatosis peritonealis, is a rare disease that can mimic peritoneal carcinomatosis. The tumors may appear together with other leiomyomatous lesions or with endometriosis. These lesions consist of small, rubbery nodules, appear to be hormone-sensitive, and develop during pregnancy or estrogen therapy. They can cause pain or gut bleeding, and they may regress with hormone withdrawal.

172 **A.** (S&F, ch31)

The most common causes of physiologic hypergastrinemia include atrophic gastritis, *H. pylori* infection, pernicious anemia, the use of potent acid suppressant drugs, chronic renal failure, and after gastric acid-reducing surgery. In these patients, which include 60% of those with

ZES, a secretin test and basal acid output (BAO) measurement should be performed. Eighty-seven percent of patients with ZES will have a 200 pg/mL increase in fasting gastrin with secretin provocation. The BAO is elevated in more than 90% of patient with ZES, being about 15 mEq/hour in patients who have not previously undergone gastric surgery and about 5 mEq/hour in patients who have undergone acid-reducing surgery.

173 D. (S&F, ch20)

Cutaneous manifestations are more common, and more specific in Crohn's disease than in ulcerative colitis. The most common cutaneous complication of Crohn's disease is granulomatous lesion of the skin, which can occur by direct extension of the underlying bowel disease. Pyostomatitis vegetans is characterized by pustules, erosions, and vegetations involving the buccal mucosa, gingival mucosa, and skin of the axilla, scalp, genitalia, and trunk. Diagnosis of pyostomatitis vegetans is by biopsy and treatment is by local or systemic steroids. Pyoderma gangrenosum presents as painful ulcerations and is more common in those with ulcerative colitisthan in those with Crohn's disease.

174 C. (S&F, ch33)

Pain near the anal canal in a granulocytopenic patient is treated as if it were due to bacterial infection until proved otherwise. Extensive supralevator and intersphincteric abscesses may be present without being apparent on external examination. Perineal herpes simplex virus (HSV) infection may also lead to painful ulcerations. Perianal infections must be treated before HCT.

175 A. (S&F, ch38)

This patient has chronic radiation proctitis. Coagulation with an argon plasma or yttrium-aluminum-garnet (YAG) laser decreases bleeding episodes and subsequent need for transfusion in these patients. Surgery is reserved for patients with intractable symptoms.

176 B. (S&F, ch31)

According to present knowledge, the key to diagnosing the somatostatinoma syndrome is to be aware of its clinical features and to consider measuring plasma levels of somatostatin-like immunoreactivity (SLI) on any patients with diabetes without a family history, with gallbladder disease with a pancreatic mass, or with a history of unexplained diarrhea.

177 C. (S&F, ch27)

Protein-losing enteropathy is the excessive leakage of plasma proteins into the lumen of the GI tract. Mechanisms for increased protein loss include increased mucosal permeability to protein secondary to cell damage or cell loss, mucosal erosions or ulcerations, or lymphatic obstruction. There is no evidence of maldigestion, malabsorption, or defect in protein or amino acid metabolism.

178 A. (S&F, ch24)

Within seconds of caustic exposure, necrosis develops. Twenty-four to 72 hours after the exposure, ulceration develops. Fibrosis can be seen after 2 to 3 weeks. Stricture takes weeks to years to develop. The most feared complication, carcinoma, takes decades to develop.

179 D. (S&F, ch20)

Serologic tests show that 40% to 80% of adults have been infected by CMV. However, symptomatic disease occurs mainly in immunocompromised patients. Retinitis and mucosal ulcers are the main features and skin is rarely affected. Biopsy of ulcers in patients with CMV will show intracytoplasmic and intranuclear inclusions. Treatment consists of administering ganciclovir, vanganciclovir, cidofovir, and foscarnet.

180 C. (S&F, ch33)

This patient has symptoms of gastroparesis. GERD and gastroparesis are particularly problematic after liver transplant or HLT and may be related to medications and vagal nerve injury during the operation. Symptomatic gastroparesis has been described in 25% of liver transplant recipients and up to 80% of HLT recipients. The course is often waxing and waning, suggesting a neuropathic, infectious (CMV), or medication-induced etiology, but ultimately there is partial or complete remission.

181 C. (S&F, ch24)

If removal of the disc battery is accomplished and no tracheoesophageal fistula is suspected, one should still consider a barium swallow within 48 hours to rule out a fistula. If a tracheoesophageal fistula is present, complete esophageal rest and enteral tube feeding may result in spontaneous closure of the fistula in 4 to 12 weeks. If there is no fistula, a second barium examination is recommended 2 weeks later to evaluate for stricture formation. Blood and urine mercury levels should be monitored if the cell is observed to have split or radiographic droplets are evident.

182 **A.** (S&F, ch36)

The pain of peritonitis can be reduced or even absent in elderly patients, in patients receiving glucocorticoids, in diabetics with advanced neuropathy, and in those under the influence of alcohol. Patients with cirrhosis and ascites may deny any pain during episodes of spontaneous bacterial peritonitis. Analgesics typically will not relieve the pain of peritonitis and it has been shown that early provision of analgesia to patients with undifferentiated abdominal pain does not affect diagnostic accuracy.

183 **B.** (S&F, ch28)

A heavy chain lymphoma is considered an immunoproliferative small-intestine disease (IPSID) lymphoma with secretion of a typical monoclonal alpha heavy chain protein from the abnormal plasma cells.

184 **C.** (S&F, ch22)

Cameron ulcer on the lesser curvature folds of a large hiatal hernia at the diaphragmatic indention occurs in approximately 5%. These ulcers are not always present to identify the hernia as the cause of blood loss, especially after empiric proton-pump inhibitor (PPI) therapy for heartburn. Other occult sites of small bowel bleeding could be identified by capsule endoscopy. Large hiatal hernias significantly increase the risk for iron deficiency anemia.

185 **E.** (S&F, ch34)

All three of these factors can contribute. Infiltration with tumor is most likely. Amyloidosis with light chain deposition occurs in about 10% of myelomas. Extramedullary hematopoiesis may contribute.

186 **E.** (S&F, ch36)

For all of the reasons listed, there has been a drastic increase in laparoscopic abdominal procedures when operating within the abdomen where the goal is to minimize or eliminate inflammation.

187 **A.** (S&F, ch22)

Spigelian hernias are difficult to palpate because they lie within the abdominal wall, covered by external oblique muscle. Only 75% are diagnosed preoperatively, and the pain can be mistaken for other acute intra-abdominal processes. Use of

ultrasound (US) and computed tomography (CT) are extremely helpful to confirm the diagnosis.

188 **C.** (S&F, ch20)

This patient has pemphigus vulgaris, which is a blistering disorder characterized by bullae and ulcers affecting the mucosa of the oral cavity, pharynx, esophagus, anus, conjunctiva, and skin. Half of these patients will present with oral ulcerations, and ulcerations will develop in virtually 100% during the course of the illness. Patients with IgG and IgA antibodies are more likely to respond to treatment. Treatment consists of oral and topical glucocorticoids, sometimes in conjunction with immunosuppressant agents.

189 **E.** (S&F, ch34)

Amyotrophic lateral sclerosis frequently involves the pharynx to the extent that terminal aspiration pneumonia can occur. Parkinsonism is associated with dysmotility in the body of the esophagus as well as the pharynx. Multiple sclerosis is associated with constipation due to failure of relaxation of pelvic muscles involved in defecation. Myotonic dystrophy is associated with abnormal GI motility and dilation in multiple areas of the GI tract, including the esophagus.

190 **D.** (S&F, ch38)

A clinical syndrome of acute esophagitis with esophageal ulceration is often seen in the second or third week of standard fractionated thoracic radiotherapy. Patients often complain of dysphagia and odynophagia. Patients may develop persistent chest pain unrelated to swallowing. The most common late complication of radiotherapy is esophageal stenosis or stricture, which appear 4 to 6 months after a course of radiotherapy. Esophageal dysmotility may be seen within 4 to 12 weeks after radiotherapy but may develop earlier in patients undergoing concurrent chemotherapy.

191 **B.** (S&F, ch33)

Eosinophilic colitis with diarrhea has been reported with the use of both tacrolimus and cyclosporine. Histologically, this is characterized by eosinophilic colonic infiltrates and peripheral eosinophilia. Elevated serum immunoglobulin E (IgE) may be present in some patients.

192 **C.** (S&F, ch28)

Although 25% of patients with MALT lymphomas test negative for *H. pylori*, administration of an antibiotic to eradicate the bacteria should still be the initial step: Many patients in this group who do not improve can be demonstrated to have one of three mutations involving chromosomal translocations. Tumors can also be refractory to therapy if they are at a more advanced stage than was indicated by initial staging procedures.

193 D. (S&F, ch31)

To differentiate hypoglycemia from insulinoma and factitious use of insulin, measurement of plasma proinsulin, C-peptide, and insulin levels are used. In patients with surreptitious use of insulin, the proinsulin level is either normal or decreased, plasma insulin level is high, and the C-peptide level is low.

194 E. (S&F, ch23)

Up to 33% of infants and children are asymptomatic after foreign body ingestion. Symptoms without a history of ingestion can include choking, vomiting, blood-stained saliva, respiratory distress, and stridor. Less commonly, children may simply refuse to eat or demonstrate failure to thrive.

195 1-C, 2-D, 3-A, 4-B, 5-E (S&F, ch20)

Dermatitis herpetiformis is a very pruritic skin disorder characterized by vesicular or bullous lesions on the scalp, shoulders, elbows, knees, and buttocks. It is seen in association with celiac sprue. Porphyria cutanea tarda is a metabolic disorder characterized by skin fragility, blisters, hypertrichosis, and hyperpigmentation in sun-exposed skin. It is associated with hepatitis C infection. Glucagonoma of the pancreas is associated with necrolytic migratory erythema of the skin, which is a rash seen around orifices, flexural regions, and the fingers. The rash is typically papulovesicular but may be in the form of erosions with fissures and crusting. Sister Mary Joseph's nodule is an umbilical metastasis of a GI carcinoma, most often a gastric cancer. Erythema nodosum appears as shiny, tender, deep, red nodules 1 cm or larger in diameter. They are seen typically in patients with IBD, in particular Crohn's disease. They are generally seen over the shins.

196 C. (S&F, ch35)

This young woman has most likely developed superior mesenteric artery (SMA) syndrome, also called Wilkie's syndrome, a condition that is usually seen after rapid weight loss. It presents as postprandial abdominal pain, vomiting, and further weight loss. It is more common in women than men. An upper GI series will show a

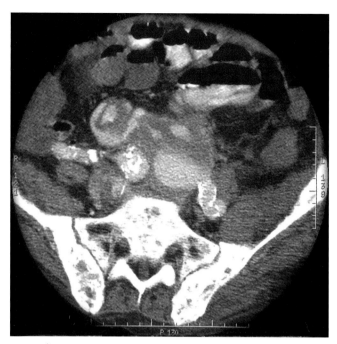

Figure for answer **196**

cutoff in the third portion of the duodenum with proximal dilatation. The cutoff is due to compression of the duodenum by the superior mesenteric artery. Symptoms usually improve after weight gain; surgical intervention is rarely needed. Esophageal stricture is unlikely in the absence of dysphagia. This patient could have recurrent lung cancer but it does not explain her symptoms. Linitus plastica is unlikely based on the results of the upper endoscopy performed 2 weeks ago.

197 E. (S&F, ch39)

All of these statements are true.

198 E. (S&F, ch31)

All of these are characteristics of glucagonoma. Hypoaminoacidemia occurs in 26% to 100% of patients with glucagonoma and essential fatty acid deficiencies have also been reported. Weight loss is a prominent feature; there was a mean weight loss of 20 kg in one study. The anemia is usually not severe and is usually normochromic and normocytic.

199 A. (S&F, ch33)

Anorexia, nausea, and/or vomiting are common following liver transplant, particularly early in the post-transplant course. These symptoms are often related to herpesvirus infections and to medications, and thus endoscopic evaluation is necessary for diagnosis in most patients. Tacrolimus is a macrolide lactone that causes nausea, abdominal pain, and diarrhea. These side effects are dose-dependent and can be managed with dose reduction or, more rarely, drug discontinuation. Mycophenolate mofetil (MMF) has a similar side effect profile. Because herpes simplex virus (HSV) infection can be a serious complication, endoscopy should be performed prior to attributing the symptoms to a medication.

200 **C.** (S&F, ch31)

This patient has a tumor that is secreting growth hormone–releasing factor (GRF) and causing acromegaly, as evidenced by enlargement of hands and feet. Skin changes, headache, and peripheral nerve entrapment also occur with acromegaly. Hyperproloactinemia is observed in 70% of patients with GRF-secreting tumors as compared to 50% of patients with somatotroph adenomas. The diagnosis is established by demonstrating elevated plasma levels of growth hormone and insulin-like growth factor-I (IGF-I). Octreotide is the agent of choice for treating patients with these tumors.

201 **E.** (S&F, ch37)

Resting LES pressures progressively decrease during gestation and then return to normal after delivery. This finding is likely due to the inhibition of smooth muscle contraction by progesterone. Transit time of intestinal contents is prolonged during gestation. In the small bowel, delayed transit time is most pronounced in the third trimester. Colonic transit time has also been shown to be prolonged in animals. Animal experiments have shown increases in small intestinal weight and villus height, changes that may have an effect on absorptive capacity. Pregnancy causes alterations in bile composition, including cholesterol supersaturation, decreased chenodeoxycholic acid and increased cholic acid concentration, and increase in the bile acid pool.

202 **B.** (S&F, ch31)

This patient's worsening symptoms of acid-peptic disorder while on twice a day proton pump inhibitor therapy leads to the suspicion that he has ZES. Clues that MEN1 is also present are (a) a history of nephrolithiasis and/or renal colic is much more frequent in patient with ZES with MEN1 than with sporadic ZES (47% vs. 4%), (b) patients with MEN1 present at a younger age with ZES (34 years vs. 43 years), and (c) 72% of those with MEN1 have a family history of endocrinopathies.

203 **E.** (S&F, ch35)

Dieulafoy's lesion can result in a massive GI bleed, usually from the stomach, but the bleed

can occur anywhere in the GI tract or even outside the GI tract such as the bronchus. The vascular abnormality consists of an artery of large caliber in the submucosa, and in some cases the mucosa, with a small overlying mucosal defect. These lesions are twice as common in men as in women and present at a mean age of 52 years. The diagnosis is best made by early endoscopy.

204 **D.** (S&F, ch39)

Although the most feared complication of colonoscopy is perforation, cardiorespiratory complications arising from sedation are more common.

205 **C.** (S&F, ch26)

Although GERD and eosinophilic esophagitis (EE) may both be associated with eosinophils in the mucosa, an eosinophil count of more than 7 per high-power field (HPF) helps to differentiate EE from GERD. In one study, a count of fewer than 7 cells/HPF was associated with 85% response to anti reflux treatment, whereas EE is refractory to such therapy. Other ways in which EE differs from GERD are that with EE there is:

1. Younger (adolescent) age at presentation
2. Associated history of atopy (present in 50% to 80% of cases)
3. More frequent location of strictures in mid or proximal esophagus
4. Greater tendency for a family history of atopy (in 39% of cases)
5. Predominately male occurrence

206 **A.** (S&F, ch24)

This patient presents with classic symptoms of antral stenosis that has caused gastric outlet obstruction. Antral stenosis usually develops 1 to 6 weeks after ingestion but may not appear for several years. It appears to occur with equal frequencyafter acid and alkali ingestions. Endoscopic dilation has been used successfully and should be considered as an initial maneuver in patients with antral stenosis. Other options are reserved for refractory cases or patients with severe injury.

207 **A.** (S&F, ch31)

MEN2a and MEN2b do not have pancreatic endocrine tumors, only MEN1s are characterized by hyperparathyroidism and PETs without the presence of medullary thyroid carcinoma, pheochromocytoma, or unusual phenotypes.

208 **D.** (S&F, ch34)

A typical case of systemic mastocytosis is described. In 40% of cases there is duodenal ulcer and 60% of patients have diarrhea, sometimes with malabsorption due to diffuse mucosal disruption of proliferating mast cells. Although there is a mutation in the *c-KIT* gene with stimulation of tyrosine kinase, Gleevac does not help because it fails to bind to sites of this particular mutation.

209 **D.** (S&F, ch36)

Fungal peritonitis can be due to gut perforation, especially perforation of the upper gastrointestinal tract. The most common isolate is *Candida* spp. This can be treated with fluconazole.

210 **C.** (S&F, ch30)

Patients with a new diagnosis of carcinoid tumor should undergo cross-sectional imaging at the level of the tumor and liver, where metastatic disease is most likely to be located. Positron emission tomography (PET) is useful in these cases because it can identify disease throughout the body. Visualization of the primary tumor is more difficult than delineation of metastatic disease and therefore, **C** is an incorrect statement.

211 **C.** (S&F, ch24)

Symptoms of caustic ingestion include persistent salivation, vomiting, hematemesis, dysphagia, odynophagia, and chest or epigastric pain. Hoarseness and stridor indicate upper airway involvement. Airway management and resuscitation should be the first priority and only when the airway is thought to be secured should further evaluation be initiated.

212 **C.** (S&F, ch22)

The triad of pain, unproductive retching, and resistance to passage of a nasogastric (NG) tube is called Borchardt's triad and is typical of gastric volvulus. Esophageal symptoms due to obstruction by a cancer would be more chronic in onset. Perforated ulcer or ruptured aneurysm would present with signs of acute abdomen and no obstruction to NG tube passage.

213 **D.** (S&F, ch22)

The chest x-ray of an "obstruction" series would show the incarcerated segment of stomach in the chest. CT and a barium study would also confirm the diagnosis but would require more time and be more costly than the plain radiographic series. EGD may be contraindicated, especially if there is ischemia.

214 1-**E**, 2-**A**, 3-**D**, 4-**C**, 5-**B** (S&F, ch20)

215 **E.** (S&F, ch35)

The correct way to manage incidental telangiectasias of the colon, as in this 54-year-old white man, is to do nothing.

216 **E.** (S&F, ch37)

Cholestasis of pregnancy usually presents in the third trimester but may be seen earlier in gestation. Serum alkaline phosphatase increases by 7- to 10-fold along with the levels of AST, ALT, and direct bilirubin. There is no evidence of hemolysis. Severe pruritus is the most common manifestation. Intense cholestasis is associated with steatorrhea that is usually subclinical but can be caused by deficiencies of fat-soluble vitamins, most notably deficiency of vitamin K. Improvement of symptoms begins with the delivery of the infant. Women with cholestasis of pregnancy have no residual hepatic defect, but are at increased risk for development of gallstones. Cholestasis of pregnancy has serious implications for fetal well-being and risk of morbidity and mortality may be reduced by close monitoring. Management is primarily palliative. Ursodeoxycholic acid is helpful in relieving symptoms and is well tolerated by both mother and fetus.

217 **D.** (S&F, ch31)

Because glucagonomas are generally malignant and it is not possible to predict in a given patient when metastases may develop, surgical resection should be performed in all patients if it is feasible.

218 **F.** (S&F, ch29)

The statements listed provide a brief outline of the mechanism of normal function and aberrant function of the *KIT* gene in GISTs.

219 **B.** (S&F, ch33)

220 **E.** (S&F, ch34)

The dysphagia common in persons with Sjögren's syndrome is aggravated by xerostomia and frequently not associated with esophageal motility disturbance. Gastric antral vascular ectasia (GAVE) is present in 25% of these patients. Among patients with primary biliary cirrhosis, Sjogren's syndrome is common.

221 **C.** (S&F, ch34)

This patient has cholestatic hepatitis related to severe extrahepatic infection/sepsis. This syndrome is frequently seen with pneumococcal infections. In the absence of ductal dilation or extrahepatic obstruction, liver function should become normal with clearing of the infection. Normalization of liver function usually occurs within several days but may take weeks if cholestasis is severe.

222 **A.** (S&F, ch36)

It is important to note that not all patients with peritonitis require laparotomy or laparoscopy. Examples of conditions that do not require these interventions include diverticulitis, acute pancreatitis, and contained perforation of appendicitis with abscess.

223 **B.** (S&F, ch30)

The rectum is a common site for the occurrence of carcinoids and the incidence appears to be rising. Rectal carcinoids appear at a younger age compared to other colonic tumors. Men and women are equally affected but the incidence in African Americans is 3-fold that in whites. More than 80% of rectal carcinoids are still localized at the time of diagnosis. They can be treated endoscopically, by local excision, and by radical excision with either low anterior or abdominoperineal resection. Rectal carcinoids greater than 2 cm in diameter have a 60% to 80% chance of metastasis.

224 **D.** (S&F, ch27)

SLE is a systemic autoimmune disease associated with protein-losing gastroenteropathy. Mesenteric vasculitis can result in intestinal ischemia and edema and altered intestinal vascular permeability. Protein losing gastroenteropathy may be the initial clinical presentation of SLE. Treatment with glucocorticoids, as well as other immunomodulatory agents such as azathioprine and cyclophosphamide, can lead to remission with resolution of symptoms.

225 **E.** (S&F, ch23)

A small bezoar may be managed conservatively with a clear liquid diet and administration of a prokinetic agent such as metoclopramide. Nasogastric lavage may effectively dissolve small phytobezoars. Cellulase, administered in tablet form or as a liquid instilled via a nasogastric tube or injected through an endoscope, can result in chemical dissolution of the bezoar. Mechanical disruption can be accomplished with standard endoscopic tools such biopsy forceps or polypectomy snares. Surgery is indicated when the methods just discussed fail or when there is a bezoar-associated complication such as perforation, obstruction, or gastrointestinal bleeding.

226 **D.** (S&F, ch34)

Although Hodgkin's disease can, rarely, produce enlarged periportal nodes and extra hepatic obstruction, the hallmark feature of this disease is an idiopathic cholestasis with no overt obstruction. This can regress with administration of systemic chemotherapy. The liver lesions associated with Hodgkin's disease include idiopathic elevation of alkaline phosphatase levels, hepatic granulomas (25%), or actual tumor infiltration. These syndromes with no tumor invasion must be recognized to correctly stage the tumor.

227 **E.** (S&F, ch30)

Most appendiceal carcinoids are less than 1 cm in diameter, and very few are more than 2 cm. Most authors recommend simple appendectomy for tumors less than 1 cm and right hemicolectomy for carcinoid tumors of the appendix that are more than 2 cm. Therefore, the correct answer is **E**. Appendiceal carcinoids have a good prognosis and have an overall 5-year survival rate of 71%. Distant metastasis is seen in 9.6% of cases at the time of diagnosis.

228 **D.** (S&F, ch36)

The absence of percussible hepatic dullness suggests the presence of free air in the peritoneal cavity, a sign of a perforated gastric ulcer.

229 **A.** (S&F, ch31)

Hypergastrinemia can be detected in 50% of patients with ovarian cancer. Gastric symptoms occur in some patients with bronchogenic carcinoma, acoustic neuroma, pheochromocytoma, or colorectal cancer; however, hypergastrinemia is not seen.

230 **C.** (S&F, ch30)

The most distinctive feature of carcinoid syndrome is flushing, which is present in 30% to 94% of the patients at some time during the course of the disease. Flushing similar to carcinoid syndrome can be seen in all of the conditions listed except **C**.

231 **E.** (S&F, ch28)

Chemotherapy plus radiation therapy gives survival rates at least as good as surgery. Rituximab is a monoclonal antibody that blocks the CD-20 receptor on B-cells.

232 **C.** (S&F, ch26)

It is important to remember that incidental or secondary infiltration of the GI tract can occur in patients with a variety of inflammatory conditions, including those without an allergy or primary cause for eosinophilic proliferation. Other main causes for secondary eosinophilic infiltration include parasitosis, systemic vasculitis, connective tissue disease, and hypereosinophilic syndrome (a hematologic disorder).

233 **C.** (S&F, ch31)

Thromboembolic phenomena were reported to have occurred in 13% to 35% of patients with glucagonoma in various series. In one series, venous thrombosis occurred in 24% of patients and pulmonary emboli in 12%. Because pulmonary embolus is life-threatening, it should be suspected in any patient with shortness of breath with glucagonoma. Weight loss is seen even in patients with small tumors without metastatic spread. Anemia, although common, is usually not severe enough to cause the symptoms listed.

234 **C.** (S&F, ch28)

Anemia occurs in 68% and perforation in 23%. Perforation has been reported after therapy as well.

235 **E.** (S&F, ch32)

This patient, as is typical of those with AIDS cholangiopathy, presented with subacute right upper quadrant pain, fever, nausea, and vomiting. Often diarrhea is present as well. Jaundice is rare because biliary obstruction is incomplete. Endoscopic sphincterotomy is performed for AIDS-related papillary stenosis and typically relieves the pain dramatically but does not affect the biochemical indices. Survival of patients with AIDS cholangiopathy is linked to the severity of immunodeficiency.

236 **C.** (S&F, ch34)

Laparoscopy should be avoided in patients with "acute abdomen." such as occurs with this disease, because adhesive obstruction often occurs after surgery. Colchicine is the therapy that has most often proven helpful. When used long-term it not only decreases the frequency of attacks but helps prevent progression of amyloidosis.

237 **B.** (S&F, ch28)

Part of the pathogenesis of this lymphoma is uncontrolled proliferation of Epstein-Barr virus (EBV) with suppression of immune system function. Stopping immunosuppressant drugs may help to control viral proliferation, and some tumors respond to this approach. Acyclovir and ganciclovir have been tried to decrease viral proliferation. Alpha interferon and rituximab have also proven somewhat beneficial. Surgery or radiation have been used if disease is documented to be localized.

238 **D.** (S&F, ch30)

False-positive elevations of urinary excretion of 5-HIAA can occur with dietary intake of foods that are rich in serotonin such as walnuts, pecans, bananas, and tomatoes; dietary supplements such as melatonin or serotonin (5-HT); or medications such as guaifenesin, methyldopa, and isoniazid (INH). Rifampin is not one of the medications that can cause false-positive elevations of 5-HIAA in the urine.

239 **E.** (S&F, ch31)

This patient has secretory diarrhea as confirmed by the low osmolar gap. Some of the laboratory abnormalities seen in patients with vipoma include hypercalcemia, hyperglycemia, hypokalemia, hypochlorhydria, and hypomagnesemia.

240 **B.** (S&F, ch29)

The level of CD-34, which originates from stem cells in the gut wall, is neither a sensitive nor a specific indicator of a GIST. Smooth muscle actin is a marker for smooth muscle cells and S-100 is a marker for nerve cells but neither is consistently present in GISTs.

241 **B.** (S&F, ch37)

Most women of child-bearing age with chronic hepatitis B infection are healthy carriers of the virus with a very low risk of developing complications of their disease during gestation. The importance of maternal hepatitis B infection during pregnancy is related to its role in the perpetuation of chronic infection through vertical transmission: maternal-fetal transmission of hepatitis B virus is responsible for most cases of chronic hepatitis B infection worldwide. Mothers with a reactive serum test for hepatitis B e-antigen have more circulating virus and higher rates of perinatal transmission than do mothers without detectable levels of serum hepatitis B e-antigen or a reactive serum test for hepatitis B e-antibody, although the latter individuals are still a source of neonatal infection. The infants of mothers with a reactive serum test for hepatitis B surface antigen should receive hepatitis B immunoglobulin at birth and also hepatitis B vaccine during the first day of life and at ages 1 and 6 months. Women with chronic hepatitis B are not treated with interferon during pregnancy. Therapy with the nucleoside analog, lamivudine, is safe in pregnant patients and has been reported to reduce the incidence of neonatal vaccination failure.

242 **C.** (S&F, ch32)

The patient has CMV infection. The clinical manifestations of this infection can vary greatly and include no symptoms in those who are carriers. The most common presentation is abdominal pain and chronic diarrhea. The infection usually occurs after the CD4 count falls below 100/L. Infection is most common in the colon; however, the esophagus, stomach, or small bowel can be involved. The most commonly used agent for treatment is ganciclovir. Because CMV primarily develops in those with severe immunodeficiency, recurrences are common following withdrawal of therapy; however, improvement in immune function with HAART will obviate the need for long-term therapy with ganciclovir.

243 **E.** (S&F, ch34)

Acute liver failure occurs with adult Still's disease. It resembles autoimmune hepatitis and may respond to immunosuppressant drug therapy. It is the most common cause of death in patients with Still's disease, in contrast to the more benign disease seen in an uncomplicated case of rheumatoid arthritis.

244 **D.** (S&F, ch31)

Calcium infusion may increase the release of hormones from insulinomas, vasoactive intestinal polypeptide (VIP)-secreting tumors, pancreatic polypeptide (PP)-secreting tumors, glucagonomas, growth-related factor (GRF)-secreting tumors, or somatostatinomas.

245 **D.** (S&F, ch30)

The etiology of diarrhea in carcinoid syndrome is not very clear. It is thought to occur as a result of partial small bowel obstruction (SBO), accelerated small bowel and colonic transit, reduced colonic capacitance, and exaggerated postprandial colonic tone. However, unlike flushing, which does not respond to serotonin antagonists, diarrhea can be well controlled by these agents. This indicates a prominent role for serotonin in the pathogenesis of this feature of carcinoid syndrome. Glucocorticoids are given to a patient with carcinoid syndrome who develops hypotension.

246 **B.** (S&F, ch29)

Two large cooperative studies involving 1700 patients with GISTs found different responses to increasing the dose of imatinib from 400 mg/day to 800 mg/day. Neither study showed improvement in overall patient survival rates. One study showed no benefit in progression-free survival while the other showed a modest but statistically significant benefit in favor of 800 mg/day dosing. Certainly a 50% improvement in nonresponse rate cannot be expected with the larger dose although increased drug toxicity was clearly seen.

247 **D.** (S&F, ch28)

Diffuse large B-cell lymphomas most always involve the muscularis propria or deeper. The finding of low-grade MALT in these tumors suggests a transition from a less-aggressive to more-aggressive cell type. The P53 and P16 mutations may be the additional factors that allow the large-cell tumors to escape their dependence on growth of *H. pylori,* which is indicated by the finding that in very early stages, these tumors may still respond to eradication of *H. pylori.*

248 **A.** (S&F, ch25)

The aerobes most often found in intra-abdominal abscesses are *Escherichia coli* and *Enterococcus* spp. The most common anaerobe is *Bacteroides fragilis.* Most abscesses contain both aerobic and anaerobic flora. The bacteria associated with intra-abdominal abscesses in patients in intensive care units are different. The most common organisms in this group of patients were *Candida, Enterococcus, Enterobacter,* and *Staphylococcus epidermidis.*

249 **D.** (S&F, ch31)

Somatostatinoma is characterized by distinct clinical syndrome of diabetes mellitus, gallbladder disease, diarrhea, and weight loss. Gallbladder disease may be a result of somatostatin inhibition of gallbladder emptying, as demonstrated by the occurrence of cholelithiases or biliary sludge in patients taking octreotide.

250 **C.** (S&F, ch33)

EBV reactivation generally presents in patients in the early post-transplant stage as a mononucleosis-like syndrome with diffuse adenopathy and fever; detection of EBV DNA in the bloodstream may allow pre-emptive therapy, with lower doses of immunosuppressant agents or treatment with rituxan.

251 **B.** (S&F, ch32)

In HIV-infected patients, *Cryptosporidium*, a cause of self-limited diarrhea in healthy hosts, is the most frequent protozoa identified. The small bowel is the most common site of infection, although the organisms can be recovered from all regions of the gut. Diarrhea is typically severe, with stool volumes of several liters per day. Borborygmi, nausea, and weight loss also frequently occur. Currently, the most effective therapy for cryptosporidiosis is HAART, because improvement of immune function results in a clinical remission of diarrhea and clearance of cryptosporidia from the stool.

252 **D.** (S&F, ch34)

This case illustrates the presentation of typhlitis (acute cecal inflammation) associated with acute leukemia. Typhlitis is especially likely to occur after the nadir of cytopenia induced by chemotherapy. The thick wall of the cecum and bloody diarrhea are confirmatory. Conservative treatment is advised unless abdominal findings suggest a perforation.

253 **E.** (S&F, ch31)

Organic hypoglycemia is generally defined as a fasting blood glucose level of less than 40 mg/dL. After an overnight fast only 53% of patients with insulinoma in one study had a blood glucose level of more than 60 mg/dL, and 39% had levels of less than 50 mg/dL. However, if a blood glucose determination is combined with a concomitant plasma insulin level, results will be positive in 65% of patients. A ratio of plasma insulin (in uU/mL) to glucose (in mg/dL) is considered positive for insulinoma if the ratio is more than 0.3.

254 **C.** (S&F, ch28)

Treatment of *H. pylori* in patients with MALT lymphoma results in resolution of lymphoma in most cases (75%).

255 **A.** (S&F, ch30)

The biochemical basis of flushing is not completely understood. The role of serotonin in flushing is unclear, because elevated levels of serotonin have not been consistently associated with flushing. Flushing is, however, worsened with stress. Norepinephrine levels have been found to be elevated during flushing episodes. At present, the best explanation for flushing is that it is due to the release of polypeptide hormones.

256 **A.** (S&F, ch33)

Gastric antral vascular ectasia (GAVE) is also a cause of severe upper intestinal bleeding in HCT recipients. Diffuse areas of hemorrhage are seen in the gastric antrum and proximal duodenum, but the underlying mucosa is intact. Histopathologic findings or abnormal dilated capillaries, thromboses, and fibromuscular hyperplasia in the lamina propria are diagnostic. Endoscopic laser therapy is the treatment of choice to control bleeding, but multiple laser treatments may be required to obliterate ectatic lesions.

257 **C.** (S&F, ch34)

The hypercalcemia of hyperparathyroidism is associated with constipation. The mechanism of diarrhea in Addison's disease is not clear. The mechanism in **B**, **D**, and **E** is hormonal.

258 **B.** (S&F, ch31)

Parathyroidectomy in patients with ZES and MEN1 with hyperparathyroidism decreases fasting gastrin levels, decreases the increase in gastrin seen after secretin injection, decreases basal acid output (BAO), and increases sensitivity to antisecretory drugs. This latter effect is particularly important because MEN1 and ZES with hyperparathyroidism can be relatively more resistant to PPIs, and patients with these conditions require higher and more frequent doses of PPIs. Surgical exploration is not indicated in those with MEN1.

259 **D.** (S&F, ch28)

The alpha heavy chain immunoglobulin secreted is always monoclonal. As such it can be detected by protein electrophoresis (it is located in the alpha 2 or beta band) or by immunoelectrophoresis. The secretion of IgA is blocked by this process and allows infestation by *Giardia*. The association of Mediterranean lymphoma with living under conditions of poor sanitation suggests that the lymphoma develops due to chronic immunostimulation by overgrowth of intestinal bacterial.

260 **A.** (S&F, ch29)

Myelotoxicity is noted more frequently in patients being treated for chronic myelogenous leukemia but it can occur in patients treated for GISTs.

261 **E.** (S&F, ch30)

The rectum is a common site for carcinoids, and the incidence appears to be rising. They usually appear at a younger age compared to other tumors of the colon and the male-to-female ratio is about 1:1. There is a 3-fold higher incidence in African Americans compared to white Americans. Carcinoid syndrome due to rectal lesions is very uncommon despite the fact that low rectal carcinoids can secrete the hormones directly into the bloodstream. Rectal carcinoids can be treated in different ways: endoscopically, by local excision, or by low anterior or abdominoperineal resection. Because the primary determinant of outcome in patients with rectal carcinoid is the underlying tumor biology, radical surgery is not always indicated. The overall 5-year survival rate is 87%.

262 **E.** (S&F, ch29)

Clinical studies have validated **A**, **B**, and **C** as indicative of malignancy. An additional sign on endoscopic ultrasound (EUS) is the presence of echogenic foci or cystic spaces in the tumor mass (indicative of central necrosis).

263 **C.** (S&F, ch33)

The abrupt onset of severe retrosternal pain, hematemesis, and painful swallowing suggests a hematoma in the wall of the esophagus, a result of retching when platelet counts are very low. Endoscopy is relatively contraindicated, because many intramural hematomas represent contained perforations. The course of intramural hematomas is one of slow resolution over 1 to 2 weeks.

264 **E.** (S&F, ch23)

Bowel perforation and obstruction are the most common significant complications associated with foreign body ingestions. Other complications include bleeding, respiratory compromise, fistulization (esophagorespiratory and esophagoaortic fistulas may present months to years after foreign body ingestion), and abscess formation. Esophageal perforation is associated with the highest mortality and morbidity. Complications include mediastinitis, lung abscess, pneumothorax, pericarditis, and cardiac tamponade.

265 **B.** (S&F, ch29)

GISTs become symptomatic when they become large enough to rupture or cause ulceration with bleeding or obstruction. They rarely spread through the lymphatics, which is the mechanism of metastasis of a Virchow's node.

266 **D.** (S&F, ch31)

Neurotensin is a 13-amino acid peptide that has a number of biologic effects, including

tachycardia, hypotension, and cyanosis; change in intestinal motility; increase in jejunal and ileal fluid and electrolyte secretion; and increase in pancreatic protein and bicarbonate secretion. Patients with neurotensinomas may present with hypokalemia, weight loss, diabetes mellitus, cyanosis, hypotension, and flushing.

267 **D.** (S&F, ch28)

268 **E.** (S&F, ch30)

Most physicians rely on the clinical features and the level of 5-HIAA in a 24-hour urine collection for the diagnosis of carcinoid syndrome. This test has its limitations; false-positive results may occur with dietary intake of foods that are high in serotonin and with certain medications. Excretion rates greater than 25 mg/day are diagnostic. Excretion rates of 5-HIAA correlate well with tumor mass and with symptoms. Midgut carcinoid tumors are associated with high rates of 5-HIAA excretion in the urine whereas foregut carcinoid tumors may have normal rates of urinary excretion of 5-HIAA.

269 **E.** (S&F, ch31)

Regarding PPomas, which are nonfunctioning pancreatic endocrine tumors, elevated plasma levels of chromogranin A and B are found in 69% to 100%, neuron-specific enolase in 31%, PP in 50% to 75%, α-HCG in 40%, and β-HCG in 20%.

270 **D.** (S&F, ch31)

PETs frequently produce chromogranins or the alpha or beta subunit of human chorionic gonadotropin. Plasma chromogranin A levels are found elevated in more than 90% of patients with various PETs and carcinoid tumors.

271 **D.** (S&F, ch33)

This patient has signs and symptoms of cholangitis and the ERCP shows anastamotic stricture. Strictures and leaks in patients with duct-to-duct anastomoses are often amenable to endoscopic therapy, while those with choledochojejunostomies may need to undergo percutaneous surgery for correction.

272 **E.** (S&F, ch34)

All of the conditions listed are more common in persons with SLE. Budd-Chiari syndrome is identified by the presence of anti-cardiolipin antibody or lupus anticoagulant. Mesenteric ischemia can be severe, causing bowel infarction.

Pancreatitis is also due to ischemia. The peritonitis of polyserositis is well known.

273 **A.** (S&F, ch31)

Overall, abdominal ultrasound, CT, and MRI are not very sensitive in localizing a primary tumor, being positive in only 10% to 40% of cases. Of the standard imaging studies, selective abdominal angiography is the most sensitive for localizing the primary tumor. SRS is now the method of choice to localize metastatic disease.

274 **B.** (S&F, ch29)

Positive staining for CD-117 can be expressed by cells harboring normal (wild type) KIT. It can also be found in normal cells, such as interstitial cells of Cajal and mast cells. It can be found in other tumors listed in **A** and **C**. The 5% of GISTs that do not stain positive for CD-117 have another mutation in the platelet-derived growth factor receptor alpha (PDGFRA), a structurally related kinase.

275 **C.** (S&F, ch27)

The gold standard for diagnosing protein-losing gastroenteropathy, measurement of the fecal loss of radiolabeled, intravenously administered Cr-albumin, is cumbersome to perform. Alpha-1 antitrypsin is a useful marker of intestinal protein loss. Enteric protein loss can be demonstrated by quantifying the concentration of alpha-1 antitrypsin in the stool or by measuring its clearance from the plasma. The optimal test is to measure alpha-1 antitrypsin from the plasma during a 72-hour stool collection.

276 **C.** (S&F, ch31)

Cutaneous lesions are one of the most common manifestations of the disease, occurring in 64% to 90% of cases. These lesions often appear long before diagnosis of the syndrome. The figure shows typical cutaneous lesions, referred to as necrolytic migratory erythema. Characteristically, the lesions start as erythematous areas, usually around the mouth or in intertriginous areas such as the groin, buttocks, thighs, or perineum, and then spreads laterally. The lesions subsequently become raised with superficial central blistering. Healing is associated with the development of hyperpigmentation.

277 **C.** (S&F, ch36)

This patient has tuberculous peritonitis, which can cause ascites in the absence of cirrhosis. The ascites fluid has a high protein content, low level of glucose, and low serum-to-albumin gradient.

Patients with this condition almost always have ascitic fluid, with an elevated WBC count, with lymphocyte predominance. The algorithm for evaluation of patients with high-lymphocyte count ascites includes cytologic evaluation of the fluid and consideration of laparoscopy. Patients with lymphocytic ascites and fever, such as this patient, usually have tuberculosis, whereas afebrile patients usually have malignancy-related ascites. Laparoscopy is 100% sensitive in detecting tuberculous peritonitis. The level of CA-125 may be elevated in tuberculous peritonitis. Cytology is positive when peritoneal carcinomatosis is present.

278 **B.** (S&F, ch25)

This patient's history is suggestive of Crohn's disease with an intra-abdominal abscess. CT with intravenous and oral contrast is the imaging modality of choice for the diagnosis of most abdominal abscesses. Administration of IV contrast is useful because it will demonstrate the wall of an abscess as an area of enhancement. The symptoms of intra-abdominal abscess are nonspecific and include abdominal pain, tenderness to palpation, distension, and in some cases, a palpable mass.

279 **D.** (S&F, ch34)

The patient probably has intestinal pseudo-obstruction due to a paraneoplastic syndrome associated with small-cell lung cancer. The pseudo-obstruction is caused by cross-reactivity of an antibody to both tumor cells and neurons in the mesenteric plexus of the bowel. Hypergastrinemia and serotonin secretion by a carcinoid would both cause diarrhea. Hypercalcemia would produce constipation but not the radiologic picture of pseudo-obstruction.

280 **A.** (S&F, ch31)

In all studies of this condition, the most important prognostic factor was found to be the development of liver metastases.

281 **B.** (S&F, ch24)

Posteroanterior and lateral radiographs from mouth to anus should be obtained after physical examination. If the battery is lodged in the esophagus, immediate endoscopy with removal is performed, often with the patient under general anesthesia. The blind passage of a Foley catheter balloon or magnetic retrieval device is not recommended.

282 **C.** (S&F, ch23)

In the United States, the foods that most often become impacted are larger pieces of beef, pork, chicken, and hot dog, which is why food impaction in the United States is often referred to as "steakhouse syndrome" or "backyard barbecue syndrome." During the evaluation of a patient with suspected food impaction, anteroposterior and lateral chest radiographs should be obtained to assess mediastinal or peritoneal free air and the presence of bones or other radio-opaque foreign material in the food bolus. Urgent management is indicated when patients are in severe distress, excessively salivating, or unable to manage their secretions. This consists of flexible endoscopy, performed using intravenous sedation, rather than rigid endoscopy, because flexible endoscopy has a high success rate, permits thorough examination, and is more safe, available, and cost-effective than rigid endoscopy. Food boluses may pass with intravenous administration of glucagon. Trial of sips water should only be attempted when bolus passage is thought to have occurred.

283 **E.** (S&F, ch31)

Patients with MEN2b have a characteristic phenotype with multiple mucosal neuromas, Marfanoid habitus, puffy lips, prominent jaw, pes cavus, and medullated corneal nerves. Pheochromocytomas, when they occur, are bilateral in 70% of cases.

284 **C.** (S&F, ch33)

An early sign of acute GVHD is loss of appetite, followed by nausea and vomiting. When symptoms occur on day 20 or later after transplant, more than 80% of patients with intractable anorexia, nausea, or vomiting will be found to have gastric and duodenal GVHD. Endoscopy will reveal edema of the gastric antral and duodenal mucosa, patchy erythema, and bilious gastric fluid, and histologic examination of a biopsy specimen will reveal epithelial cell apoptosis and dropout, often with localized lymphocytic infiltrates. Immunosuppressant drug therapy (a 10-day course of prednisone 1 mg/kg plus oral beclomethasone dipropionate 8 mg/day) is an effective therapy.

285 **D.** (S&F, ch23)

Bezoars can be classified into four types: phytobezoars, composed of vegetable matter; trichobezoars, composed of hair or hair like fibers; medication bezoars (pharmacobezoars), consisting of medications or medication vehicles; and lactobezoars, or milk curd bezoar, in infant formula reconstituted from powder. Gastroparesis is commonly seen in patients with bezoars. Patients with comorbid illnesses such as diabetes, end-stage renal disease on dialysis, or mechanical ventilation are at increased risk of bezoar

formation. Of numerous medications responsible for pharmacobezoars, cardiovascular medications such as nifedipine, procainamide, and verapamil are common.

286 **E.** (S&F, ch33)

Typhlitis occurs in granulocytopenic patients but is not common after HCT. Symptoms include fever, right lower quadrant pain, nausea and vomiting, diarrhea, occult blood in stool, and shock. The diagnosis of typhlitis is usually made on the basis of the history and physical exam, laboratory test, and imaging study findings; laparotomy is rarely necessary. If typhlitis is a possibility, imipenem and oral vancomycin therapy should be started along with an antibiotic with activity against bacteria and fungi typically found in the intestinal lumen.

287 **B.** (S&F, ch21)

Patients with large and symptomatic Zenker's diverticula should be offered surgical treatment, whereas those with small asymptomatic or minimally symptomatic diverticula can be treated by observation alone, because progressive enlargement is uncommon. Open surgical treatment may be considered in any symptomatic patient who has no contraindication to surgery. An open surgical approach is the safest alternative for patients with large (more than 5 cm) diverticula that extend into the thorax. Upper esophageal sphincter (UES) myotomy should always be part of the procedure. In general, compared to endoscopic techniques, open surgical procedures result in a lower recurrence rate and a greater proportion of patients obtaining symptom relief. However, risk of complications is higher with open surgery than with endoscopic techniques.

288 **B.** (S&F, ch20)

Pellagra is characterized by symmetrical, brown red blistering or scaling plaques, usually in sun-exposed areas of the body. It can occur with any of the above-mentioned conditions except vipoma.

289 **B.** (S&F, ch33)

A syndrome of hyperammonemia and coma has been described in patients who received high-dose chemotherapy, including conditioning for HCT. Patients present with progressive lethargy, confusion, weakness, loss of coordination, vomiting, and hyperventilation. The diagnosis is confirmed by a plasma ammonia concentration exceeding 200 μmol/L in the absence of evidence of liver failure. This syndrome is rare, but it is associated with a high mortality.

290 **C.** (S&F, ch34)

Options **A, B,** and **D** have been associated with autonomic neuropathy. Insulin-dependent diabetics also are more prone to this complication.

291 **B.** (S&F, ch31)

PETs are thought to originate from cells that are part of the diffuse neuroendocrine cell system. These cells share certain cytochemical properties and tumors of these cells have been referred to as APUDomas (amine precursor uptake and decarboxylation tumors). Ultrastructurally these cells often have electron-dense granules and produce multiple regulatory hormones and amines, including neuron-specific enolase, synaptophysin, and chromogranin A or C.

292 **C.** (S&F, ch28)

Because bacterial infection is believed to be a major stimulant of the immune cells in this tumor, antibiotics should be tried first if the tumor is confined to the mucosa. Response rates range from 33% to 71%. If no response has been noted by 6 months after a course of antibiotic therapy or the patient has advanced disease at presentation, chemotherapy with CHOP is preferred.

293 **C.** (S&F, ch32)

Drug-induced liver injury has emerged as the most prevalent cause of liver function test abnormalities in HIV-infected patients, largely due to the increasing array of antiretroviral medications used in their care. The protease inhibitors, especially ritonavir, are the most common causes of abnormal liver function tests in these patients. The major risk factors for drug-induced hepatotoxicity include coexistent viral hepatitis, older age, and greater increase in CD4 cells after HAART. The abnormalities usually follow a hepatocellular pattern.

294 **A.** (S&F, ch33)

Lung transplant (LT) recipients may develop giant gastric ulcers (more than 3 cm in diameter), even with routine use of medications to suppress acid secretion. These ulcers have significant morbidity and mortality. They are more often associated with bilateral LT, administration of high-dose NSAIDs after transplant, acute rejection requiring high-dose

glucocorticoid therapy, and cyclosporine immunosuppression.

295 **C.** (S&F, ch22)

Medial thigh paresthesias and pain in the hip and thigh with extension and medial rotation comprise the Howship-Romberg sign that is typical in those with an obturator hernia.

296 **E.** (S&F, ch34)

When granuloma of the liver progresses to a more advanced stage or with longer duration of sarcoidosis, periportal fibrosis and ductopenia with associated granulomas may be difficult to distinguish from primary biliary cirrhosis (PBC). Fibrosis with dense granulomatosis has been reported to cause cirrhosis in about 6% of those with sarcoidosis and is characterized by all of the complications of portal hypertension.

297 **E.** (S&F, ch39)

Use of cutting current during sphincterotomy has not been definitely shown to decrease the risk of post-ERCP pancreatitis. The other statements are true.

298 **A.** (S&F, ch20)

This young woman has a condition called blue rubber bleb nevus syndrome, which is a rare disorder of the skin and GI tract. Its features include a constellation of cutaneous and GI tract malformations. In patients such as the woman described here, blue, compressible nodules develop subcutaneously. GI tract vascular malformations are very common, especially in the small intestine or colon, and GI bleeding is almost always present. The malformations may be treated surgically or with photocoagulation.

299 **E.** (S&F, ch34)

Hepatitis B and C infection is more prevalent in patients who received a blood transfusion prior to 1992. It has been reported that one third of those with sickle cell disease test positive for HCV antibody. Ischemic damage from crises can lead to perisinusoidal fibrosis. Chronic iron load from transfusion is a well-known cause of cirrhosis.

300 **D.** (S&F, ch37)

HELLP syndrome is seen in 20% of women with severe pre-eclampsia. In addition to the diagnostic abnormalities of hemolysis, elevated serum aminotransferase levels and thrombocytopenia in conjunction with hypertension and proteinuria, patients with typical HELLP syndrome frequently have complaints of chest, epigastric, and right-upper quadrant abdominal pain. These symptoms often are accompanied by some combination of nausea, vomiting, headache, and blurred vision. The diagnosis of HELLP syndrome is based on an assessment of the clinical features of the illness at the time of presentation. Fragmented red blood cells are seen on smears, and the serum lactate dehydrogenase (LDH) level is elevated. Serum aminotransferase levels also are elevated, sometimes minimally and other times over a thousand. Serum bilirubin levels often are elevated, but in most patients only mildly. A diagnosis of fatty liver of pregnancy also should be considered in patients with clinical findings of HELLP syndrome, but acute fatty liver usually is associated with signs of more significant liver disease and possibly liver failure.

301 **E.** (S&F, ch31)

In addition to MEN1, there is an increased incidence of PETs in phacomatoses: von Hippel-Lindau disease, von Recklinghausen's disease (neurofibromatosis-1, NF-1), and tuberous sclerosis (Bourneville's disease).

302 **A.** (S&F, ch34)

Elevation in alkaline phosphatase in the average patient with rheumatoid arthritis is usually to no more than twice normal, fluctuates with activity of the disease, and is not associated with severe liver histopathology (usually only with fatty change).

303 **D.** (S&F, ch36)

This patient has developed bacterial peritonitis while undergoing CAPD. This complication occurs about 1.4 times per patient-year of CAPD treatment. The complication is most likely due to inadvertent contamination of the indwelling catheter. The most common isolates in patients treated with CAPD are *Staphylococcus epidermidis* and other skin flora. Vancomycin and a second- or third-generation cephalosporin are good options for treatment.

304 **E.** (S&F, ch25)

When to discontinue percutaneous abscess drainage and obtain follow-up imaging studies depend on the clinical response, catheter drainage, and presence of an enteric communication (fistula). If the clinical response is good and catheter output has diminished to less than 20 mL/day, the catheter can safely be removed. If the clinical response is inadequate, repeat imaging is warranted. Persistently high catheter output raises the suspicion of a fistula. A catheter study performed by instilling water-soluble contrast through the catheter under fluoroscopy is the best method to assess for an internal fistula.

305 1-**B**; 2-**C** and **D**; 3-**C**. (S&F, ch28)

In stage I disease, antibiotics should be used primarily. With nodal involvement (stage II) chemotherapy and radiation therapy must be ordered. Surgery is a poor second choice for these patients because it involves total gastrectomy, which frequently results in poor quality of life. With distant disease (stage IV) chemotherapy is used with remissions but no expectation of cure. (See Table 28-3.)

306 **C.** (S&F, ch30)

Periumbilical pain, borborygmi, and periumbilical tenderness all point to a disorder involving the small bowel. These symptoms, in association with weight loss, a sudden feeling of warmth, and heme-positive stools, make carcinoid tumor the most likely diagnosis. Therefore, the first best test for definitive diagnosis is UGI with SBFT. This young man is unlikely to have mesenteric angina. Although PET may be useful if he has carcinoid tumor, that is not the next best test. Enteroclysis is a good test for the small bowel but is seldom performed today.

307 **A.** (S&F, ch33)

Myeloablative conditioning regimens damage hepatic sinusoids, leading to hepatomegaly, fluid retention and weight gain, and elevated serum bilirubin. Individual variability in cyclophosphamide metabolism, irradiation dose, use of gemtuzumab ozogamicin, and pre-existing liver inflammation and fibrosis are risk factors. The diagnosis may be made from clinical signs if they develop before day 20 post-transplant, but Doppler ultrasound, measurement of the wedged hepatic venous pressure gradient, and liver histology may be needed in difficult cases. Treatment of severe sinosoidal obstruction syndrome (SOS) is unsatisfactory; the best results are currently obtained from intravenous administration of defibrotide (25 mg/kg/day), a porcine oligonucleotide that has effects on microvascular endothelial cells.

308 **D.** (S&F, ch20)

This woman has lichen planus, which is a common, chronic, inflammatory disorder involving the oral mucosa and skin. The white, lace-like oral lesions may occur with or without erythema and ulcerations. The disease usually begins in adulthood, and two thirds of all patients are women. Odynophagia or dysphagia may develop years after disease onset. Characteristic endoscopic findings include erythema, ulcerations, proximal esophageal web, or erosions at any location in the esophagus. Oral lichen planus is associated with an increased risk of squamous cell carcinoma, regardless of treatment.

309   A. (S&F, ch38)

Clinical symptoms of acute radiation enteritis usually appear during the third week of standard fractionated radiotherapy. Radiation-induced enteritis is rarely life-threatening except when chemotherapy is administered concurrently. Increased intestinal motility can lead to abdominal cramping, diarrhea, and nausea. These symptoms usually subside after the discontinuation of radiation. Malabsorption can occur due to the loss of intestinal crypt cells and decreased surface area for absorption. The diagnosis of acute radiation enteritis is based on the history and no specific diagnostic tests are required. Colonoscopy should be avoided unless necessary, because it poses risk of perforation.

310   A. (S&F, ch31)

Diazoxide is a nondiuretic benzothiazide analogue that has a potent hyperglycemic effect and is the drug of choice. Therapy should be initiated with a total dosage of 150 to 200 mg/day, divided into two to three doses; if this regimen is not effective, the dosage may be increased to a maximum of 600 to 800 mg/day. There are anecdotal reports that verapamil, propranolol, phenytoin, and glucocorticoids were effective in some patients, but they may have only minor effects. Trichlormethiazide is a diuretic that is appropriate for patients with sodium retention due to diazoxide therapy.

311   C. (S&F, ch34)

Rheumatoid arthritis has developed, rarely, as a complication of hepatitis. More often, cryoglobulinemia has been associated with arthralgias and positive results of tests for rheumatoid factor. Flaring of hepatitis B infection has been reported with administration of immunosuppressant medications to patients with rheumatoid arthritis. Progression of hepatitis C infection and autoimmune hepatitis have also been reported in patients with rheumatoid arthritis.

312   E. (S&F, ch23)

Surgery is indicated for patients with evidence of perforation, hemorrhage, fistula formation, or small bowel and colonic obstruction secondary to foreign body ingestion. Surgery is also indicated when an ingested foreign body fails to progress and/or cannot be retrieved endoscopically. Finally, surgery may be considered in patients with abnormal gastrointestinal anatomy or pathology that makes uneventful passage of the foreign body unlikely.

313   C. (S&F, ch28)

PCR or fluorescence staining can reveal a specific mutation in B-lymphocytes in the tumor but this information is of little value in the average case, although it may be of benefit if the tumor is refractory to treatment. Biopsy of all areas of the stomach is suggested, because MALT may be multifocal. EUS, bone marrow biopsy, and CT are valuable in determining the extent of lymphoma for staging.

314   A. (S&F, ch23)

Most patients with food bolus impactions have a predisposing factor. Esophageal pathology is present in 75% to 100% of patients with acute food impactions. Although food bolus impactions may occur in patients with surgical anastomoses, tight fundoplication wraps, bariatric gastroplasties, or esophageal cancers, they are most likely to occur in those with benign esophageal stenoses such as Schatzki's ("B") rings, peptic strictures, webs, and extrinsic compression.

315   E. (S&F, ch32)

Patients who are infected with both HIV and hepatitis C virus are more likely to be found to have active cirrhosis on biopsy and an accelerated course to clinical cirrhosis and liver failure. Factors that predict fibrosis and progression to cirrhosis in coinfected patients include: older age at infection, higher ALT levels, higher levels of inflammatory activity, alcohol consumption of more than 50 g/day, and CD4 count of less than 500 cells/mm³. The mechanism for this rapid disease course is unknown but it has been reported to occur in other patients who are immunocompromised.

316   A. (S&F, ch23)

If there is a suspicion of an object in the hypopharynx or cervical esophagus, anteroposterior and lateral films of the neck should be obtained. CT is also a safe and accurate technique to evaluate such foreign bodies. Also, metal detectors have been found to have 98% sensitivity for detecting coins and their location in the GI tract.

317 **D.** (S&F, ch34)

The incidence of pancreatitis is 2-fold the population average in young persons with type I diabetes mellitus, and pancreatic cancer also has a higher incidence in those with diabetes. Nonspecific elevation of amylase/lipase (less than 3 times normal) occurs with ketoacidosis. Abdominal pain due to circumferential radicular pain has been confused with an acute abdominal process. Inflammatory bowel disease has no reported association with diabetes.

318 **B.** (S&F, ch39)

Esophageal strictures do not need to be dilated to the size of uninvolved lumen but to a diameter that results in symptom resolution. The type of dilator used does not appear to affect the risk of perforation. Proximal esophageal strictures are the greatest risk.

319 **E.** (S&F, ch24)

The degree of injury to the gastrointestinal tract depends on the agent; its concentration, quantity, physical state; and the duration of exposure.

320 **E.** (S&F, ch23)

The esophagus has four areas of physiologic narrowing where foreign bodies or food boluses are apt to become impacted. These are at the levels of the upper esophageal sphincter and cricopharyngeal muscle; the aortic arch; the crossing of the mainstem bronchus; and the gastroesophageal junction. These areas have been characterized as sites of true luminal narrowing, having a maximal physiologic diameter of 23 mm or less in the average adult.

321 **E.** (S&F, ch27)

This patient most likely has celiac sprue. Patients with this condition usually present with weight loss and diarrhea secondary to malabsorption. On endoscopy, scalloping of the mucosal folds in the small intestine can be seen. The diagnosis is made by finding flattening of the villi on histopathologic examination of a duodenal biopsy specimen.

322 **D.** (S&F, ch31)

The diagnosis of ZES requires the demonstration of acid hypersecretion in the presence of hypergastrinemia. Therefore, to diagnose ZES,

assessments of fasting serum gastrin levels and acid secretion are required.

323 **B.** (S&F, ch27)

This patient has primary intestinal lymphangiectasias. These patients often present before 30 years of age with edema, hypoproteinemia, diarrhea, and lymphocytopenia. The mainstay of therapy is a low-fat, high-protein diet. Laboratory findings are similar to those in other forms of protein-losing enteropathy and include hypoproteinemia with decreased serum levels of albumin, IgG, IgM, IgA, transferrin, and ceruloplasmin. Clotting factors are also frequently decreased, but this rarely leads to clinical consequences. Histopathologic examination reveals markedly dilated lymphatics, which are most apparent in the tips of the villi.

324 **B.** (S&F, ch36)

Fluid resuscitation and antibiotic therapy followed by urgent laparotomy or laparoscopy are the mainstays of treatment for peritonitis. Glucocorticoids have been shown not to provide benefit for patients in septic shock. Vasopressor agents are generally to be avoided if possible.

325 **D.** (S&F, ch35)

This patient has hereditary hemorrhagic telangiectasia (HHT) or Osler-Weber-Rendu disease. This is an autosomal dominant disorder characterized by telangiectasias of the skin and mucous membranes as well as recurrent GI bleeding. Telangiectasias can occur in the colon, but they more often occur in the stomach wall and the small intestines. Vascular involvement of the liver is not uncommon and may present as high output heart failure due to right-to-left intrahepatic shunting, portal hypertension, and biliary tract disease. Giant hemangiomas in the liver are not a manifestation of HHT.

326 **A.** (S&F, ch28)

This tumor has a very poor prognosis. Response to chemotherapy is 58% with relapse in 80% of responders. Very few patients who relapse survive.

327 **D.** (S&F, ch24)

Compared with other causes, caustic esophageal strictures require more numerous and more frequent dilations to achieve and maintain adequate lumen diameter. Care must be taken to dilate slowly and carefully. PPIs should be used as an adjunct to prevent acid reflux. In an uncontrolled study, intralesional steroid injections at the time of endoscopic dilation were found to have a beneficial effect.

328 **E.** (S&F, ch32)

Mycobacterial involvement of the bowel by either *Mycobacterium tuberculosis* or MAC may lead to diarrhea, abdominal pain, and, rarely, to obstruction or bleeding. In some series of patients, MAC was the most common organism identified in patients with chronic diarrhea and low CD4 counts. Duodenal involvement is most common and may be suspected at endoscopy by the presence of yellow mucosal nodules, often in association with malabsorption, bacteremia, and systemic infection.

329 **E.** (S&F, ch33)

There is a risk for recurrence of the underlying liver disease following orthotopic liver transplant (OLT), including hepatitis C virus (HCV) infection, hepatitis B virus (HBV) infection, autoimmune hepatitis, nonalcoholic steatohepatitis (NASH), primary biliary cirrhosis (PBC), and primary sclerosing cholangitis (PSC).

330 **C.** (S&F, ch30)

The commonest site for carcinoid tumors is the ileum, not the appendix. It is true that carcinoid tumors of the esophagus are rare. The stomach is the most common location in the foregut for carcinoid tumors.

331 **D.** (S&F, ch34)

The liver is involved in 95% of patients with ALL and 75% of patients with AML. Hepatomegaly can be attributed to extramedullary hematopoiesis, leukemic infiltration, or infectious and toxic complications.

332 1-**D**, 2-**C**, 3-**A**, 4-**E**, 5-B (S&F, ch20)

333 **B.** (S&F, ch23)

Once in the stomach, 80% to 90% of all ingested objects pass spontaneously through the remaining digestive tract within 7 to 10 days with no complications. Long objects (those longer than 5 cm) are usually unable to pass through the pylorus and the duodenal sweep. Large-diameter objects (>2 cm) are usually not able to pass through the pylorus. Endoscopic or surgical retrieval is indicated when the ingested

foreign body is believed to be either longer or larger in diameter than these dimensions, either by history or by visualization on the results of a radiographic study. Because endoscopic retrieval is less invasive, it should be attempted first in these cases. Retrieval is also indicated for objects that, after observation, are not moving satisfactorily by 5 to 7 days after ingestion.

334 **D.** (S&F, ch33)

Pneumatosis intestinalis may be discovered as an incidental finding during abdominal imaging after solid organ transplant (SOT) but can also be a manifestation of life-threatening intestinal ischemia or infection with a gas-forming organism. Pneumatosis intestinalis is associated with CMV infection, *C. difficile* colitis, sepsis, and glucocorticoid therapy. The majority of patients require no specific intervention and the gas collections resolve spontaneously.

335 **C.** (S&F, ch35)

Mycotic aneurysms of the aorta and splanchnic vessels are very rare. They were so named because their appearance is similar to fungi and not because fungal infection is the commonest cause. The early symptoms are nonspecific. More often than not, these lesions must be treated surgically.

336 **E.** (S&F, ch24)

Esophageal strictures are usually located where caustic agents pool at the cricopharyngeus, the level of the aortic arch and tracheal bifurcation, and the lower esophageal sphincter. Most strictures occur in the antrum of fasting patients, as opposed to the midbody in those who have recently ingested food.

337 **B.** (S&F, ch23)

Once the esophageal food impaction has been cleared, the presence of underlying esophageal pathology, reported in as many as 86% to 97% of patients, should be assessed. However, in the acute setting there is usually considerable mural edema and mucosal erythema and abrasion, making it difficult to discriminate an acute from a chronic process. More than half of patients with this condition have abnormal results on a 24-hour pH study and nearly half have esophageal dysmotility on manometry. A proton-pump inhibitor agent may be prescribed and elective outpatient endoscopy scheduled after acute mural inflammation has had a chance to resolve. Patients should be educated on methods of reducing the risk of food bolus impactions. Instructions include eating more slowly, chewing foods thoroughly, and avoiding troublesome foods.

338 **D.** (S&F, ch32)

Patients with esophageal candidiasis generally complain of substernal dysphagia. Odynophagia, when present, is usually not severe. The definitive diagnosis is made by upper endoscopy findings of focal or diffuse plaques and biopsy findings of desquamated epithelial cells with typical-appearing yeast forms. Although CMV is the pathogen most commonly identified with AIDS, *Candida* is more often associated with esophageal disease. CMV causes ulcerations that are large and deep. Biopsy allows for demonstration of this viral cytopathic effect. Dysphagia is much less common than in patients with *Candida* esophagitis and fever is often present. HSV esophagitis is uncommon in persons with AIDS. The disease follows a predictable sequence: discrete vesicles form, then shallow ulcers, which coalesce into regions of diffuse shallow ulceration. Biopsies are likely to show epithelial cell invasion and nuclear changes typical of herpes infections.

339 **D.** (S&F, ch34)

Although hyperthyroidism is associated with diarrhea and weight loss, steatorrhea has not been reported. The malabsorption associated with Addisonian diarrhea has not been characterized. The malabsorption of abetalipoproteinemia is due to absence of this lipid transport mechanism in the mucosa of the small bowel. The malabsorption that occurs in patients with hypoparathyroidism is due to intestinal lymphangiectasia with protein-losing enteropathy. Coexistent celiac disease can also contribute if an autoimmune reaction is responsible for the hypoparathyroid state. Consequently, a gluten-free diet can benefit patients with either problem.

340 **B.** (S&F, ch21)

The most common clinical presentation of jejunal diverticulosis is that of recurrent abdominal pain, early satiety, and bloating. Loud borborygmi and intermittent diarrhea may be caused by the motility disorder. Malabsorption may result from associated bacterial overgrowth. Patients with progressive systemic sclerosis or scleroderma have small bowel dysmotility with delayed transit time and associated jejunal diverticula. Treatment includes intermittent courses of broad-spectrum oral antibiotics.

341 **B.** (S&F, ch30)

Typical carcinoid syndrome is usually caused by metastatic midgut carcinoids. In typical carcinoid syndrome, tryptophan is converted to 5-hydroxytryptophan (5-HTP) and then rapidly to 5-hydroxytryptamine(serotonin). Serotonin is then stored in granules or released into the circulation. Once in the circulation, the enzymes monoamine oxidase and aldehyde dehydrogenase convert serotonin into 5-HIAA, which is excreted in the urine. Therefore, patients with typical carcinoid syndrome will have elevated plasma and platelet serotonin levels and increased urinary excretion of 5-HIAA. On the other hand, atypical carcinoid syndrome is most often associated with foregut carcinoids. Patients with foregut carcinoids are deficient in the enzyme dopa decarboxylase, which is responsible for the conversion of 5 HTP to serotonin. Therefore, these patients have high plasma levels of 5-HTP and normal levels of serotonin. Urinary excretion of 5-HIAA may be normal or slightly elevated.

342 **C.** (S&F, ch32)

If the patient has rectal bleeding, tenesmus, or leukocytes in the stool and bacterial cultures are negative it is important to biopsy the mucosa and examine the specimen forevidence of viruses and protozoa. CMV, for example, is the most common viral cause of diarrhea and the most frequent cause of chronic diarrhea in patients with AIDS who have had no evidence of infection on multiple stool tests.

343 **A.** (S&F, ch28)

The most common site in residents of developed countries is the stomach, although the small intestine is a frequent site in residents of the Middle East.

344 **D.** (S&F, ch22)

345 **C.** (S&F, ch36)

This patient most likely has familial Mediterranean fever, which is an autosomal recessive disease. It could affect the peritoneum as well as other serous membranes. It is more frequently found in Ashkenazi Jews, Armenians, and Arabs. It is an aseptic form of recurrent peritonitis. Patients present with sporadic episodes of abdominal pain, fever, synovitis, and pleuritis. Treatment with colchicine appears to prevent attacks and can prevent fatal renal amyloidosis.

346 **D.** (S&F, ch24)

Grade I injury (superficial burn) corresponds to a first-degree burn. Grade II injury corresponds to a second-degree burn, whereas grade III injury corresponds to a transmural burn and necrosis without perforation. Grade IV injury (perforation) is usually not encountered because clinical and radiographic suspicion of perforation precludes EGD. Zargar and associates suggested that grade II burns be labeled grade IIA if the ulcerations are patchy or linear, or grade IIB if the injury is circumferential. Grade I and grade IIA (noncircumferential) injuries rarely result in strictures, whereas 70% to 100% of grade IIB (circumferential) and grade III lesions result in strictures.

347 **D.** (S&F, ch29)

The reported cases of GIST associated with neurofibromatosis type I have not demonstrated any mutation in the *KIT* gene. It is not clear whether these tumors will respond to imatinib in the same way as do tumors of the nonhereditary type with *KIT* mutation. The skin pigmentation in these cases is patchy and related to stimulation of melanocytes by the increased activity of tyrosine kinase.

348 **C.** (S&F, ch20)

FAP, with its variant Gardner's syndrome, is inherited as an autosomal dominant condition. Patients have multiple osteomas, varying in size from 1 to 10 mm, in the oral cavity. The APC gene on chromosome 5q21 is mutated in the germline of these patients. Cutaneous features of this syndrome precede the development of polyps and include multiple epidermoid cysts of the face, scalp, and extremities that appear before puberty. However, these cysts are not true sebaceous cysts, and therefore **C** is the correct answer.

349 **A.** (S&F, ch26)

Eosinophils are normally found in the lamina propria of the GI tract. The highest concentrations are found in the appendix and cecum. Normally, no eosinophils are present in the esophagus.

350 **C.** (S&F, ch33)

Cytomegalovirus (CMV) is the predominant viral pathogen occurring within the first year after SOT; the intestine and hepatobiliary tracts are the most common sites of infection. Factors predisposing to CMV infection include the type of immunosuppression used, that is, use of antilymphocyte antibody in addition to conventional immunosuppression or maintenance mycophenolate mofetil (MMF) therapy. The peak onset of symptoms is generally 6 to 8 weeks after transplantation; symptoms include fever, malaise, myalgia, and, occasionally, cough and minor elevations of serum ALT. CMV DNA or antigen is generally detected in the bloodstream, but CMV can be recovered from intestinal biopsy tissue in the absence of detectable virus in the bloodstream. Post-transplant antiviral prophylaxis with either ganciclovir significantly reduces the risk of CMV disease.

351 **B.** (S&F, ch23)

Estimation of the suspected site or level of impaction by the patient is generally not reliable. The one area where patients may be able to accurately localize the object is at the cricopharyngeal muscle, but localization becomes progressively less accurate for distally impacted foreign bodies, with an accuracy of 30% to 40% for those in the esophagus and close to 0% for those in the stomach.

352 **D.** (S&F, ch38)

Prostaglandins have been investigated for their ability to protect patients from the side effects of radiation therapy. Misoprostol suppositories reduce symptoms of acute radiation enteritis in patients undergoing radiotherapy. Radiation therapy techniques play an important role in reducing the rate of complications. Use of only anterior and posterior fields should be avoided because of the high dose and large volume of bowel irradiated. Patients should be instructed to maintain a full bladder during radiation of the pelvis, because the full bladder mechanically displaces the small intestine out of the pelvis. Treatment in the prone position allows the small intestines to drop out of the radiation field.

353 **E.** (S&F, ch33)

The risk of cancer in long-lived transplant recipients is higher than in the general population, particularly for lymphomas, skin cancers, and Kaposi's sarcoma. Patients who underwent liver transplant for cirrhosis secondary to primary sclerosing cholangitis are at high risk for the development of colonic dysplasia and diffuse colon cancer related to underlying ulcerative colitis. If severe dysplasia is discovered, colectomy can be performed safely as early as 10 to 12 weeks following transplant.

354 **D.** (S&F, ch34)

Granulomatous involvement of the liver is a very frequent occurrence with sarcoidosis, occurring in as many as 95% of patients in some studies. If the diagnosis is suspected, with or without overt systemic disease, it can be confirmed by liver biopsy.

355 **D.** (S&F, ch24)

Cleaning products accounted for 225,578 ingestions in 2002, and the majority of these, 53,100, were caused by bleaches. Non-household acid/alkali solutions were second with 15,601 ingestions.

356 **C.** (S&F, ch25)

Early mortality can be hastened by inadequate fluid and electrolyte replacement, and more chronically by underlying disease such as cancer. The main cause is sepsis with multiorgan failure. This often results from inadequate drainage of complex fistulas allowing a nidus of continued infection.

QUESTIONS

357 Developmental abnormalities of the esophagus are relatively common. Which of the following statements is false?

A. Esophageal atresia and tracheoesophageal fistula are the most common developmental abnormalities.

B. Esophageal atresia most commonly occurs as an isolated abnormality of the foregut.

C. Esophageal anomalies are associated often with nonforegut anomalies of the renal, limbic, and cardiac systems.

D. Tracheoesophageal fistula may present as recurrent pneumonia in infancy.

E. Diagnosis of certain types of tracheoesophageal fistula may be delayed to adolescent or adult life.

358 Which of the following conditions are associated with esophagitis?

1. Scleroderma
2. Sjögren's syndrome
3. Zollinger-Ellison syndrome
4. Pregnancy

A. (1) and (3)
B. (2) and (4)
C. (1), (2), and (3)
D. All of the above

359 A 36-year-old woman with acquired immunodeficiency syndrome (AIDS) complains of persistent severe odynophagia despite a 10-day course of oral antifungal therapy. The most appropriate diagnostic test would be:

A. Barium swallow

B. Computed tomography of the chest
C. Endoscopy with brushings and biopsies
D. Cytomegalovirus titers

360 A 64-year-old man undergoes pneumatic balloon dilation for achalasia. The patient has severe chest pain and fever after the procedure. A Gastrografin swallow shows a small perforation with contrast flowing into the pleural space. Management should consist of the following steps.

A. Intravenous (IV) antibiotics, parenteral alimentation, and observation

B. IV antibiotics and placement of a removable stent

C. IV antibiotics and immediate thoracotomy

D. IV antibiotics and placement of a chest tube for drainage

361 A 52-year-old man is referred for evaluation. The patient has typical heartburn symptoms. His response to a standard dose of a proton-pump inhibitor (PPI) drug is excellent. Endoscopy revealed a 6.0-cm area of Barrett's esophagus without dysplasia. The following recommendation should be made:

A. Endoscopic surveillance and continued maintenance PPI

B. Laser ablation plus fundoplication

C. Surveillance and step down to maintenance doses of H_2-receptor antagonists

D. Endoscopic surveillance only

362 A 36-year-old man presents with a 4-year history of dysphagia. Barium swallow and esophageal manometry results are normal. Endoscopy reveals multiple rings throughout the length of the esophagus. Biopsy may show the following.

A. Active esophagitis with mucosal disruption
B. A dense infiltrate of lymphocytes
C. Eosinophilic infiltration
D. Columnar metaplasia with dysplasia
E. None of the above

363 Which of the following statements regarding the treatment of esophageal abnormalities is not correct?

A. Pill-induced esophagitis is most often treated by a surface coating agent such as sucralfate suspension in conjunction with acid suppressive therapy.
B. *Candida* esophagitis is usually treated with fluconazole or clotrimazole troche.
C. Severe herpetic esophagitis may be treated with orally administered acyclovir or valacyclovir.
D. Routine treatment of human papillomavirus involving the esophagus involves bleomycin or interferon.

364 A 76-year-old patient is referred for evaluation of dysphagia. Symptoms began after a cerebrovascular accident (CVA) and have not progressed over the past 3 months since the CVA. A barium swallow with video images was ordered by the speech therapy department. The barium swallow would be expected to show which of the following features?

A. Diffuse esophageal dilation with aperistalsis
B. A prominent cricopharyngeal muscular contraction with obstruction
C. Vallecular pooling with nasopharyngeal regurgitation
D. Asymmetric cervical esophageal contractions opposite the side of the stroke

365 A 61-year-old man is found to have an "inlet patch" of hypertrophic mucosa during endoscopy. The mucosa is gastric in type. Which step is now recommended?

A. Yearly surveillance with multiple biopsies
B. Argon plasma coagulation with high-dose proton pump inhibitor drug therapy
C. No further tests
D. pH monitoring with proximal electrode placement

366 Which of the following statements is true regarding the effect of sclerotherapy on the esophagus?

A. Wall damage or neural effects may lead to abnormalities in esophageal motor function.
B. Strictures commonly occur as the result of sclerotherapy.

C. Ulcers occur at the site of sclerotherapy injection in a minority of patients.
D. H_2-receptor antagonists or proton pump inhibitors may be effective in preventing esophageal damage from sclerotherapy.

367 A 45-year-old patient with dysphagia for liquids and solids and a prominent history of regurgitation over a 6-month period is referred for evaluation. The barium swallow shows a minimally dilated esophagus with poor emptying in the supine position. The endoscope is easily passed into the stomach. Because of the minimal esophageal dilation, the diagnosis is questioned. Which study would be of greatest value?

A. A methacholine (mecholyl) challenge
B. Serologic studies for scleroderma
C. An endoscopic ultrasound of the distal esophagus
D. Routine esophageal manometry
E. A 24-hour pH study

368 Regarding therapy for gastroesophageal reflux disease (GERD), which statement is correct?

A. PPI therapy is effective because PPIs generally keep pH above 4 for 24 hours.
B. Eight weeks of PPI therapy may lead to healing of ulcerative esophagitis in more than 80% of patients.
C. H_2-receptor antagonists (H_2Raf) are as effective in healing esophagitis as are PPIs.
D. An H_2Raf medication should not be taken at bedtime with a PPI drug.

369 Which of the following factors has/have been demonstrated to alter lower esophageal sphincter (LES) pressure?

A. The migrating motor complex
B. Circulating of gut neuropeptides
C. Ingested foods
D. Intra-abdominal pressure
E. Respiration
F. All of the above
G. None of the above

370 The pathogenesis of peptic esophagitis secondary to gastroesophageal reflux is most dependent upon which of the following factor or factors?

A. Gastric acidity
B. Pepsin
C. Gastric acid plus pepsin
D. Gastric acid plus bilirubin

371 A 74-year-old man has marked odynophagia. Endoscopy reveals white plaques along the entire esophagus. The oropharynx is normal in appearance. Which statement best characterizes this condition?

A. *Candida tropicalis* is the fungal organism usually responsible for this clinical picture.
B. Most esophageal cases are seen with oropharyngeal infection.
C. Topical antifungal drugs may be effective agents.
D. Achalasia is an established risk factor for esophageal candidiasis.
E. Topical administration of glucocorticoids has been shown not to be a risk factor.

372 A 37-year-old man with intermittent solid food dysphagia undergoes barium swallow, which shows a ring-like narrowing at the distal esophagus. The diameter of the ring is 12 mm. Which of the following therapies is indicated at this time?

A. Careful food preparation with the avoidance of meat and bread
B. Endoscopy followed by bougie dilation
C. Laser ablation
D. Proton pump inhibitor drug therapy
E. Observation only

373 Which of the following statements regarding Barrett's esophagus is most accurate?

A. Patients with Barrett's esophagus may have a 50-fold increased risk of developing adenocarcinoma of the esophagus.
B. The incidence of adenocarcinoma in patients with Barrett's esophagus has risen rapidly over the last several years while the incidence of squamous cell carcinoma of the esophagus is rapidly decreasing in the United States.
C. The risk of adenocarcinoma in patients with short-segment (<3 cm) Barrett's esophagus is the same as the incidence in those with long-segment Barrett's esophagus.
D. Severe heartburn is seen in almost all patients with Barrett's esophagus.
E. Barrett's esophagus is diagnosed endoscopically by the appearance of columnar epithelium above the esophagogastric junction.

374 A 32-year-old man has an esophageal stricture on barium swallow. Dysphagia has been present since childhood. The stricture is suspected to be congenital. Which statement best characterizes this abnormality?

A. The stenotic segment varies in length, but is usually located within the middle or lower third of the esophagus.
B. The stenotic segment is usually short (<2 cm long).
C. The stenotic segment usually shows mucosal abnormalities.

D. Esophageal dilation is generally easily accomplished with through-the-scope balloons.
E. Congenital stenosis is often associated with congenital vascular abnormalities.

375 A 37-year-old woman is referred for evaluation of recurrent aspiration. She has frontal baldness, cataracts, and evidence of myotonia. Her mother had a similar illness. On manometry, she had markedly decreased contraction pressure of the pharynx and upper esophagus. The diagnosis is:

A. Myotonia dystrophica
B. Amyotrophic lateral sclerosis
C. Oculopharyngeal dystrophy
D. Myasthenia gravis

376 Which statement is correct regarding the pathogenesis of GERD?

A. Hiatal hernia is not important in the pathogenesis of GERD.
B. Acid alone in the absence of pepsin causes severe esophageal damage.
C. Gastric acid output is normal in most patients with GERD.
D. *Helicobacter pylori* infection worsens GERD.

377 An 86-year-old woman ingests tetracycline before going to sleep. The next morning, she has severe chest pain, odynophagia, and salivation. Which statement best characterizes the condition causing her symptoms?

A. The lesion is superficial and will heal within 48 hours.
B. The endoscopic appearance of this condition is pathognomonic.
C. Hematemesis is common.
D. The abnormality generally occurs at a site of an anatomic or physiological narrowing or a stricture.

378 Which of the following statements is correct regarding the routine use of endoscopy in patients with esophageal abnormalities?

A. Endoscopy is important for the diagnosis of esophageal injury due to medications.
B. Routine endoscopy is suggested shortly after blunt trauma to the chest suffered in an automobile accident.
C. Multiple "volcano like" vesicles are characteristic of herpetic esophagitis.
D. Gastrografin contrast studies are contraindicated in patients who have severe traumatic injuries.
E. All of the above

379 Which of the following is the least common complication of esophagitis?

A. Stricture formation
B. Barrett's esophagus
C. Hemorrhage
D. Perforation

380 A 47-year-l woman with prominent heartburn carries the diagnosis of CREST syndrome or limited scleroderma. Esophageal manometry would be expected to show which of the following patterns?

A. Reduction in peristaltic contraction amplitude in the distal esophagus along with LES hypotension
B. Forceful esophageal contractions with impaired LES relaxation
C. Pharyngeal and upper esophageal hypomotility
D. LES hypotension with normal esophageal peristalsis

381 Which of the following statements are true regarding pill-induced esophagitis?

1. Dysphagia and odynophagia are common clinical symptoms.
2. Double-contrast radiographic barium swallow or endoscopy are the preferred diagnostic modalities.
3. Substernal chest pain or heartburn after ingestion of small amounts of orange juice are typical symptoms.
4. Moderately severe erythema is the usual endoscopic finding.

A. (1) and (3)
B. (2) and (4)
C. (1), (2), and (3)
D. All of the above

382 A 56-year-old man has biopsy-proven intestinal metaplasia at the gastric cardia. The recommendation should be:

A. Surveillance plus PPI medication
B. Surveillance alone
C. Evaluation for *H. pylori* infection and eradication if present
D. Coagulation of the site with an argon plasma laser

383 The most accurate statement regarding transient lower esophageal sphincter relaxation (TLESr) is:

A. TLESr is a predominant mechanism of gastroesophageal reflux in patients with GERD, but not in those without this condition.
B. All transient LESr episodes are accompanied by gastroesophageal reflux.

C. TLESr episodes are vagally mediated and occur in response to gastric distention.
D. Transient TLESr episodes generally occur after swallowing and are usually accompanied by esophageal peristalsis.

384 Antireflux surgery for chronic gastroesophageal reflux disease has been shown to have the following benefit:

A. Reduction of the need for esophageal stricture dilation
B. Reduction of the risk for developing esophageal adenocarcinoma in patients with Barrett's esophagus
C. Promotion of regression of Barrett's tissue in the esophagus
D. Allowance of step-down to an H_2-receptor antagonist medication

385 Which of the following statements is most accurate regarding testing for GERD?

A. An empiric test of high-dose proton pump inhibitor therapy is a reliable test for suspected GERD.
B. A barium esophagogram is helpful in detecting mild esophagitis.
C. Inspection of the esophagus at upper endoscopy is a reliable way to diagnose most cases of GERD.
D. Esophageal manometry is a valuable and important part of the evaluation of uncomplicated GERD.
E. Impedance testing is valuable in that it detects only nonacid gastroesophageal reflux.

386 Which of the following statements concerning esophageal A and B rings is false?

A. The A ring is most common.
B. The B ring is thin, being comprised of only mucosa and submucosa.
C. The A ring is broad, being comprised of hypertrophied muscle.
D. Both types of rings may cause dysphagia.

387 Which of the following statements regarding pill-induced esophagitis is true?

A. An anatomic defect or motility disorder of the esophagus is almost always present in cases of pill-induced esophagitis.
B. Tetracycline or its derivatives cause pill-induced esophagitis by production of a caustic alkaline solution.
C. Antibiotics as a class are uncommon causes of medication-induced esophagitis.
D. Esophageal damage from a bisphosphonate medication, such as alendronate, can be

minimized by ingestion of a full 8-oz. glass of water taken in the upright position.

E. Chemotherapeutic agents are unlikely causes of pill-induced esophagitis.

388 A 27-year-old patient with herpes simplex infection is suspected of having esophageal involvement. Which of the following conditions may be found concurrent with this viral infection?

A. Gastrointestinal blood loss
B. Deep linear ulcerations
C. Esophageal stricture
D. Occasional dysphagia

389 Which of the following statements regarding the clinical course of GERD is most appropriate?

A. The clinical course is uncertain and nonerosive disease tends to progress to erosive esophagitis over time.
B. Once effective treatment has been administered and healing has occurred, most patients will remain asymptomatic without need for maintenance therapy.
C. Gastrointestinal bleeding is a common complication of reflux esophagitis.
D. Barrett's esophagus is predominantly a disease of middle-aged white men.

390 A 54-year-old man is referred by a radiologist because of suspected dysphagia lusoria. Which of the following best describes the suspected clinical abnormality?

A. Any esophageal obstruction related to muscular compression of the esophageal wall
B. A benign esophageal ring
C. Symptoms arising from vascular compression of the esophagus caused by an aberrant right subclavian artery
D. Difficulty in swallowing related to abnormal proximal esophageal spastic contractions

391 The pathogenesis of GERD may include which of the following?

1. Decreased lower esophageal sphincter (LES) pressure
2. Decreased acid clearance
3. Decreased esophageal mucosal resistance to acid
4. Peristaltic dysfunction

A. (1) and (3)
B. (2) and (4)
C. (1), (2), and (3)
D. All of the above

ANSWERS

357 **B.** (S&F, ch40)

Esophageal atresia is usually associated with a tracheoesophageal fistula. It occurs as an isolated abnormality in only 7% of cases.

358 **C.** (S&F, ch42)

Pregnant women typically suffer from gastroesophageal reflux disease (GERD) but rarely have histologically proven esophagitis. The two conditions are not the same. GERD encompasses all aspects of gastroesophageal reflux, whereas esophagitis specifically indicates mucosal injury. Esophagitis can complicate Sjögren's syndrome because patients with this syndrome have xerostomia and therefore inability of the saliva to neutralize normally refluxed acid. Patients with scleroderma have severe esophageal dysmotility with resultant poor acid clearance and consequent esophagitis. They may also be troubled with Sjögren's syndrome, compounding the problem. Hypersecretory states of Zollinger-Ellison syndrome are often complicated by esophagitis.

359 **C.** (S&F, ch43)

Patients with acquired immunodeficiency syndrome who have persistent odynophagia after empirical antifungal therapy merit endoscopic evaluation to exclude cytomegalovirus infection, herpes simplex virus infection, other fungal diseases, and large esophageal ulcers.

360 **C.** (S&F, ch40–44)

Perforation after pneumatic dilation in patients with achalasia requires immediate surgery for closure of the perforation if the patient is febrile and if contrast extends into the pleural or peritoneal cavity. Limited or contained perforation can be managed conservatively.

361 **A.** (S&F, ch40–44)

This patient has long-segment Barrett's esophagus and has an increased risk of esophageal adenocarcinoma. Treatment is with continuous acid suppressive therapy. Discontinuation of acid suppression will result in recurrent esophagitis in the majority of patients. Endoscopic surveillance with biopsy to detect dysplasia is indicated every 1 to 2 years.

362 **C.** (S&F, ch40–44)

Eosinophilic esophagitis is a cause of solid food dysphagia. It is generally seen in young men. The cause is not known. Dilation may result in perforation or mucosal tears.

363 **D.** (S&F, ch43)

Surface acting agents are generally effective with acid suppression for pill-induced esophagitis. Effective therapy for other forms of infectious esophagitis are described. Infection with the human papillomavirus often does not require treatment; however, if the lesions are large, they may need to be removed by an endoscopic or even a surgical procedure. Routine medical treatments, including interferon and bleomycin administration, have not had consistently effective results and therefore are not commonly used.

364 **C.** (S&F, ch40–44)

The classical radiographic features of oropharyngeal dysphagia following a stroke are vallecular pooling, tracheal aspiration, and nasopharyngeal aspiration.

365 **C.** (S&F, ch40–44)

The inlet patch is comprised of gastric fundic or antral mucosa. It is not Barrett's-type metaplastic tissue. The patch may secrete acid and is rarely associated with a web, stricture, or ulcer. It may be infected with *H. pylori*. There are no data to indicate that ablation therapy is needed.

366 **A.** (S&F, ch43)

Ulcerations after sclerotherapy have been noted in approximately half of patients. Strictures, on the other hand, are uncommon, occurring in only 15% or fewer of such patients. Esophageal motor function may be affected by sclerotherapy; the mechanism of damage may be vagal nerve damage or wall injury. Only liquid sucralfate suspension has been shown to prevent or treat postsclerotherapy ulcerations and acid suppression is generally not considered an effective form of therapy.

367 **D.** (S&F, ch40–44)

Routine esophageal manometry will show aperistalsis and a hypertensive, nonrelaxing LES. In early achalasia, the esophagus is only minimally dilated.

368 **D.** (S&F, ch42)

Standard once-a-day dosing with a PPI generally maintains pH levels above 4 for approximately 10 to 14 hours per day. Double doses or increased amounts of medication may further decrease acid production. H$_2$Rafs may be used, especially in the evening, for patients with nocturnal acid breakthrough as an additive form of therapy to decrease acid production. H$_2$Rafs are not as effective as PPIs in the therapy of esophagitis. PPIs will lead to healing after 2 months of therapy in more than 80% of patients.

369 **F.** (S&F, ch40–44)

LES pressure varies with many factors, including respiration, foods, and peptide hormones. The role of each of these factors in gastroesophageal reflux is unclear.

370 **C.** (S&F, ch40–44)

Esophagitis requires that the mucosa be exposed to both acid and pepsin.

371 **D.** (S&F, ch40–44)

Esophageal candidiasis occurs in most patients without oral disease (*candida albicans* is most common). It is seen with esophageal stasis in patients with scleroderma, achalasia, and other motility disorders. Oropharyngeal disease is most common patients being treated wth inhaled glucocorticoids and in immunosuppressed patients. Odynophagia or dysphagia is the most common presentation. Systemic antifungals are used for treatment.

372 **B.** (S&F, ch40–44)

A Schatzki's ring is a frequent cause of intermittent dysphagia for solids. The ring diameter is critical, with constriction to a diameter of 13 mm or less causing frequent symptoms. Dilation is effective, but repeat dilation may be required in about a third of cases.

373 **A.** (S&F, ch42)

The risk of adenocarcinoma is much higher in patients with Barrett's esophagus than among those in the general population. The incidence of squamous cell carcinoma, however, is stable. Long-segment Barrett's esophagus is believed to confer a 3- to 5-fold increased risk of adenocarcinoma compared to short-segment Barrett's esophagus. With the development of columnar epithelium in Barrett's esophagus, acid sensitivity may be lost and as many as 25% to 30% of patients with Barrett's esophagus may no longer exhibit heartburn. A biopsy showing intestinal metaplasia with goblet cells is required to make the diagnosis, because not all columnar epithelium in the esophagus represents Barrett's tissue.

374 **A.** (S&F, ch40–44)

Congenital stenosis of the esophagus is usually seen in the distal or middle third of the esophagus. The length of stenosis varies from 2 to 20 cm. The mucosa is usually normal. The wall may contain cartilaginous structures of tracheobronchial origin. Dilation may be difficult, because mucosal tears are common.

375 **A.** (S&F, ch40–44)

The patient's history, physical exam, and manometry results are classic for individuals with this dominantly inherited skeletal muscle condition.

376 **C.** (S&F, ch42)

The presence of *H. pylori* infection may lessen the risk of GERD by decreasing hydrogen ion production by the gastric antrum. A hiatus hernia is, at the very least, a cofactor or promoter in the production of GERD. Pepsin, even in small amounts, is required for increasing the severity of gastroesophageal reflux on esophageal mucosa.

Overall, gastric acid secretion is normal in patients with GERD.

377 **D.** (S&F, ch40–44)

Pill-induced esophagitis may occur with many types of pills. Pain is the usual presentation. The endoscopic appearance varies from that of a discreet ulcer to that of a pseudomembrane to a tumor-like appearance.

378 **A.** (S&F, ch43)

Endoscopic evaluation is considered the most effective means of evaluating suspected pill esophagitis in patients with odynophagia or dysphagia. Routine endoscopy after blunt trauma to the chest is relatively contraindicated, but Gastrografin contrast studies may be quite useful as a noninvasive means of evaluating the esophagus after such trauma. Herpetic esophagitis is characterized by multiple small vesicles in the esophagus.

379 **D.** (S&F, ch42)

Spontaneous perforation secondary to esophagitis is quite rare. Strictures develop in 8% to 20% of patients with esophagitis. Barrett's metaplasia is seen in approximately 10% of patients with esophagitis. Significant gastrointestinal hemorrhage complicates esophagitis in 2% to 5% of cases.

380 **A.** (S&F, ch40–44)

Patients with scleroderma have diminished esophageal contractions in the smooth muscle (distal) portion of the esophagus, along with LES hypotension. Similar changes are seen in patients with the generalized and limited (CREST) form of the disease.

381 **C.** (S&F, ch43)

Pill-induced esophagitis leads to disruption of the mucosal integrity of the esophagus and dysphagia (difficulty swallowing) or odynophagia (pain on swallowing) are commonly seen after ingestion of small amounts of even mildly caustic liquids such as citrus juice drinks or alcohol. Endoscopic findings include mucosal disruption; most commonly seen are ulcerations, single or multiple. These findings may be noted on double-contrast radiography images or at endoscopy (the latter is the preferred evaluation technique).

382 **C.** (S&F, ch40–44)

The lesion is considered benign and not associated with an increased risk of cancer. *H. pylori* infection may play a role and should be eradicated if present.

383 **C.** (S&F, ch42)

Transient LES relaxations are the predominant form of gastroesophageal reflux in both patients with GERD and in individuals without GERD. Not all TLESr episodes are accompanied by reflux. Transient LES relaxations occur independently of swallowing and are not accompanied by esophageal peristalsis.

384 **A.** (S&F, ch40–44)

Stricture dilation is consistently reduced after fundoplication but other changes are not consistently seen after this procedure.

385 **A.** (S&F, ch42)

A barium esophagogram is generally only useful in cases of severe reflux esophagitis. The results of upper endoscopy are generally normal in patients with GERD. A biopsy may assist in making the diagnosis, but inspection alone is not adequate. Impedence testing helps, both in cases with acid and those with non-acid reflux.

386 **A.** (S&F, ch40–44)

The A ring is rare compared to the B ring or Schatzki's ring. The A ring is comprised of hypertrophied muscle of the upper end of the LES. It may cause dysphagia.

387 **D.** (S&F, ch43)

While there may be an increased risk of pill-induced esophagitis in individuals with an esophageal stricture, another anatomic defect, or a motility disorder such as scleroderma or achalasia, many if not most of the patients with pill-induced esophagitis have normal esophageal function and the condition is caused by inadequate intake of liquid with oral ingestion of a pill while in a recumbent position. Tetracycline causes direct esophageal toxicity. Toxicity from bisphosphonate or any pill-induced esophagitis can be minimized by taking the medication with copious liquid in an upright position. Both antibiotics and chemotherapeutic agents are frequent causes of pill-induced esophagitis.

388 **A.** (S&F, ch40–44)

Herpes esophagitis generally presents with odynophagia, heartburn, or fever. Endoscopically, the condition is characterized by diffuse friability and ulceration of the mucosa and presence of an exudates, usually in the distal esophagus. Discrete circumscribed ulcers with raised edges are usual, not deep linear ulcers.

Bleeding and perforation may occur, and dysphagia is persistant.

389 **D.** (S&F, ch42)

Barrett's esophagus is two to three times more common in men than women, and it is rare in African-American and Asian populations. Up to 85% of patients with GERD will suffer a relapse within 6 months after treatment stops. In most patients with nonerosive disease, the disease will *not* progress to erosive esophagitis. Gastrointestinal hemorrhage is a rare complication of reflux esophagitis and is generally associated with deep ulcers or severe esophagitis.

390 **C.** (S&F, ch40–44)

Dysphagia lusoria is a specific disorder. It is caused by an aberrant right subclavian artery that arises from the left side of the aortic arch and crosses the esophagus, compresses the esophageal lumen. The result is a pencil-like indentation in the esophagus. Confirmation of this condition is made by seeing these anatomic aberrations on computed tomography or magnetic resonance arteriography.

391 **D.** (S&F, ch42)

The pathogenesis of gastroesophageal reflux is complex and may involve each or all of the mechanisms listed.

Stomach and Duodenum

QUESTIONS

392 Regarding chronic use of nonsteroidal anti-inflammatory drugs (NSAIDs) and acid/peptic ulceration, all of the following statements are true *except:*

A. Gastric mucosal blood flow is compromised.
B. Gastric injury may be visible endoscopically within a few days of daily use.
C. Long-term substitution with an enteric-coated NSAID can prevent ulcerations.
D. Serious gastrointestinal (GI) complications occur in 1% to 4% of such cases each year.

393 Which of the following stimulate gastrin?

(1) Amino acids in the gastric lumen
(2) Somatostatin
(3) Gastric distention
(4) Gastric pH less than 3.0

A. (1) and (3)
B. (2) and (4)
C. (1), (2), and (3)
D. All of the above

394 A 1-week-old girl who was born preterm with polyhydramnios is brought to the hospital with bilious emesis. Abdominal radiography reveals a "double-bubble" sign corresponding to air in the stomach and first portion of the duodenum. Contrast radiography rules out midgut volvulus and confirms duodenal atresia. Which is the definitive treatment of choice?

A. Gastrojejunostomy
B. Pancreaticoduodenostomy
C. Duodenoduodenostomy

D. Jejunostomy tube placement
E. Pyloromyotomy

395 A 53-year-old African-American woman undergoes upper endoscopy for evaluation of epigastric symptoms. A 1.5-cm polypoid mass is seen in the proximal stomach and biopsied. Histopathologic evaluation of biopsy tissue reveals well-differentiated adenocarcinoma. Which of the following is the most appropriate next step?

A. Resection with snare polypectomy
B. Endoscopic ultrasound (EUS)
C. Computed tomography (CT) of the abdomen
D. Positron emission tomography (PET)
E. Transabdominal ultrasound

396 A 72-year-old man with a remote history of gastrojejunostomy for peptic ulcer disease presents with chronic typical indigestion. Esophagogastroduodenoscopy (EGD) reveals a normal esophagus, but there are multiple exophytic masses at the gastroenteric anastomosis. Biopsies show foveolar hyperplasia and cystic glands, which extend through a disrupted muscularis mucosa into the submucosa. Which is the most clinically important association with this patient's condition?

A. *H. pylori* infection
B. Polycystic kidney disease
C. Osler-Weber-Rendu disease
D. Gastric adenocarcinoma
E. Pancreatic mucinous cystadenoma

397 Each of the following stimulates gastric acid secretion *except:*

A. Decaffeinated coffee
B. Wine
C. Milk
D. Gin
E. Tea

398 A 60-year-old African-American man is referred for evaluation of a 3-month history of upper abdominal discomfort and 5-pound weight loss. An upper GI series reveals thickening of the gastric folds involving the fundus and the body of the stomach. Which of the following is the least likely diagnosis?

A. Ménétrier's disease
B. Lymphoma
C. Gastric adenocarcinoma
D. Granulomatous gastritis
E. Zollinger-Ellison syndrome

399 A 79-year-old man whose rheumatoid arthritis is being treated with anti-tumor necrosis factor (TNF) and prednisone reports having epigastric pain, nausea, and fever 2 months ago after a caving trip in Kentucky. EGD reveals enlarged, reddened gastric folds. Which findings are most likely on gastric biopsy?

A. Pseudohyphae with necrotic fibrinoid debris
B. Hyphae branching at 90-degree angles
C. Macrophages infiltrated with yeast in the lamina propria and submucosa
D. Basophilic organisms in the superficial mucous layer
E. Eosinophilic abscesses with a 0.3-mm diameter worm identified in one section

400 Testing to confirm eradication of *H. pylori* would include all of the following *except:*

A. Urea breath test 2 weeks after completion of a course of antibiotic therapy
B. Endoscopy with biopsy for rapid-urease testing
C. Endoscopy and biopsy for histologic examination
D. Stool antigen test

401 Which of the following findings in a patient with early gastric cancer (EGC) is most likely to be associated with lymph node metastasis?

A. No lymphatic or perineural invasion
B. Tumor in the gastric cardia
C. A 1.5-cm flat, sessile mass
D. Nodular, raised mass more than 3 cm in diameter

402 A 50-year-old obese white man who denies any upper gastrointestinal symptoms undergoes upper endoscopy preoperatively for planned gastric bypass surgery. EGD reveals nonerosive antral gastritis with red streaks. Biopsy specimens obtained at EGD show a chronic infiltrate in the lamina propria and epithelium with lymphoid follicles containing germinal centers. Which of the following management options would be most appropriate?

A. Repeat endoscopy in 6 months with surveillance biopsies
B. Evaluate with computed tomography and refer to an oncologist
C. Perform genetic testing for E-cadherin mutation
D. Perform total gastrectomy
E. Prescribe triple therapy for *H. pylori* infection

403 A 2-month-old boy with a history of polyhydramnios during gestation experiences recurrent vomiting, respiratory infections, and malnutrition. Laboratory tests reveal iron and cobalamin (vitamin B_{12}) deficiency. Contrast radiography would be expected to reveal which of the following findings?

A. Tubular stomach with megaesophagus
B. Gastric diverticulum
C. Large hiatal hernia
D. Jejunal diverticula
E. Esophageal diverticula

404 The most common type of gastric lymphoma is:

A. Non-Hodgkin's lymphoma
B. Mucosa-associated lymphoid tissue (MALT) lymphoma
C. Hodgkin's lymphoma
D. None of the above

405 All of the following statements about the mucous layer in the stomach are true *except:*

A. Ninety-five percent of the mucous gel is water
B. Mucins have antigens corresponding to a person's blood type
C. The layer slows back-diffusion of H^+ toward the mucosa
D. Prostaglandins inhibit mucus production
E. The layer is degraded by pepsin

406 A 1-month-old boy is brought to the hospital with a 1-week history of mild spitting episodes after feeds that over the past 24 hours have progressed to projectile vomiting. A palpable "olive" is felt in the epigastrium and peristaltic waves are visible. Ultrasound confirms a 3-mm diameter sonolucent "donut" of hypertrophied circular muscle. Which of the following is the appropriate definitive therapy?

A. Partial gastrectomy with Roux-en-Y reconstruction
B. EGD with through-the-scope (TTS) dilation of the pylorus
C. Pyloromyotomy
D. Jejunal feeding tube placement
E. Nasojejunal feeding tube placement

407 The most common genetic mutation found in gastric cancer is:

A. Adenomatous polyposis coli (*APC*) gene
B. *FHIT* gene
C. *p53* gene
D. *K-Ras* and *Myc* genes

408 A 56-year-old man presents with hematemesis. On EGD the only abnormality noted is an ulcerated, compressible cystic structure on the posterior aspect of the first portion of the duodenum. Endoscopic ultrasound reveals a unilocular cystic structure with echogenic mucosa with a hypoechoic muscle layer deep to this. Doppler shows no evidence of flow. Which of the following management strategies is most appropriate?

A. Local excision
B. Gastrojejunostomy
C. Pancreaticojejunostomy
D. Choledochojejunostomy
E. Transjugular intrahepatic portosystemic shunt

409 A 55-year-old man is prescribed naproxen for arthritis in his knee. He will need it daily for an indefinite period and is eager to avoid GI toxicity. He has never had peptic ulcer disease. Correct advice for this patient will include:

A. Co-treatment with glucocorticoids is permissible
B. Stop daily alcohol use
C. Test for *H. pylori* infection
D. It is safe to add 81 mg of aspirin to the daily medication regimen

410 Which of the following is true regarding metoclopramide therapy in patients with gastroparesis?

1. It can cause extrapyramidal reactions.
2. It relieves constipation.
3. It can elevate prolactin levels and cause gynecomastia.
4. It does not cross the blood-brain barrier.

A. 1 and 3
B. 2 and 4
C. 1, 2, and 3
D. All of the above

411 Which of the following patients has an increased risk of regional lymph node metastasis and thus requires more aggressive management?

A. A 60-year-old white man receiving long-term proton-pump inhibitor (PPI) therapy for GERD
B. A 55-year-old white woman with a history of pernicious anemia and atrophic gastritis who, at upper GI endoscopy, is found to have a 1-cm-diameter submucosal antral mass
C. A 45-year-old African-American woman with a history of recurrent gastric and duodenal ulcers who is found to have a fasting gastrin level of 1000
D. A 70-year-old healthy African-American man who undergoes EGD to evaluate symptoms of chronic reflux; on endoscopy, a 2-cm submucosal mass is found in the body of the stomach and endoscopic ultrasound (EUS) shows that the mass is confined to the submucosa

412 The optimal treatment regimen for *H. pylori* infection would be:

A. Amoxicillin, clarithromycin, and a PPI for 7 days
B. Metronidazole and a PPI for 14 days
C. Metronidazole, tetracycline, bismuth, and a PPI for 14 days
D. Ciprofloxacin and amoxicillin for 14 days
E. Amoxicillin and a PPI for 14 days

413 Peptic ulcer is a common complication of treatment with NSAIDs. Choose the correct statement regarding prophylactic therapy:

A. H_2-receptor antagonists do not lower the risk.
B. Misoprostol has not been shown to reduce GI complications.
C. Patients with *H. pylori* infection should undergo eradication therapy.
D. Ulcer bleeding can be prevented in high-risk patients by administration of omeprazole.

414 Gastric emptying of liquids has all of the following characteristics *except:*

A. Liquids rapidly disperse throughout the stomach
B. There is no lag period
C. Emptying follows an exponential pattern
D. Emptying rate is not affected by nutrient content
E. Carbonation delays emptying of fluids

415 A 68-year-old African-American man was found to have a proximal adenocarcinoma of the stomach. Based on the results of CT and EUS, the lesion was staged to be T3N1M0. The 5-year survival rate for this tumor is:

A. More than 80%
B. Less than 5%
C. Less than 20%
D. About 50%

416 A 34-year-old man with no chronic medical illnesses presents with syncope soon after vomiting bright red blood. In the emergency department, red hematemesis is documented. The patient is awake but agitated and has cool extremities, dry mucous membranes, a heart rate of 130 beats/minute, and supine blood pressure of 90/60 mmHg. There is no scleral icterus. The abdomen is soft and nontender, without hepatomegaly, but there is black stool in the rectum that tests positive for occult blood. Laboratory studies reveal hemoglobin of 11.0 mg/dL, blood urea nitrogen (BUN) of 40 mg/dL, creatinine of 0.9 mg/dL, prothrombin (PT) and partial thromboplastin (PTT) times that are normal, aspartate aminotransferrase (AST) level of 119 U/L, alanine aminotransferase of 42 U/L, and alcohol level of 280 mg/dL.

The first intervention for this patient should be:

A. A bolus dose followed by an infusion of octreotide
B. A bolus dose followed by an infusion of a proton pump inhibitor
C. Insertion of a nasogastric tube
D. Emergency upper endoscopy
E. Placement of a large-bore intravenous (IV) catheter to allow for vigorous fluid resuscitation

417 An 86-year-old man with severe coronary artery disease and recently diagnosed gastric cancer has elected to forego further treatment. He presents now complaining of intense epigastric pain with fever and requests endoscopy. Esophagogastroduodenoscopy (EGD) reveals an ulcerated mass with purulent material draining from a small opening. Histopathologic examination and culture of the purulent material show that gram-positive filamentous anaerobic bacteria are present. Which is the most appropriate treatment?

A. High-dose penicillin for 6 to 12 months
B. Intravenous vancomycin for 14 days
C. Paromomycin for 3 months
D. Linezolid for 3 months
E. Unasyn for 14 days

418 A 71-year-old white woman underwent upper endoscopy to evaluate dyspepsia and findings of heme-positive stool. Upper endoscopy revealed a 1.5-cm sessile mass in the mid-body greater curvature of the stomach. It was biopsied and on histologic examination it was revealed to be adenomatous tissue with high-grade dysplasia. Initially the mass was staged based on no

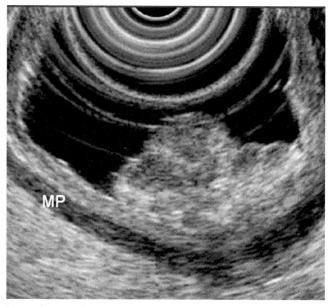

Figure for question **418**

abnormal findings on CT of the abdomen and pelvis. Based on these findings and the results of EUS (see figure), what would be the most effective treatment for this patient?

A. Chemotherapy and radiation therapy
B. Photodynamic therapy (PDT)
C. Subtotal gastrectomy
D. Endoscopic mucosal resection

419 Which of the following tests can be used to diagnose gastroparesis?

1. Electrogastrography (EGG)
2. Gastric emptying of technetium-labeled eggs
3. 13C-octanoic acid breath test
4. Ultrasonography

A. (1) and (3)
B. (2) and (4)
C. (1), (2), and (3)
D. All of the above

420 A 34-year-old woman with a history of cholecystectomy complains of 5 years of epigastric burning that is worse after meals. The results of laboratory tests and ultrasound are normal. EGD demonstrates a normal esophagus; however, the antrum and body of the stomach contain areas of erythema, erosions, and bile staining. Which is the most appropriate therapy?

A. Cholestyramine
B. Proton pump inhibitor
C. Ursodiol
D. Roux-en-Y choledochojejunostomy
E. Nissen fundoplication

421 Which of the following structures are located adjacent and posterior to the stomach?

A. Pancreas, transverse colon, diaphragm, spleen, left kidney, and left adrenal gland
B. Pancreas, diaphragm, spleen, right kidney, and right adrenal gland
C. Pancreas, spleen, right kidney, and right adrenal gland
D. Pancreas, diaphragm, right kidney, and right adrenal gland
E. Pancreas, transverse colon, diaphragm, spleen, and right adrenal gland

422 The role of photodynamic therapy (PDT) in the treatment of gastric cancer remains controversial. Cutaneous complications related to PDT include all of the following *except:*

A. Phototoxicity (first-, second-, and third-degree burns)
B. Erythema nodosum
C. Photosensitivity
D. Erythema multiforme

423 Regarding duodenal ulcer caused by *H. pylori* infection, all of the following statements are true *except:*

A. Antrum-only biopsies are not adequate for diagnosis when antisecretory medication has been taken within one week of EGD.
B. After 1 to 2 weeks of eradication therapy, an additional 4 weeks of antisecretory therapy are required.
C. Noninvasive confirmation of eradication is advised for all complicated ulcers.
D. After treatment, maintenance therapy with an antisecretory drug is not needed.

424 All peptic ulcerations of the stomach and duodenum have use of NSAIDs or *H. pylori* infection as a predisposing factor. True or False?

425 A 2-cm submucosal mass is identified in the fundus of the stomach. Based on the findings at endoscopy and EUS (see figures), what is the likely diagnosis?

A. Gastric adenocarcinoma
B. Gastric lipoma
C. Pancreatic rest
D. Gastric carcinoid
E. Gastrointestinal stromal tumor (GIST)

426 The increased prevalence of *H. pylori* infection in older Americans is due to reinfection. True or False?

427 Gastric distention, vagal stimulation, and luminal protein stimulate gastric G cells. Which of the following statements best describes the physiologic interplay between gastric G cells and D cells?

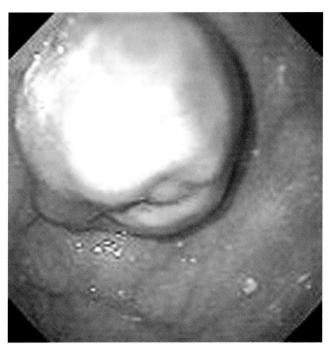

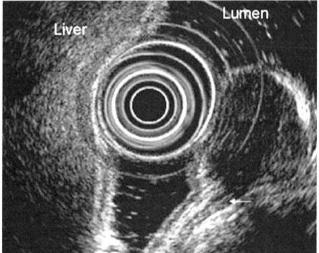

Figures for question **425**

A. G cells produce gastrin, while D cells secrete somatostatin, which inhibits gastrin secretion.
B. G cells produce gastrin, while D cells produce bicarbonate, which indirectly inhibits acid secretion.
C. G cells produce gastrin, while D cells produce bicarbonate, which directly neutralizes luminal acid.
D. G cells produce mucus and bicarbonate, while D cells produce histamine, which stimulates acid production.
E. G cells produce gastrin, while D cells produce serotonin, which inhibits acid production.

428 Which of the following findings increase(s) the likelihood that a gastric ulcer is associated with a gastric adenocarcinoma?

A. Smaller size (diameter <1.0 cm)
B. Intestinal metaplasia
C. Nodular folds in the adjacent mucosa that radiate to the edge of the ulcer
D. Simultaneous occurrence of a duodenal ulcer
E. All of the above

429 EGD for the evaluation of peptic ulcer disease (PUD) symptoms:

A. Should be performed after upper GI (UGI) radiographic studies
B. Is less sensitive, although more specific, than UGI radiography
C. Can, with appropriate biopsy and brushing of the ulcer margins, lead to diagnosis of 85% of malignant gastric ulcers
D. Is not mandatory to repeat to confirm ulcer healing when malignancy has been excluded by the results of pathology and cytology studies

430 Diffuse corporal atrophic gastritis (DCAG) has the following oncologic association(s):

A. Gastric adenocarcinoma only
B. Gastric adenocarcinoma and carcinoid
C. Gastric metaplasia only
D. Esophageal adenocarcinoma
E. Gastric lymphoma

431 At diagnosis, more than 75% of gastric adenocarcinomas are found to have metastasized to lymph nodes. Which therapy provides the best adjuvant therapy after surgical resection?

A. Chemotherapy alone
B. Observation
C. Radiation therapy alone
D. Combined chemotherapy and radiation therapy

432 A newborn boy with Down syndrome has forceful, nonbilious emesis at his first feeding. Radiographs reveal a stomach distended with gas and a "gasless intestine." Contrast radiography demonstrates a complete obstruction at the antrum. Which is the most appropriate plan for management?

A. Gastric decompression, rehydration, and gastroduodenostomy
B. Gastric decompression, rehydration, and gastrojejunostomy
C. Gastric decompression, rehydration, and endoscopic mucosal resection
D. Rehydration and pyloroplasty
E. Rehydration and endoscopic mucosal resection

433 During endoscopy, active bleeding begins. The best course of treatment at this point is:

A. Administration of a bolus dose, followed by infusion of a proton pump inhibitor
B. Epinephrine injection
C. Argon plasma coagulation (APC)
D. Contact thermal therapy (heater probe or multipolar electrocautery)
E. Combination therapy with B and D

434 A 64-year-old white woman undergoes upper endoscopy to evaluate midepigastric pain. Markedly abnormal rugal folds without ulceration are identified. Multiple biopsy specimens are obtained using a jumbo biopsy forceps. Histopathologic evaluation reveals no malignancy (see figure). EUS reveals thickening of the muscularis propria. Which of the following is least likely to be the diagnosis?

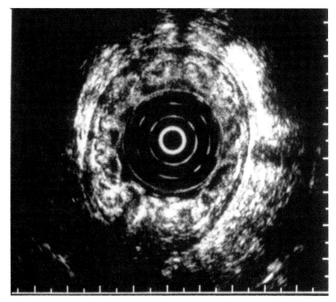

Figure for question **434**

A. Metastatic melanoma
B. Lymphoma
C. Ménétrier's disease
D. Metastatic breast cancer
E. Gastric carcinoma

435 A patient is evaluated within minutes of onset of acute, severe epigastric pain (an acute abdomen). Upright plain films demonstrate pneumoperitoneum. The treating physician should:

A. Give IV fluids and a clear liquid diet
B. Inquire about NSAID or crack cocaine use
C. Perform an emergency EGD
D. Request a routine surgical consultation

436 The location of *H. pylori* gastritis determines the clinical sequelae. Chronic gastritis in the body and fundus is associated with all of the following *except:*

A. Gastric ulcer
B. Gastric adenocarcinoma
C. Duodenal ulcer
D. Gastric lymphoma
E. Chronic nonatrophic superficial gastritis

437 Treatment of *Helicobacter pylori* infection should lead to improvement in all of the following conditions *except:*

A. Gastric and duodenal ulcers
B. Gastric and duodenal inflammation
C. Gastric adenocarcinoma
D. Gastric B-cell lymphoma/mucosa-associated lymphoid tissue (MALT) lymphoma
E. None of the above

438 A 39-year-old alcoholic man complains of an episode of epigastric pain followed by three episodes of moderate-volume hematemesis. He has early satiety and has lost 20 pounds over the past 3 months. Endoscopy demonstrates an ulcerated mass in the antrum, which is partially obstructing the pylorus. No signs of recent bleeding are noted. Which of the following diagnostic plans is most appropriate?

A. Tissue sampling for *Campylobacter*-like organism (CLO) analysis
B. Multiple biopsies of the mass and ulcer to send for histopathologic analysis
C. Multiple biopsies of the mass, sparing the ulcer to avoid bleeding
D. Multiple biopsies for histopathologic and acid-fast bacteria (AFB) evaluation
E. Multiple biopsies for histopathologic and cytomegalovirus (CMV) evaluation

439 All of the following statements about cephalic-vagal stimulation are true *except:*

A. Cephalic-vagal stimulation accounts for 1/3 of acid secretion
B. The smell, sight, and thought of food stimulate dorsal motor nuclei of vagus nerves
C. Acetylcholine activates postganglionic gastric neurons
D. Atropine abolishes cephalic-vagal stimulation of acid secretion
E. The sight of food is a more potent stimulus than taste

440 Abdominal pain, which is almost always present in PUD, has which of the following clinical features?

A. There is no difference between gastric and duodenal ulcer pain.

B. The pain description can be used to distinguish between benign and malignant ulcer.
C. It is always present prior to perforation or major bleeding.
D. PUD pain can be mimicked by reflux esophagitis.

441 According to American Gastrointestinal Association (AGA) guidelines, which of the following patients should undergo upper endoscopy promptly?

A. A 25-year-old African-American woman complaining of a 1-week history of midepigastric pain
B. A 50-year-old white man complaining of midepigastric pain that was responsive to a 2-week course of proton pump inhibitor therapy
C. A 70-year-old African-American man complaining of a 6-week history of midepigastric pain associated with a 10-pound weight loss, nausea, and vomiting
D. A 62-year-old asymptomatic white woman with normal hemoglobin level, heme-positive stool, and normal results of colonoscopy

442 Which of the following statements regarding the prevalence of *H. pylori* infection is true?

A. About 80% of American children are infected by age 10.
B. The risk for infection is related to socioeconomic status of the family during childhood.
C. In developed countries, the prevalence is higher in children.
D. Genetic susceptibility is not a factor in infection.
E. Animals are important reservoirs of *H. pylori*.

443 A 45-year-old woman presents with chronic recurrent abdominal pain followed by bilious emesis. Transabdominal ultrasound demonstrates an annular pancreas. Magnetic resonance cholangeopancreatography (MRCP) reveals an annulus containing a duct encircling the duodenum. There is no evidence of malignancy. Which of the following procedures would be optimal in this case?

A. Pancreaticojejunostomy
B. Duodenoduodenostomy
C. Surgical diversion of pancreatic tissue
D. EGD with dilation
E. Insertion of a nasojejunal tube

444 Screening for gastric cancer is indicated for patients with any of the following conditions *except:*

A. Hyperplastic/fundic gland polyps
B. Low-grade gastric dysplasia
C. Familial adenomatous polyposis (FAP) syndrome
D. Gastric adenoma

445 Duodenal ulcer pathophysiology is usually associated with:

A. Gastric acid hyposecretion
B. Elevated fasting serum gastrin levels
C. Delayed emptying of gastric acid into the duodenum
D. Increased duodenal bicarbonate production

446 The accuracy of C13 urea breath tests for the presence of *H. pylori* can be compromised by all of the following *except:*

A. Recent use of a PPI
B. Recent use of antibiotics
C. Prior partial gastrectomy
D. Recent use of H_2-receptor antagonists
E. Small numbers of organisms in the stomach

447 Which environmental and/or dietary factors are least likely to trigger the development of an intestinal-type gastric cancer?

A. *H. pylori* infection
B. High intake of fresh fruits and vegetables
C. High intake of pickled foods, soy sauce, salted fish and meats
D. Cigarette smoking
E. High intake of preserved foods high in nitrates and polycyclic aromatic amines

448 A 48-year-old man recently had an episode of binge alcohol intake. He presents 1 day after acute onset of epigastric abdominal pain, nonbloody vomiting, and fever. In the emergency department his tachycardia and hypotension both respond to administration of 1 L of saline. He has severe epigastric tenderness, and rectal exam is negative for blood. Abdominal radiographs reveal gas bubbles conforming to the contour of the stomach. Which is the most appropriate management course?

A. Broad-spectrum antibiotic therapy, CT, and surgical consultation
B. Broad-spectrum antibiotic therapy with intravenous hydration
C. Intravenous hydration and nasogastric tube suction
D. Emergency endoscopy
E. Administration of charcoal via nasogastric tube

449 The process of B_{12} absorption includes all of the following except:

1. Release of cobalamin from dietary protein by pepsin in acidic stomach
2. Binding of cobalamin by R protein
3. Cleaving of R-cobalamin complexes by pancreatic trypsin
4. Attachment of intrinsic factor-bound cobalamin to receptors on ileal mucosa

A. (1) and (3)
B. (2) and (4)
C. (1), (2), and (3)
D. All of the above

450 Which of the following statements is true regarding *H. pylori* infection?

A. PUD will develop in approximately 50% of patients infected with *H. pylori*.
B. Successful treatment does not eliminate the associated gastritis.
C. Serologic testing is useful to confirm eradication.
D. Ulcer disease is more common in cagA-positive patients.

451 Substances that may protect against gastric cancer include all of the following *except:*

A. Fresh fruits and vegetables
B. Aspirin
C. Green tea
D. All of the above

452 Choose the correct set of associations for gastric chief cells, parietal cells, and enterochromaffin (EC) cells:

A. Chief cells–histamine, parietal cells–intrinsic factor, EC cells–serotonin
B. Chief cells–pepsinogen, parietal cells–HCl, EC cells–serotonin
C. Chief cells–bicarbonate, parietal cells–intrinsic factor, EC cells–histamine
D. Chief cells–serotonin, parietal cells–HCl, EC cells–histamine
E. Chief cells–pepsinogen, parietal cells–intrinsic factor, EC cells–histamine

453 A 40-year-old man with HIV infection and chronic recurrent gastric ulcer has fever, diarrhea, and weight loss. On EGD a gastric ulcer and fine, white duodenal nodules are seen. CT reveals mesenteric lymphadenopathy. Which findings are most likely on histologic evaluation of a biopsy specimen?

A. Basophilic stippling at the epithelial cell–apical membrane
B. Numerous mucosal foamy histiocytes containing acid-fast bacilli
C. Multiple mucosal spirochetes visible on silver stained sections
D. Fibrinoid debris and pseudohyphae
E. Foveolar hyperplasia

454 Which of the following early gastric cancers is most amenable to endoscopic mucosal resection?

A. A stage T2N0M0 gastric cancer in a 40-year-old white man
B. A 4-cm mass in the gastric cardia with pathology revealing intestinal type of gastric adenocarcinoma in a 75-year-old African-American man
C. A 2-cm stage T1N0M0 tumor along the lesser curvature, posterior midbody of the stomach associated with a well-differentiated adenocarinoma in the gastric antrum in a 50-year-old African-American woman
D. A 1.5-cm stage T1N0M0 tumor in the midbody greater curvature of the stomach in an 85-year-old white man

455 A male patient has rebleeding after endoscopy and requires 3 units of packed erythrocytes to maintain his hemoglobin level above 10 g/dL. Two days later, while on a diet of clear liquids and twice-daily administration of a PPI, he develops melena. His pulse increases to 100 beats/minute although without orthostatic hypotension, and his hemoglobin level drops to 9 g/dL.

The next best step is:

A. Consult a surgeon regarding operative treatment of this patient's ulcer
B. Consult a surgeon to perform vagotomy and oversew the bleeding vessel
C. Consult a surgeon to oversew the bleeding vessel
D. Repeat EGD for possible endoscopic therapy
E. Transfuse additional packed red blood cells and observe

456 A 34-year-old African-American woman has chronic postprandial epigastric discomfort. Endoscopy reveals pale, shiny mucosa with prominent submucosal vessels. Gastric antral biopsies show mucosal atrophy and intestinal metaplasia. Which of the following statements about her condition is true?

A. Genetic factors have not been implicated in the pathogenesis of this condition.
B. *H. pylori* is seen in 85% of cases.
C. Her metaplasia carries risk of progression to gastric carcinoid.
D. Pernicious anemia is strongly associated with this condition.
E. Hashimoto's disease has been associated with this condition.

457 A patient with cancer in the gastric antrum but without any evidence of metastasis on CT undergoes endoscopic ultrasonography (EUS) for staging of the cancer. EUS reveals a 2-cm hypoechoic mass (see figure). Based on these findings, this tumor is most appropriately classified as:

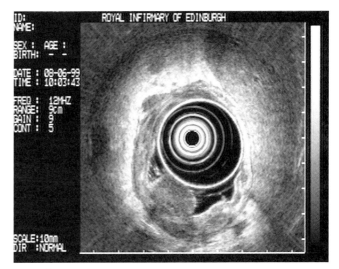

Figure for question **457**

A. T2N1M0
B. T2N2M0
C. T2N3M0
D. T3N0M0
E. T3N2M0

458 The incidence of hospital admission for bleeding or perforated peptic ulcer has gradually decreased over the past 40 years, coincident with the decline in the prevalence of *H. pylori* infection. True or False?

459 A 40-year-old man with a remote history of duodenal ulcer presents with chronic epigastric burning that is partially alleviated by taking a proton pump inhibitor agent. Endoscopy reveals mild diffuse gastritis and normal duodenal mucosa. Biopsy specimens should be obtained from the antrum and which of the following regions?

A. Gastric cardia
B. Distal esophagus
C. Duodenal bulb
D. Body of stomach
E. Mid-esophagus

460 To reduce the risk of complications, patients with PUD should be advised to:

A. Stop alcohol use completely
B. Adopt a bland diet
C. Discontinue smoking
D. Reduce emotional stress

461 All of the following paraneoplastic syndromes are associated with gastric cancer *except:*

A. Acanthosis nigricans
B. Disseminated intravascular coagulation
C. Thrombophlebitis (Trousseau's sign)
D. Pyoderma gangrenosum
E. Nephrotic syndrome

462 A 32-year-old woman with a history of cervical cancer reports having two episodes of hematemesis and epigastric pain for 6 months, without weight loss. On a previous upper GI barium study, thickened folds with serpiginous ulcerations and a stricture were seen in the mid-stomach ("hourglass" stomach). She has not been following recommendations made at that time. EGD is performed and shows serpiginous gastric ulcerations without stigmata of GI bleeding and a mid-body ulcerated stricture. Which of the following is the most appropriate next step?

A. Biopsy the stricture and ulcer edges
B. Biopsy the stricture and central aspect of the ulcerations
C. Biopsy the stricture and ulcer and examine sections stained with Warthin-Starry silver stain
D. Biopsy the stricture and ulcer and examine sections stained for acid-fast bacteria
E. Biopsy the stricture and ulcer and evaluate specimens by flow cytometry

463 The major factor in the speed at which solids are emptied from the stomach is:

A. Meal volume
B. Calorie density
C. Particle size
D. Food temperature

464 A patient undergoes urgent endoscopy. No active bleeding or old blood is seen, although a few erosions are noted in the gastric antrum. Inspection of the duodenal bulb reveals a raised red protuberance in the center of an ulcer. The duodenal ulcer measures 15 mm in diameter.

The approximate likelihood of rebleeding from this ulcer is:

A. <10%
B. 20%
C. 40%
D. 80%

465 A 39-year-old woman with celiac disease has been noncompliant with her gluten-free diet. Endoscopy performed for abdominal pain reveals thickened gastric mucosal folds, along with nodularity and aphthous erosions (varioliform gastritis). Which is the most appropriate next step?

A. Directed gastric biopsies with CLO test for *H. pylori*
B. Directed gastric biopsies
C. Directed gastric biopsies with brush cytology
D. Directed gastric biopsies with random cardia biopsies
E. Directed biopsies with staining for acid-fast bacteria (AFB)

466 All of the following are true about pepsin *except:*

A. It is secreted as a proenzyme into the gastric lumen
B. It is activated by gastric acid in the lumen
C. Pepsins can convert pepsinogens
D. Pepsins cleave peptide bonds
E. Pepsins are inactivated at a pH of about 3

467 Which of the following statements is true regarding gastric cancer?

A. Patients younger than age 40 have a better prognosis.
B. Depth of invasion is the primary prognostic indicator.
C. Survival rates are worse for men than women.
D. Early gastric cancer is defined as penetration through the muscularis propria.
E. Serum carcinoembryonic antigen (CEA) levels greater than 5 ng/mL are found in nearly 50% of patients with resectable gastric cancer.

468 Proton pump inhibitor therapy is better than misoprostol or H_2-receptor antagonists in the treatment of NSAID-associated PUD. True or False?

469 A 47-year-old man presents with a 2-month history of epigastric pain, nausea, and nonbloody vomiting. The results of laboratory tests and ultrasound are normal. EGD demonstrates diffuse, edematous hypertrophic folds. Gastric biopsies show foveolar hyperplasia with cystic dilations and minimal inflammation. There are no intranuclear inclusions or signs of malignancy. A CLO assay is negative. The gastrin level is normal. Which of the following treatments is most appropriate?

A. Proton pump inhibitor and octreotide
B. Proton pump inhibitor
C. Octreotide
D. Glucocorticoids and octreotide
E. Partial gastrectomy

470 Bloating and nausea in a diabetic may be signs of gastroparesis or they could indicate all of the following *except:*

A. Acute hyperglycemia
B. Functional dyspepsia
C. Anorexia nervosa
D. Gastric ulcer
E. *H. pylori* infection

471 The most accurate procedure to stage gastric cancer is:

A. Transabdominal ultrasound
B. Magnetic resonance imaging
C. Helical CT
D. Endoscopic ultrasound

472 A 57-year-old man with metastatic colon cancer involving his lungs has recently undergone chemotherapy and radiation therapy. He develops epigastric discomfort, fever, and intermittent nonbloody emesis. Endoscopy reveals multiple small, linear, superficial ulcers that impart a cobblestone appearance to the stomach. The most appropriate endoscopic diagnostic procedure would be:

A. Directed biopsies and brush cytology
B. Directed biopsies and tissue collection for CLO analysis
C. Brush cytology
D. Directed gastric biopsies and random duodenal biopsies
E. Directed biopsies

473 The rate of gastric emptying is slowed by all of the following *except:*

A. Duodenal distension
B. Acidification of the duodenum
C. Perfusion of fat
D. Colonic distension
E. Hypoglycemia

474 Worldwide, which country has the greatest incidence of gastric cancer?

A. United States
B. Korea
C. Japan
D. Australia

475 The gastric and duodenal mucosa is protected from acid/peptic injury by all of the following *except:*

A. Epithelial mucous coat
B. Paracellular tight junctional complexes
C. Parietal proton pumps
D. Mucosal blood flow

476 Which structures are located immediately posterior to the first portion of the duodenum?

A. Gastroduodenal artery, hepatic vein, common bile duct
B. Common bile duct, portal vein, gallbladder
C. Common bile duct, gastroduodenal artery, portal vein
D. Left hepatic duct, portal vein
E. Portal vein, common bile duct, splenic artery

477 Histamine-receptor antagonists have never been shown to decrease bleeding rates or mortality in patients with bleeding duodenal ulcer. True or False?

478 A 70-year-old man has midepigastric pain that is unresponsive to proton pump inhibitor therapy. Upper endoscopy is performed (see figure) and histopathologic evaluation of a biopsy specimen shows high-grade dysplasia. Optimal management of this patient's condition would be:

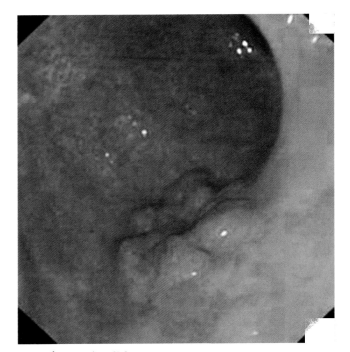

Figure for question **478**

A. Perform endoscopy yearly
B. Perform endoscopic mucosal resection
C. Continue proton pump inhibitor therapy
D. Evaluate for *H. pylori* infection and if present, treat and repeat endoscopy in 3 months
E. Perform subtotal gastrectomy

479 A pathologist evaluating biopsy specimens from the gastric wall of a patient with a clinical history consistent with *H. pylori* infection will expect to find organisms in which tissue layer or region of cells?

A. Lamina propria
B. Superficial mucous layer
C. Submucosa
D. Epithelial cell cytoplasm
E. Muscularis propria

480 Slow waves in the duodenum occur at the same frequency as gastric slow waves. True or False?

481 True statements regarding the pathophysiologic effects of NSAID use include all of the following *except*:

A. COX-2 is the predominant cyclooxygenase in the stomach
B. The effect on cyclooxygenase activity is systemic, not topical
C. Prostaglandin concentration in the mucosa is reduced
D. Neutrophil adherence to the gastric vascular endothelium affects mucosal blood flow

482 A 45-year-old African-American woman with pulmonary sarcoidosis presents with abdominal pain and weight loss. Which is the most likely site of gastrointestinal involvement with her disease?

A. Esophagus
B. Stomach
C. Duodenum
D. Ileum
E. Colon

483 Which of the following *most* accurately describes histamine H$_2$-receptor antagonists?

A. Tolerance is not seen with oral or intravenous dosing.
B. They should not be used at all in patients in liver failure.
C. They have side effects profiles comparable to those of placebo.
D. They have clinically significant interactions with other drugs.

484 In the United States, gastric cancer is most often located in which region of the stomach at diagnosis?

A. Proximal third
B. Middle third
C. Distal third
D. Entire stomach

485 A 34-year-old man has colonic Crohn's disease that has been kept in remission for 3 years with a 5-aminosalicylic acid (5-ASA) compound. He now presents with a 1-month history of severe epigastric abdominal pain without diarrhea, bleeding, or weight loss. The results of laboratory tests and ultrasound are normal, but EGD reveals serpiginous erosions in the antrum and biopsies show noncaseating granulomas. Which is the most appropriate therapy?

A. Oral prednisone
B. Intravenous glucocorticoids
C. Budesonide
D. Proton pump inhibitors
E. Sulfasalazine

486 Proton pump inhibitors are very effective in treating acid peptic disease. Which of the following statements about these agents is true?

A. Hypergastrinemia due to profound acid suppression may lead to the development of gastric carcinoids.
B. Optimal dosing has been achieved when most of the pumps are inactivated.
C. Rebound acid hypersecretion after cessation of therapy may last 2 months.
D. Hepatic and renal insufficiency require dose adjustments.

487 Peptic ulcer in the pyloric channel is the most common cause of gastric outlet obstruction. True or False?

488 A 47-year-old white woman with type 1 diabetes mellitus presents with a 5-year history of epigastric burning. Gastroscopy reveals gastric fold effacement and thin mucosa in the fundus. Biopsies show intestinal metaplasia in the fundus and laboratory tests reveal hypergastrinemia. These findings lead to suspicion of which of the following hematologic abnormalities?

A. Antiphospholipid antibody syndrome
B. Iron deficiency anemia
C. Pernicious anemia
D. Hyperhomocysteinemia
E. Myelodysplasia

489 The incidence of gastric cancer is *least* likely to be elevated in patients with:

A. Familial adenomatous polyposis (FAP)
B. Hereditary nonpolyposis cancer (HNPCC)
C. Juvenile polyposis syndrome
D. Family history of a second-degree relative with gastric cancer

490 Regarding PUD bleeding, it is correct to state that:

A. It carries a 5% to 10% risk of death
B. Therapeutic endoscopy benefits all patients
C. It may present with hematochezia alone
D. It accounts for 50% of all cases of UGI bleeding

491 In comparison to all causes of upper GI bleeding, his mortality is higher than average. True or False?

492 A 47-year-old East Asian woman received a stem cell transplant last year to treat acute myelogenous leukemia (AML). She now presents with a 1-week history of fever, epigastric pain, and nausea. EGD demonstrates edematous, erythematous, ulcerated mucosa in the gastric antrum. Analysis of biopsy specimens would most likely lead to identification of:

A. Noncaseating granulomas
B. Birefringent crystals under polarized light
C. Pancreatic acinar cells
D. Foveolar hyperplasia with absence of parietal cells
E. Epithelial cell intranuclear and intracytoplasmic inclusions

493 Which of the following is a correct statement about perforated peptic ulcers?

A. Surgical therapy is always required.
B. For a duodenal ulcer, omental patching without an acid-lowering procedure is inadequate therapy.

C. Perforated gastric ulcer in the elderly is often associated with NSAID use.
D. The majority of perforated ulcers originate in the stomach.

494 Patients with gastric ulcers limited to the prepyloric antrum are typically acid hyposecretors. True or False?

495 Which of the following are true about gastric acid secretion in healthy elderly persons?

1. It decreases with age.
2. It remains constant with age.
3. Fasting gastric pH is less than 3.0.
4. Gastric HCO3 secretion declines with age.

A. (1) and (3)
B. (2) and (4)
C. (1), (2), and (3)
D. None of the above

496 An 84-year-old man with cardiovascular disease needs treatment for a painful, osteoarthritic joint. He is taking a low dose (81 mg/day) of aspirin and warfarin for therapeutic anticoagulation. He should be advised to:

A. Avoid NSAIDs altogether
B. Begin NSAIDs only after stopping the aspirin
C. Start a COX-2 inhibitor
D. Start a COX-2 inhibitor with a PPI

ANSWERS

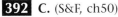

392 **C.** (S&F, ch50)

Although enteric-coated NSAIDs may have fewer topical effects on the gastric mucosa, they have all the same adverse *systemic* effects as noncoated formulations of these drugs. Decreases in gastric mucosal blood flow may be the most significant of these effects. Hemorrhagic erosions are topical manifestations and are seen early in the course of treatment. Ulcer perforation, outlet obstruction, and hemorrhagic complications are seen annually in 1% to 4% of patients treated with NSAIDs.

393 **C.** (S&F, ch47)

The major stimulant of gastrin is luminal amino acids, especially phenylalanine and tyrosine, derived from peptic hydrolysis of dietary proteins. Distension of the gastric body/fundus stimulates gastrin release. A pH below 3.0 decreases secretion of gastrin.

394 **C.** (S&F, ch45)

Duodenal atresia refers to congenital obstruction of the duodenum; it may occur as a blind-ending pouch, a pouch with a fibrous cord, or an obstructing membrane. The treatment of choice is duodenoduodenostomy with a diamond-shaped anastomosis.

395 **C.** (S&F, ch52)

Once the diagnosis of gastric adenocarcinoma is made, proper staging of the tumor should occur prior to therapeutic intervention. CT of the abdomen should be performed first, with or without PET to exclude distant metastasis. If the results of these examinations are negative, EUS is used to determine the T (depth of tumor invasion) and N (nodal status) stage of the tumor. Decisions regarding endoscopic resection, surgical resection, or combined modality therapy (CMT) are based on the tumor stage.

396 **D.** (S&F, ch49)

Gastritis cystica profunda can, rarely, complicate partial gastrectomy with gastroenterostomy. The lesions have been associated with gastric stump adenocarcinoma and should prompt a concerted search for synchronous or metachronous gastric malignancy.

397 **D.** (S&F, ch47)

All stimulate acid production except gin.

398 **D.** (S&F, ch52)

Thickening of the gastric folds with normal overlying mucosa indicates an infiltrative process such as Menetrier's disease, lymphoma, or gastric adenocarcinoma. Zollinger-Ellison syndrome will cause hypertrophic gastric folds secondary to hypergastrinemia, but granulomatous gastritis will cause mucosal disease with submucosal thickening.

399 **C.** (S&F, ch49)

Histoplasmosis is endemic in the Midwest: Ohio, Kentucky, Tennessee, and Illinois. *Histoplasma capsulatum* organisms invade macrophages, especially in immunocompromised individuals (i.e., those receiving anti-TNF therapy, glucorticoid therapy, or post-transplant immunosuppression). The history in the case presented is less compatible with candidiasis, mucormycosis, cryptosporidiosis, or anisakiasis.

400 **A.** (S&F, ch48)

One should wait a minimum of 4 weeks after completion of a course of antibiotic therapy before performing follow-up testing.

401 **D.** (S&F, ch52)

Multivariate analyses have shown that lymphatic or perineural vessel invasion, histologic ulceration of the tumor, and larger size (more than 3 cm in diameter) are independent risk factors for regional lymph node metastasis. The incidence of lymph node metastasis from an intramucosal early gastric cancer not associated with any of these three risk factors is 0.36%.

402 **E.** (S&F, ch49)

Patients with diffuse antral-predominant gastritis (DAG) are often asymptomatic. Chronic lamina propria inflammation accompanied by neutrophilic infiltration and lymphoid follicles with germinal centers are characteristic of *H. pylori* infection.

403 **A.** (S&F, ch45)

Microgastria can present with all of the features described. Iron deficiency can be caused by gastric acid hyposecretion. B_{12} deficiency is due to decreased secretion of intrinsic factor. Gastric histology will be normal. Treatment options include frequent, small feedings, jejunostomy feedings, or a Hunt-Lawrence jejunal pouch, which is anastomosed to the greater curvature of the stomach. The other abnormalities listed would not be expected to result in this patient's constellation of symptoms.

404 **A.** (S&F, ch52)

Gastric lymphomas comprise 3% to 6% of all gastric malignancies. More than 95% of gastric lymphomas are non-Hodgkin's lymphomas. Gastric lymphoma is the most common form of extranodal non-Hodgkin's lymphoma, accounting for over 30% of all cases of primary non-Hodgkin's lymphoma.

405 **D.** (S&F, ch47)

Prostaglandins stimulate mucous production; 95% of mucus is water and 5% is mucin glycoprotein. The mucous layer prevents back-diffusion of H^+ and is degraded by pepsin at an acidic pH.

406 **C.** (S&F, ch45)

Infantile hypertrophic pyloric stenosis (IHPS) can present with marked metabolic alkalosis. Initial differential diagnostic considerations with mild spitting episodes are GERD and formula allergy. However, projectile vomiting with the classic physical findings described in this case are highly suggestive of IHPS. The treatment of choice after fluid and electrolyte replacement is Weber-Ramstedt pyloromyotomy. This procedure is low risk and can be performed laparoscopically. The other options are not treatments of choice.

407 **C.** (S&F, ch52)

A p53 mutation is the most common genetic mutation found in patients with gastric cancer; it has an incidence of 60% to 70%. The FHIT genetic mutation is found in 60% of cases, the APC genetic mutation in 50% of cases, and the K-Ras/Myc genetic mutations in 10% to 15% of cases of gastric cancer.

408 **A.** (S&F, ch45)

A duodenal duplication cyst can present with gastrointestinal bleeding if the cyst becomes ulcerated. Malignancy in these lesions has also been reported. Local incision is an accepted therapy for this condition. The lesion is not located in the second portion of the duodenum and does not require biliary or pancreatic bypass. Enteral bypass is similarly unnecessary if a less extensive surgery can be performed. Transjugular intrahepatic portosystemic shunt (TIPS) would not be valuable in these cases because there is no evidence of portosystemic hypertension.

409 **B.** (S&F, ch50)

Glucocorticoids increase the risk of ulcer and complications in patients being treated with NSAIDs, as does daily alcohol consumption. Testing for *H. pylori* infection in those who take NSAIDs but who have never had an ulcer is controversial. There is good evidence for increased toxicity when low-dose ASA is combined with an NSAID.

410 **A.** (S&F, ch46)

The medication works in the foregut only, so it is of little help in managing constipation. It crosses the blood-brain barrier and causes central nervous system (CNS) side affects.

411 **D.** (S&F, ch52)

Gastric carcinoid tumors account for 2% of all gastrointestinal carcinoids and 0.3% of all gastric neoplasms. Answers **A**, **B**, and **C** are related to enterochromaffin-like (ECL) hyperplasia secondary to hypergastrinemia. ECL lesions do not have malignant potential. An isolated gastric carcinoid, not related to hypergastrinemia, should be surgically resected if greater than 1 to 2 cm. Gastric carcinoids tend to have a good prognosis: when the disease does not metastasize, more than 95% of patients survive 5 years or longer, and even those with metastases have a greater than 50% chance of surviving 5 years.

412 **C.** (S&F, ch48)

Single-antibiotic regimens are not recommended because of concerns about antibiotic resistance. The regimen described in **A** is good but the shorter course is less effective than the 14-day course.

413 **C.** (S&F, ch51)

High-dose H_2-receptor blocker therapy reduces the risk that gastric ulcers will develop with NSAID use. The prostaglandin analog misoprostol has been shown to decrease NSAID complications by 40%. Patients infected with *H. pylori* who are long-term users of NSAIDs have a 6-fold

increased risk for GI bleeding. Eradication of the infection lowers the risk of ulcer formation in patients who are planning long-term therapy with NSAIDs. High-risk patients ideally will avoid NSAIDs altogether. Even high-dose PPI therapy poses increased risk of bleeding in these patients.

414 **D.** (S&F, ch46)

Nutrient-containing liquids are retained longer than non-nutrient fluids.

415 **B.** (S&F, ch52)

T3N1M0 adenocarcinoma of the stomach corresponds to stage IIIA disease. The likelihood of 5-year survival for those in the United States with this stage tumor is less than 20%.

416 **E.** (S&F, ch51)

Fluid resuscitation is the most important intervention for this patient who is severely volume-depleted from GI bleeding. Pharmacotherapy (with octreotide or a PPI) is a less urgent need. Documented red emesis obviates the need to insert a nasogastric tube for diagnostic purposes; if there is repeated vomiting, a nasogastric tube may be passed to decompress the stomach and decrease the risk of aspiration. EGD should be performed as an emergency procedure after fluid volume has been restored.

417 **A.** (S&F, ch49)

Actinomyces israelii is part of the normal oropharyngeal flora. Invasion of the stomach, and more commonly the ileum and colon, can occur as a consequence of trauma, surgery, or neoplasia. Sinus tracts and abscesses can involve the abdominal wall as well. The treatment of choice is a 6- to 12-month course of penicillin or amoxicillin.

418 **D.** (S&F, ch52)

The EUS image shows a T1 lesion (tumor confined to the mucosa measuring less than 2 cm in diameter), and such lesions are amenable to endoscopic mucosal resection (EMR). Subtotal gastrectomy, chemotherapy, and radiation therapy are also therapeutic options. Photodynamic therapy has yet to be adequately studied and no definitive recommendations can be made about this treatment.

419 **D.** (S&F, ch46)

All of the tests can assess gastric emptying but problems in performance or interpretation limit their clinical usefulness.

420 **B.** (S&F, ch49)

Bile reflux gastropathy can occur after gastric surgery, cholecystectomy, sphincteroplasty, or in patients with no history of surgery. Bile reflux can cause gastric atrophy and is thought to increase the risk of gastric intestinal metaplasia, gastric adenocarcinoma, and Barrett's esophagus. Proton pump inhibitors and sucralfate have both been shown to provide symptomatic relief and improve the appearance of the mucosa at endoscopy. Roux-en-Y choledochojejunostomy without gastric resection has also provided improvement but should be used only after medical treatment options have been exhausted.

421 **A.** (S&F, ch45)

The pancreas, transverse colon, diaphragm, spleen, apex of the left kidney, and left adrenal gland are located adjacent and posterior to the stomach.

422 **B.** (S&F, ch52)

Cutaneous complications of PDT include photosensitivity, phototoxicity, and erythema multiforme. Erythema nodosum is found in patients with inflammatory bowel disease; the incidence is higher in those with Crohn's disease than in those with ulcerative colitis.

423 **B.** (S&F, ch51)

False-negative antral biopsies may be seen in patients undergoing antisecretory therapy, notably with PPIs. Proximal migration of the bacteria into the gastric body occurs even after 1 week of treatment; in such cases, both the antrum and corpus should be biopsied. Combination eradication therapy alone can result in healing of the ulcer; additional antisecretory therapy is not definitely needed in uncomplicated cases. Complicated duodenal ulcers caused by *H. pylori* should be treated with antimicrobial therapy and eradication of the pathogens should be confirmed. After successful eradication, acid-lowering therapy can be discontinued.

424 **False.** (S&F, ch50)

Although infection with *H. pylori* or use of NSAIDs is common among patients with PUD, some patients have neither risk factor.

425 **E.** (S&F, ch52)

The endoscopic image shows a submucosal mass with normal overlying mucosa. The endosonographic image reveals that the mucosa and submucosa are intact. The tumor arises from the muscularis propria and is well-circumscribed, characteristics consistent with a gastrointestinal stromal tumor (GIST). Adenocarcinomas of the stomach arise in the mucosa, and lipomas, pancreatic rest, and gastric carcinoids arise in the submucosa.

426 **False.** (S&F, ch48)

The higher prevalence in older persons is a cohort phenomenon, reflecting the age of acquisition. Re-infection is rare among Americans.

427 **A.** (S&F, ch45)

Gastric G cells produce gastrin, which stimulates parietal cells to secrete HCl. The gastric D cells secrete somatostatin, which inhibits gastrin secretion and acid secretion through paracrine and/or endocrine pathways.

428 **B.** (S&F, ch52)

The relative risk of developing gastric cancer in patients with intestinal metaplasia can be as high as 20%. In addition, 42% of patients develop gastric cancer early (within 5 years of follow-up). Gastric ulcers less than 2 cm in diameter, coexisting duodenal ulcers, and a gastric ulcer with endoscopic features of "radiating folds" are less likely to be associated with gastric cancer.

429 **D.** (S&F, ch50)

EGD is more sensitive than UGI, especially for detecting superficial lesions, and in the modern era, a pre-EGD radiograph is not necessary. Brushings and biopsies of an ulcer, when properly obtained, can exclude cancer in 98% to 100% of cases. Once malignancy has been ruled out, a low-risk gastric ulcer need not be re-evaluated solely to confirm healing.

430 **B.** (S&F, ch49)

Both carcinoid and gastric adenocarcinoma have been associated with DCAG.

431 **D.** (S&F, ch52)

Patients found to have cancer cells in lymph nodes after resection of the primary tumor have a 49% risk of local recurrence, 17% risk of peritoneal recurrence, 21% risk of local-regional disease, and 17% risk of hematogenous spread. Combined modality therapy (CMT) with chemotherapy consisting of 5-fluorouracil (5-FU) and leucovorin and radiation therapy had mean survivals of 36 months compared to 27 months for patients treated with surgery alone.

432 **A.** (S&F, ch45)

Gastric atresia presents with gastric outlet obstruction and can eventually progress to dehydration, metabolic acidosis, shock, and gastric perforation. Both Down syndrome and epidermolysis bullosa are associated with gastric atresia. The exact type of lesion (complete segmental defect, segmental defect bridged by fibrous cord, or a membrane) is diagnosed at surgery. Management should include gastric decompression, rehydration, and a surgical procedure such as gastroduodenostomy. Gastrojejunostomy is avoided due to the risk of marginal ulcer.

433 **E.** (S&F, ch51)

Although high-dose PPI infusion may decrease the risk of rebleeding after endoscopic treatment, drug therapy alone is probably insufficient. Injected epinephrine is absorbed from the duodenal submucosa and provides only short-term hemostasis. Argon plasma coagulation lacks the mechanical component of therapy present in the contact-thermal modalities. Multiple trials have shown the highest rates of permanent hemostasis with epinephrine injection followed by application of either heater probe or multipolar electrocautery.

434 **C.** (S&F, ch52)

This endosonographic image shows thickening of the muscularis propria, which would indicate infiltration by a tumor such as a gastric cancer, lymphoma, metastatic melanoma, or breast cancer. EUS imaging in a patient with Ménétrier's disease would show diffuse thickening of the submucosa.

435 **B.** (S&F, ch50)

Patients with suspected perforation should be allowed nothing by mouth. NSAIDs and crack cocaine are associated with perforated ulcers. EGD is contraindicated in patients who may have a perforation. Surgical consultation should be obtained without delay.

436 **C.** (S&F, ch48)

Antral gastritis is associated with duodenal ulcer. The other conditions are related to hypochlorhydria from infection by acid-producing cells in the body and fundus.

437 **C.** (S&F, ch52)

Helicobacter pylori infection has been associated with gastric/duodenal ulcers, MALT lymphomas, and gastric adenocarcinomas. Treatment should lead to improvement of ulcer disease and MALT lymphoma. Gastric adenocarcinoma can potentially be prevented by eradication of *Helicobacter pylori,* but it cannot be treated.

438 **D.** (S&F, ch49)

Mycobacterium tuberculosis can produce ulcerations, masses, and even gastric outlet obstruction. This infection should be suspected with a history of incarceration, alcoholism, and weight loss.

439 **E.** (S&F, ch47)

Thought and taste are more important than sight and smell. All other statements are true.

440 **D.** (S&F, ch50)

Epigastric pain provoked by fasting, reliably relieved by meals, and frequently awakening the patient is classically seen in duodenal ulcer, whereas gastric ulcer pain often worsens postprandially and rarely causes symptoms at night. Gastric cancer and benign PUD may have identical pain patterns. Major complications of peptic ulcer may present without antecedent pain. Reflux disease, especially with erosive disease in the intra-abdominal esophagus, can present with PUD-type pain.

441 **C.** (S&F, ch52)

AGA recommendations for prompt endoscopy include the following: age older than 45 years with new-onset dyspepsia, age under 45 years with alarm symptoms (weight loss, recurrent vomiting, dysphagia, bleeding, anemia), and dyspepsia not responsive to empiric therapy with a proton pump inhibitor. Recommendations for upper endoscopy for an asymptomatic patient with a heme-positive stool sample and normal colonoscopy are less clear.

442 **B.** (S&F, ch48)

The major risk factor is socioeconomic status in childhood. The prevalence among middle- or upper-class children in the United States is 10% to 15%. The higher incidence in adults is a birth-cohort phenomenon. Host genetics play a role, as shown by the results of studies in twins. Human beings are the primary reservoirs.

443 **B.** (S&F, ch45)

Diversion or disruption of pancreatic tissue often results in complications such as pancreatitis and pancreatic fistula. Nasojejunal intubation and pancreaticojejunostomy do not reverse the primary abnormality. Duodenoduodenostomy or duodenojejunostomy are the procedures of choice.

444 **A.** (S&F, ch52)

Malignant transformation of a hyperplastic/fundic gland polyp occurs in less than 1% of cases. Patients with gastric adenomas, FAP syndrome, and polyps with low-grade dysplasia have an approximately 11% risk of developing carcinoma in situ within 4 years.

445 **B.** (S&F, ch50)

Patients with duodenal ulcer are usually *hypersecretor*s of acid. Serum gastrin levels are elevated. Gastric acid emptying into the duodenum is generally accelerated, and bicarbonate production decreased.

446 **D.** (S&F, ch48)

All of the others reduce the accuracy of the breath test. H_2-receptorblockers can be used up to the day before the breath test.

447 **B.** (S&F, ch52)

H. pylori infection, pickled foods, soy sauce, salted fish and meats, cigarette smoking, and preserved foods high in nitrates are clearly associated with an increased risk of developing gastric cancer. Fresh fruits and vegetables contain antioxidants and have been associated with a decreased risk of gastric cancer.

448 **A.** (S&F, ch49)

Emphysematous gastritis, a variant of phlegmonous gastritis, is caused by gas-forming organisms such as *Clostridium welchii*. Treatment of phlegmonous gastritis involves broad-spectrum antibiotics and surgical resection or drainage.

449 **D.** (S&F, ch47)

Cobalamin is released from dietary protein by acid-activated pepsin and most of the cobalamin is bound to R protein. In the upper small bowel, R-cobalamin complexes are cleaved by pancreatic trypsin. The free cobalamin binds to intrinsic factor and is absorbed in the ileum.

450 **D.** (S&F, ch50)

The incidence of PUD in *H. pylori*–infected individuals is less than 20%. *H. pylori* gastritis is eliminated by successful antimicrobial therapy. The patient's serum may continue to test positive for *H. pylori* antibodies for years despite

eradication of the infection. The cagA mutation appears to increase the risk for ulcer.

451 **D.** (S&F, ch52)

Fresh fruits and vegetables are rich in antioxidants and appear to have a chemoprotective effect for gastric cancer. Aspirin inhibits cyclooxygenase and may be able to inhibit cell growth and apoptosis and increase angiogenesis. Green tea, which contains polyphenols, has a variety of antitumor effects, including antioxidant activity, induction of apoptosis, and inhibition of tumor cell proliferation.

452 **B.** (S&F, ch45)

The chief cells secrete pepsinogen I and II, while parietal cells secrete both HCl and intrinsic factor. Enterochromaffin cells contain mostly serotonin and should be differentiated from enterochromaffin-like (ECL) cells, which are the only enteroendocrine cells that contain histamine.

453 **B.** (S&F, ch49)

Refractory or recurrent gastric ulceration in patients with HIV infection with fever, weight loss, and lymphadenopathy is consistent with *Mycobacterium avium* intracellulare complex (MAC).

454 **D.** (S&F, ch52)

Intramucosal tumors less than 2 to 3 cm in diameter are most amenable to endoscopic mucosal resection. The tumors described in answers **A**, **B**, and **C** are deep to the mucosa, larger than 2 to 3 cm, and with synchronous areas of tumor within the stomach.

455 **D.** (S&F, ch51)

The patient has bled again, despite endoscopic and antisecretory therapy. Although the risks of surgery in this case are probably low, repeating the endoscopy would confirm the clinical suspicion and allow retreatment. If surgery is ultimately needed the best option is vessel ligation and postoperative PPI therapy. The more limited operation would avoid the morbidity of vagotomy and gastric resection.

456 **C.** (S&F, ch49)

This patient has demographic characteristics, endoscopic findings, and histology findings consistent with multifocal atrophic gastritis (MAG). Predisposing factors include genetic background (risk is higher among African-

American individuals, Scandinavians, Asians, and Hispanics) and *H. pylori* infection (found in 85% of those with MAG). Inflammation of the antrum and body leads to destruction of epithelial cells and replacement with metaplastic epithelium, predisposing to intestinal-type gastric cancer. Carcinoids and autoimmune diseases such as pernicious anemia and Hashimoto's disease are associated with the separate entity of diffuse corporal atrophic gastritis (DCAG), also called autoimmune gastritis.

457 **D.** (S&F, ch52)

The T stage signifies depth of tumor invasion, N identifies the nodal status, and M indicates the extent of metastasis. The lack of evidence of metastasis on CT leads to designation of this tumor as M0. The tumor extends beyond the serosa of the stomach, so it is stage T3. No evidence of malignancy in perigastric lymph nodes results in a nodal status of N0. Thus, the stage for this tumor is T3N1M0.

458 **False.** (S&F, ch50)

Although the incidence of *H. pylori* infection has been declining for nearly a century, complications of PUD have not decreased in frequency. The popularity of NSAID therapy is the likely cause.

459 **D.** (S&F, ch49)

This patient's history suggests *Helicobacter pylori* infection. Obtaining a biopsy sample from the gastric body can improve diagnostic accuracy in patients who have been treated with proton pump inhibitors.

460 **C.** (S&F, ch50)

Although alcohol can cause clinically insignificant gastric erosions, there is no good pathophysiologic evidence for an association between drinking and PUD. No specific diet has been shown to prevent or treat peptic ulcers. Cigarette smoking increases the risk of PUD, interferes with normal ulcer healing, and increases the relapse rate. Emotional stress may be an associated co-morbidity, but has never been shown to be an independent risk factor.

461 **D.** (S&F, ch52)

Acanthosis nigricans, disseminated intravascular coagulation (DIC), thrombophlebitis, and nephrotic syndrome are all paraneoplastic syndromes that may be associated with gastric cancer. Pyoderma grangrenosum is most commonly associated with inflammatory bowel disease, ulcerative colitis more often than Crohn's disease.

462 **C.** (S&F, ch49)

A history of cervical cancer at an early age suggests infection with human papilloma virus and the possibility that the patient may also be infected with other sexually transmitted diseases. Hematemesis is the most common gastric complaint in patients with secondary or tertiary syphilis involving the stomach. Serpiginous ulcerations with an "hourglass" stomach evident on a barium exam are characteristic of syphilis. Warthin-Starry silver stain and modified Steiner silver impregnation stain will demonstrate numerous spirochetes. Penicillin is effective therapy in such patients. Tuberculosis and lymphoma would be less likely to have caused such extensive gastric disease without significant weight loss.

463 **C.** (S&F, ch46)

Only particles less than 1 mm pass through the pylorus.

464 **C.** (S&F, ch51)

There is a non-bleeding visible vessel in the duodenal ulcer. In most clinical studies, the risk of a rebleed in such cases was more than 40%.

465 **A.** (S&F, ch49)

Lymphocytic gastritis has been associated with celiac disease and *H. pylori* infection. Both a gluten-free diet and *H. pylori* eradication have led to improvement in symptoms of lymphocytic gastritis. Intestinal metaplasia and gastric adenocarcinoma are also more common in patients with lymphocytic colitis. Biopsies of the gastric antrum and/or body reveal infiltration of lymphocytes and plasma cells in the lamina propria.

466 **E.** (S&F, ch47)

Pepsins are active in a pH range of 1.8 to 3.5. They are activated by gastric acid and once this reaction starts, pepsin converts pepsinogens to pepsins. Pepsin preferentially cleaves peptide bonds formed by aromatic amino acids, phenylalanine, and tyrosine.

467 **B.** (S&F, ch52)

The most important prognostic indicator for gastric cancer is the depth of tumor invasion—the T stage. The prognosis is worse in patients younger than age 40, equal among men and women, and worse for high CEA levels, which appear to correlate with unresectability. Early gastric cancer is defined as tumor confined to the mucosa.

468 **True.** (S&F, ch51)

NSAID-associated peptic ulcers can be treated with misoprostol or an H_2-receptor antagonist, but healing rates are higher with PPI therapy. PPIs are clearly superior if NSAID therapy must be continued.

469 **B.** (S&F, ch49)

The differential diagnoses for hypertrophic gastric folds include Ménétrier's disease, hyperplastic/hypersecretory gastropathy, Zollinger-Ellison syndrome, lymphoma, carcinoma, granulomatous gastritides, eosinophilic gastritis, gastric varices, and infectious gastritis (i.e., by cytomegalovirus or *H. pylori*). This patient's findings suggest a variant of Ménétrier's disease, known as hyperplastic/hypersecretory gastropathy. This condition is characterized by increased or normal acid secretion, parietal and chief cell hyperplasia, and normogastrinemia. (Ménétrier's disease, in contrast, is associated with hypochlorhydria). Antisecretory agents are the first-line therapy for hyperplastic/hypersecretory gastropathy. Glucocorticoids, octreotide, and antifibrinolytic agents have been used to treat Ménétrier's disease; partial gastrectomy is reserved for severe complications such as refractory bleeding, obstruction, cancer, or severe hypoproteinemia.

470 **E.** (S&F, ch46)

H. pylori infection does not affect gastric emptying but all of the other conditions can decrease emptying and mimic gastroparesis.

471 **D.** (S&F, ch52)

EUS is the best modality to stage gastric cancer. Imaging can provide one with T (depth of tumor invasion) and N (nodal status) with an accuracy of 80%. Helical CT scan and MRI can provide information regarding distant metastases.

472 **A.** (S&F, ch49)

This immunocompromised patient is at risk for reactivation of prior herpes simplex virus (HSV) or CMV, among other disorders. The cobblestone appearance on endoscopy is compatible with HSV and diagnostic methods should include biopsies and brush cytology to obtain cells from a wider sampling surface area.

473 **E.** (S&F, ch46)

Hypoglycemia enhances gastric contractility. All of the other conditions slow emptying time.

474 **C.** (S&F, ch52)

The highest incidence rates for gastric cancer are in the Far East. Japan ranks first worldwide followed by Korea, South America, Costa Rica, and Equador. The lowest risk areas include North America, Africa, South Africa, and Australia.

475 **A.** (S&F, ch50)

Hydrochloric acid secretion via proton pumps is the sine qua non for all peptic ulcers. The mucous coat and tight junctional complexes are important defense mechanisms. Preserved mucosal blood flow maintains epithelial integrity and facilitates clearance of acid that has diffused through.

476 **C.** (S&F, ch45)

The first portion of the duodenum is bordered by the common bile duct, gastroduodenal artery, and the portal vein posteriorly. The gallbladder is positioned anterior to the duodenal bulb.

477 **True.** (S&F, ch51)

Clinical studies of the effectiveness of parenteral H_2-receptor antagonist therapy in treating bleeding PUD demonstrate a benefit for this therapy in patients with gastric ulcer alone. Tachyphylaxis to the effect of H_2-receptor blockers in other patients may explain the absence of benefit in those with a typically increased acid state of duodenal ulcer disease.

478 **B.** (S&F, ch52)

Early gastric cancer (EGC) is defined as cancer that does not invade beyond the submucosa regardless of lymph node involvement. This can be confirmed by endoscopic ultrasonography (EUS). An EGC less than 2 cm in diameter can best be removed via endoscopic mucosal resection (EMR), sparing the patient a subtotal or total gastrectomy. Candidates for EMR include those with mucosal involvement but without lymph nodes involved, who have a tumor of maximum size less than 2 cm, who have no evidence of multiple gastric cancers, and who have the intestinal type of gastric cancer.

479 **B.** (S&F, ch49)

H. pylori organisms are highlighted in the superficial mucous layer along the surface of the mucosa and in the gastric pits with the following stains: Acridine orange fluorescent stain, Giemsa's stain, Warthin-Starry silver stain, Gram's stain, and immunocytochemical stains.

480 **False.** (S&F, ch46)

In the duodenum, the frequency is 11 to 12 cycles/minute. In the stomach, the frequency is 3/minute and the electrical signals of the stomach do not cross the pylorus.

481 **A.** (S&F, ch50)

The cyclooxygenase isoform found in the stomach is COX-1, and the NSAID effect is systemic. Cyclooxygenase being the rate-limiting enzyme in prostaglandin synthesis, gastric mucosal concentrations of prostaglandin are reduced by COX inhibition. Expression of intercellular adhesion molecules (ICAMs) increases neutrophil adherence in the gastric microcirculation, leading to a decrease in mucosal blood flow.

482 **B.** (S&F, ch49)

Noncaseating granulomas in the gastrointestinal tract are a nonspecific finding. The differential diagnosis can include any of the following: Crohn's disease, sarcoidosis, tuberculosis, xanthogranulomatous gastritis, lymphoma, Whipple's disease, Langerhans cell histiocytosis, and Churg-Strauss syndrome. Therefore, a diagnosis of GI sarcoidosis requires documentation of sarcoidosis at another site (ie, lungs, lymph nodes, skin, or eyes). The stomach is the most common GI site of sarcoidosis involvement.

483 **C.** (S&F, ch51)

Tolerance rapidly develops with IV administration of all H2RAs. Liver disease is not a contraindication to their use, and dose modifications are not needed. H_2-receptor blockers are extremely safe, with side effect profiles similar to those of placebo drugs. Drug-drug interactions, though common, are rarely clinically significant.

484 **A.** (S&F, ch52)

In the United States, the distribution of gastric cancer within the stomach is 39% in the proximal third, 17% in the middle third, 32% in the distal third, and 12% involving the entire stomach.

485 **D.** (S&F, ch49)

This patient's presentation is compatible with gastric Crohn's disease. He is not currently experiencing diarrhea or bleeding, which would suggest colonic involvement. Proton pump inhibitors should be considered first for treatment of gastric Crohn's disease. There is no compelling evidence to support treatment of gastric Crohn's disease with glucocorticoid and/ or immunosuppressant drugs.

486 **C.** (S&F, ch51)

Carcinoid tumor of the stomach, though seen in some animal studies, has never been observed in humans. The clinical effect of PPIs is maximized by administering the drug prior to mealtimes, to coincide with activation of the proton pumps in the immediate postprandial state. Although tolerance does not develop with chronic use, there is a rebound hypersecretion of acid with PPI discontinuation that may last up to 2 months. PPIs are neither hepatotoxic nor nephrotoxic, and no dose adjustment is needed for patients with liver or renal disease.

487 **False.** (S&F, ch50)

With declining rates of peptic ulcer, pyloric channel obstruction is now most often caused by gastric cancer.

488 **C.** (S&F, ch49)

Patients with diffuse corporal atrophic gastritis (DCAG) commonly have antibodies to parietal cells or intrinsic factor, leading to impaired acid production and resultant B_{12} deficiency, classified as pernicious anemia. Type 1 diabetes and other autoimmune disorders have been associated with DCAG.

489 **D.** (S&F, ch52)

Individuals with familial adenomatous polyposis (FAP) syndrome have a 10-fold higher risk of gastric cancer compared to the general population. Patients with hereditary non-polyposis cancer (HNPCC) have an 11% chance of developing gastric cancer. Those with juvenile polyposis syndrome have a 12% to 20% risk of gastric cancer. Patients with a first-degree relative who has gastric cancer have a greater risk of developing gastric cancer, but not a second-degree relative.

490 **A, C,** and **D.** (S&F, ch50)

Despite improvements in general medical treatment and in the care of peptic ulcers specifically, the mortality for bleeding PUD has not decreased much over recent decades, and it remains at 5% to 10%. Endoscopic therapy for bleeding ulcers benefits only those with active bleeding or nonbleeding visible vessels. Brisk UGI bleeding may present without melena or hematemesis, owing to the rapid transit of large volumes of blood. Half of all cases of UGI bleeding may be explained by acid/peptic ulcerations of the stomach and duodenum.

491 **True.** (S&F, ch51)

This patient presented with red hematemesis, which has been identified as an adverse clinical prognostic factor. In addition he has signs of significant hemodynamic compromise, another adverse factor.

492 **E.** (S&F, ch49)

Immunocompromised patients with recent onset of fever, nausea, and abdominal pain should be evaluated to rule-out cytomegalovirus (CMV) infection of the upper digestive tract, among other diagnoses. "Owl-eye" intranuclear inclusions are a hallmark of this infection. Granulomatous diseases (i.e., Crohn's disease, sarcoidosis, and lymphoma), amyloid, pancreatic rest, and Ménétrier's disease are less compatible with this presentation.

493 **C.** (S&F, ch51)

In highly selected patients with small perforations that spontaneously seal, an operation is not always necessary. In the era of potent antisecretory medications, omental patching of the perforated ulcer without vagotomy is acceptable therapy. NSAIDs are probably the most common cause of perforated ulcer in this population. Although the incidence of duodenal ulcer is declining, most perforations are still caused by duodenal ulcer.

494 **False.** (S&F, ch50)

The pathophysiology of gastric ulcers in the prepyloric antrum is similar to that of duodenal ulcers. Patients with these types of ulcers are therefore predominantly acid hypersecretors.

495 **B.** (S&F, ch47)

Gastric HCO_3 secretion declines with age. Most Americans in 9th or 10th decades have fasting gastric pH less than 3.0. Acid decreases with age if there is chronic gastritis present.

496 **A.** (S&F, ch51)

This patient is at high risk because of his age, co-morbid illnesses, and concurrent therapy with aspirin and warfarin. GI bleeding would potentially be fatal, and NSAIDs should be avoided if at all possible. NSAIDs without prophylactic therapy would be risky. A COX-2 inhibitor with aspirin and without an antisecretory agent would be dangerous as well. COX-2 therapy with high-dose PPI is the next best option.

Pancreas

QUESTIONS

497 Fecal elastase may be used to diagnose chronic pancreatitis. Which of the following conditions does *not* result in abnormal levels of fecal elastase?

A. Celiac sprue
B. Crohn's disease
C. Diffuse jejunal diverticulosis
D. Diabetic diarrhea
E. Primary sclerosing cholangitis

498 The most common types of genetically inherited hyperlipidemia associated with the development of pancreatitis in adults are as follows:

A. Types I and III
B. Types II and IV
C. Types I and V
D. Types II and V

499 A 75-year-old woman is admitted to the hospital for management of dehydration. During the last week she has been unable to tolerate any oral nutrition due to recurrent nausea and vomiting. Nausea and occasional vomiting and early satiety had been present for the prior 2 months. She is started on intravenous (IV) fluids and has a nasogastric tube placed with significant relief of her symptoms. During her hospitalization she is found to have a gastric mass that is causing a gastric outlet obstruction and is started on total parenteral nutrition (TPN) for nutritional support. Three days later the patient has an episode of pulseless cardiac electrical activity that results in cardiac arrest. Laboratory analysis of blood samples obtained during resuscitation show the following values:

Sodium (Na): 135 mmol/L
Potassium (K): 2.5 mmol/L
Chloride (Cl): 102 mmol/L
Carbon dioxide (CO_2): 20 mmol/L
Blood urea nitrogen (BUN): 15 mg/dL
Creatinine (Cr): 0.9 mg/dL
Glucose: 124 mg/dL
Calcium (Ca): 8.4 mg/dL
Phosphate: 1.0 mg/dL
Magnesium (Mg): 0.8 mg/dL

What is the most likely cause of this patient's electrolyte abnormalities?

A. Dilutional effect secondary to volume repletion and TPN
B. Gastrointestinal fluid loss via the nasogastric tube
C. Increased renal excretion of electrolytes
D. Intracellular electrolyte shifts
E. Miscalculation of electrolytes that need to be supplied in the TPN feedings

500 An 8-year-old previously healthy Hispanic girl is brought to the emergency department with 1 week of diarrhea and upper respiratory symptoms, for which the pediatrician had prescribed amoxicillin. According to the patient's parents, on the day of presentation the patient had two episodes of bloody diarrhea. The patient reports having severe right upper quadrant and epigastric pain for the past day. The patient has a temperature of 99.7°F, pulse of 113 beats/minute, respiratory rate of 15 breaths/minute, and blood pressure of 82/45 mmHg. On physical exam, she has epigastric tenderness with voluntary guarding. Few bowel sounds are heard. A rectal examination reveals bright red blood per rectum.

Laboratory test results are as follows:
Hemoglobin: 10.2 g/dL
Platelet count: 60,000/mL
Serum creatinine: 3.2 mg/dL
Amylase: 840 IU/L
Lipase: 1200 IU/L
Total bilirubin: 3.9 mg/dL
Indirect bilirubin: 2.5 mg/dL

Prothrombin time (PT), activated partial thromboplastin time (aPTT), D-dimer test results, and fibrinogen level: within normal limits

Examination of a peripheral blood smear shows the presence of schistocytes.

Computed tomography (CT) of the abdomen revealed colonic wall thickening, normal bile ducts, and pancreatic parenchymal edema with stranding.

The most likely cause of the patient's pancreatitis is:

A. Sepsis
B. Acute gallstone pancreatitis
C. Cystic fibrosis
D. *Clostridium difficile* colitis
E. Hemolytic uremic syndrome

501 Which of the following is an accepted definition of severe pancreatitis?

A. Apache II score >5
B. C-reactive protein (CRP) level >100
C. Presence of three or more Ranson's criteria
D. Respiratory rate >30 breaths/minute
E. Hematocrit <50%

502 The congenital anomaly shown on this image obtained during endoscopic retrograde cholangiopancreatography (ERCP) (see figure) is most likely a result of:

A. Failure of fusion of the dorsal and ventral pancreatic ducts
B. Failure of recanalization of the duodenal lumen during the third week of embryonic development
C. Isolated agenesis of the dorsal pancreas
D. Coalescence of pancreatic ductules
E. Right ventral pancreatic bud encircling the duodenum

503 Why are serum trypsinogen levels useful in the diagnosis of chronic pancreatitis (choose the one best answer)?

A. Elevated levels of serum trypsinogen are 90% specific for the diagnosis of chronic pancreatitis.
B. In patients with chronic pancreatitis, serum trypsinogen levels are uniformly abnormal

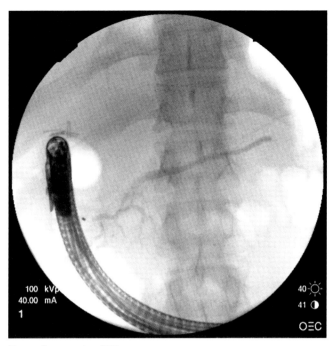

Figure for question **502**

even when the results of pancreatic imaging studies are normal.
C. The serum trypsinogen level is helpful in determining the presence or absence of exocrine pancreatic insufficiency.
D. The serum trypsinogen level is most helpful in determining the etiology of chronic pancreatitis.
E. Serum trypsinogen levels may differentiate chronic pancreatitis from malignant pancreatic duct obstruction.

504 A 42-year-old woman presents to the emergency department with an 8-hour history of severe abdominal pain that is epigastric in origin and radiates to her back. On the basis of laboratory test results and radiologic imaging studies, acute pancreatitis is diagnosed. The patient is ordered nothing by mouth and started on IV fluid therapy and an IV analgesic. Over the next several days the patient's condition worsens. Hypotension develops, requiring frequent boluses of IV fluid, followed by respiratory failure necessitating intubation and ventilator support. A decision is made to start TPN. The patient's height is 168 cm and her weight is 75 kg.

What is this patient's daily energy requirement?

A. 1858 kcal/day
B. 2043.8 kcal/day
C. 2322.5 kcal/day
D. 2787 kcal/day

505 Which of the following tests would be most appropriate for the patient described in question

504 who is on ventilator support and starting TPN (choose the one best answer):

A. Abdominal CT scan
B. ERCP
C. Endoscopic ultrasonography (EUS)
D. Gastric emptying scintigraphy
E. Small-bowel barium radiographic study

506 The total daily volume of pancreatic secretions in a healthy adult is as follows:

A. 0.5 L
B. 1.5 L
C. 2.5 L
D. 3.5 L

507 The most common mechanism of drug-induced pancreatitis is as follows:

A. Accumulation of a toxic metabolite
B. Hypersensitivity reaction
C. Alteration of acinar cell membrane permeability
D. Alterations in trypsin inhibitor
E. Induction of hypertriglyceridemia

508 Which of the following statements *best* describes the epidemiologic relationship between diabetes and chronic pancreatitis?

A. Anatomic abnormalities of the pancreatic duct occur in up to half of all patients with type 1 diabetes.
B. Chronic pancreatitis is more often seen in patients with type 2 diabetes than those requiring insulin.
C. Chronic pancreatitis with endocrine insufficiency accounts for 7% to 10% of all cases of diabetes in the population.
D. Steatorrhea resulting from exocrine pancreatic insufficiency is a common complication of chronic pancreatitis associated with pre-existing diabetes.

509 An 18-year-old African-American man presents to the emergency department with a 5-day history of periumbilical pain, early satiety, persist nausea, and periodic episodes of projectile vomiting of copious amounts of foul-smelling material. CT of the abdomen reveals findings suspicious of an annular pancreas. Definitive management would be as follows:

A. Treat conservatively with a course of antibiotic therapy and intravenous administration of fluids
B. Perform magnetic resonance imaging (MRI) of the abdomen and magnetic resonance cholangiopancreatography (MRCP) to confirm the diagnosis of an annular pancreas
C. Proceed to endoscopic ultrasonography (EUS) to evaluate for pancreatic malignancy mimicking annular pancreas

D. Surgically resect the pancreatic tissue causing duodenal obstruction
E. Perform surgical bypass of the duodenum

510 In contrast to other forms of pancreatic insufficiency, pancreatic dysfunction in patients with cystic fibrosis is characterized by:

A. A significantly higher duodenal pH
B. A significantly lower duodenal pH
C. Lower levels of secretory immunoglobulin A (IgA)
D. Elevated gastric pH
E. Lower gastric pH

511 A 66-year-old patient has been told that she has chronic pancreatitis. The history, physical examination results, and findings on abdominal MRI are nondiagnostic. Which of the following statements is true regarding the rationale for recommending ERCP in this case?

A. Biopsies of the pancreas should be performed to establish the diagnosis.
B. ERCP is superior to other modalities for establishing a diagnosis of chronic pancreatitis.
C. ERCP can differentiate age-related changes from chronic pancreatitis.
D. ERCP is much better than MRCP at determining whether there is dilation of the main pancreatic duct in the head of the pancreas.
E. ERCP allows for endoscopic management of symptoms.

512 A patient undergoes ERCP for suspected choledocholithiasis. A pancreaticogram and cholangiogram are obtained and biliary sphincterotomy is performed. A balloon biliary clearance procedure fails to produce a stone. This patient:

A. Has a 45% risk of developing asymptomatic hyperamylasemia
B. Has a 20% risk of developing procedure-related acute pancreatitis
C. Should be started on gabexate mesylate to reduce the risk of post-ERCP pancreatitis
D. Would have had a reduced risk of pancreatitis if, instead of biliary sphincterotomy, balloon sphincteroplasty had been performed
E. Would have had a reduced risk of pancreatitis if nonionic contrast had been used to obtain the pancreatogram

513 This histologic slide (see figure) shows a section of pancreas obtained at biopsy in a child with chronic pancreatitis of unknown etiology. The most probable cause of this patient's chronic pancreatitis is:

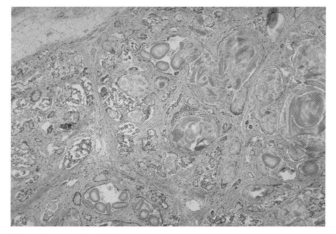

Figure for question **513**

A. Cystic fibrosis
B. Autoimmune fibrosis
C. α1 antitrypsin deficiency
D. Sarcoidosis
E. Adverse reaction to a drug

514 The major mediator of pancreatic hydrogen ion–stimulated bicarbonate and water secretion is

A. Cholecystokinin (CCK)
B. Secretin
C. Acetylcholine
D. Gastrin
E. Vasoactive intestinal polypeptide (VIP)

515 The development of diffuse pancreatic calcifications is *least* likely to occur in a patient with which of the following types of chronic pancreatitis:

A. Alcoholic chronic pancreatitis
B. Early-onset idiopathic chronic pancreatitis
C. Hereditary chronic pancreatitis
D. Late-onset idiopathic chronic pancreatitis
E. Tropical chronic pancreatitis

516 Pancreatic secretory trypsin inhibitor (SPINK1) is a 56–amino acid peptide that specifically inhibits trypsinogen activation by

A. Inhibiting vagal stimulation
B. Decreasing secretion of CCK
C. Physically blocking the active site of trypsinogen
D. Enzymatically cleaving trypsin
E. Stimulating adenosine triphosphatase (ATPase) activity

517 Which of the following tests is *most* sensitive in diagnosing early chronic pancreatitis?

A. Endoscopic retrograde pancreatography (ERP)

B. Endoscopic ultrasonography (EUS)
C. Fecal elastase test
D. Secretin stimulation test
E. Serum trypsinogen test

518 Sudan staining for fecal fat reveals 11 globules of fat per high-power field, indicating steatorrhea (normal is less than 7 globules/high-power field). The physician explains to the patient that steatorrhea is due to fat malabsorption, which in turn is *most* likely to have occurred as a result of:

A. A loss of function of 70% of pancreatic lipase secretion
B. Deactivation of lipase due to inactivation by increased secretion of gastric acid
C. Decrease in gastric lipase production
D. Increased gastric motility due to cytokines released by pancreatic inflammation
E. Precipitation of bile salts in the duodenum

519 An 8-year-old boy develops acute pancreatitis. The *most* likely cause for pancreatitis in this case is as follows:

A. Mutation of the cationic trypsinogen gene (PRSS1)
B. Mutation of the cystic fibrosis transmembrane conductance regulator (CFTR) gene
C. Trauma
D. Mumps
E. Pancreas divisum

520 The *best* therapeutic option for patients with pancreatitis secondary to pancreas divisum is as follows:

A. Endoscopic therapy directed at the minor papilla; this is successful in almost half of individuals
B. Endoscopic therapy to treat exocrine dysfunction; endoscopy is more effective for this goal than in relieving abdominal pain
C. ERCP to determine whether the patient is likely to obtain benefit from an endoscopic therapy
D. Surgical sphincteroplasty; this is associated with a 2-fold higher success rate in relieving symptoms compared to endoscopic therapy

521 A 2-year-old white boy with a new diagnosis of cystic fibrosis is referred to a neurologist for evaluation of increased muscle weakness and difficulty in walking. The neurologic examination reveals hyporeflexia, decreased proprioception, decreased vibratory sense, and distal muscle weakness. These symptoms are due to:

A. Demyelinating disease of the neurons
B. Calcium deficiency
C. Guillain-Barré syndrome

D. Vitamin E deficiency

E. Cerebral microinfarcts

522 A 53-year-old woman who chronically abuses alcohol presents for management of abdominal pain attributed to chronic pancreatitis. MRI/MRCP reveals calcification throughout the pancreas, dilation of the pancreatic duct in the body and tail, and possible stricture in the head of the pancreas. The *best* reason to perform ERCP as the next step in this patient's care is that:

A. She has a 60% likelihood of immediate relief if a stent is able to be placed across a stricture

B. If the patient does respond to therapy, it is likely that relief of pain will last at least 3 years

C. Measurements of pancreatic duct pressure will determine whether to proceed with pancreatic duct therapy

D. Post-ERCP pancreatitis is rare.

523 A 45-year-old obese diabetic man presents to the hospital with crescendo-type midepigastric pain radiating to the back and associated with nausea. He denies alcohol use. On physical exam his heart rate is 110 beats per minute. His vital signs are otherwise within normal ranges. His abdomen is remarkable for mild distention, decreased bowel sounds, and midepigastric tenderness without peritoneal signs. His serum amylase level is 370 U/L (normal is less than 132 U/L) and serum lipase is 2330 U/L (normal is less than 52 U/L). Abdominal ultrasound reveals fatty infiltration of the liver, a normal gallbladder, and a normal biliary tree. This patient's pancreatitis is most likely due to:

A. Trauma

B. Gallstones

C. Hypertriglyceridemia

D. A medication reaction

E. An autoimmune process

524 A 41-year-old man with a history of ulcerative colitis is admitted to the hospital for left upper quadrant pain. Acute pancreatitis is diagnosed, based upon elevated amylase and lipase levels and CT evidence of pancreatic enlargement and peripancreatic fat stranding. The patient states that prior to coming to the hospital he had been feeling well; there had been no flaring of his ulcerative colitis and indeed he had not been taking medications for 2 years. Except for ulcerative colitis he has no past medical history of significance, he denies alcohol use, and he says he takes no medications. There is no family history of pancreatic disease. As part of the differential diagnosis, a diagnosis of autoimmune pancreatitis is considered.

Which of the following statements is true regarding autoimmune pancreatitis?

A. A dense acinar infiltrate of neutrophils is seen in the majority of patients.

B. Autoimmune pancreatitis is more common in women than men.

C. Two thirds of patients have clinical manifestations of autoimmune disease of other organs.

D. Segmental narrowing of the pancreatic duct is a typical feature.

525 A 48-year-old man with a new diagnosis of head and neck cancer is scheduled to undergo chemotherapy and radiation therapy. The decision is made to place a percutaneous endoscopic gastrostomy (PEG) tube prior to his cancer therapy.

Which of the following is the most common complication of PEG tube placement?

A. Buried bumper

B. Colocutaneous fistula

C. Hematoma

D. Peristomal wound infection

E. Peritonitis

526 Which of the following is *most* associated with a poor quality of life in individuals with chronic pancreatitis:

A. Continuing alcohol abuse

B. Diabetes

C. Tobacco use

D. Steatorrhea

527 A patient is admitted to the intensive care unit with severe pancreatitis. A computed tomography scan obtained 72 hours after admission shows marked pancreatic and peripancreatic edema and 30% of the pancreas appears to be necrotic. How should this patient's nutritional needs be addressed?

A. Fluid resuscitation should be started but no nutrition should be provided so early in the patient's course.

B. Total parenteral nutrition without intralipids so as not to stimulate the pancreas should be started.

C. Nasojejunal feedings are preferred for nutrition of patients with severe acute pancreatitis.

D. Administration of pancreatic lipase should be initiated prior to feeding via either the oral or gastric route.

E. Nutrition via any route should be initiated at no more than 250 kcal/day.

528 A 14-year-old Bangladeshi boy with a 3-year history of periumbilical abdominal pain and weight loss appears thin and has erythematous thickening of the mucous membranes of his mouth and of his tongue. He denies fevers, chills, or diarrhea. He is found to have glycosuria and diabetes mellitus is diagnosed. The patient is suspected to be suffering from tropical pancreatitis. Which of the following findings would *most* strongly support this diagnosis?

A. A dietary history of heavy use of Betel nuts
B. Mutation of the gene encoding for cationic trypsinogen (PRSS1)
C. The patient's age
D. A lipase level two times the normal level
E. Cross-sectional images of the pancreas showing intraductal calcifications

529 A 13-year-old white girl presents to the emergency department complaining of a several-hour history of right upper quadrant pain that radiates to the back. Previous hospital records show that she has been admitted three times previously with a diagnosis of "acute pancreatitis." The patient's mother has a history of systemic lupus erythematosus. On physical examination, the girl appears to be in mild distress and has a heart rate of 95 beats/minute, blood pressure of 135/65 mmHg, and temperature of 98.9°F. The patient's amylase level is 456 IU/L (normal 25 to 125 IU/L) and lipase is 340 IU/L (normal 10 to 145 IU/L). Her serum calcium level and the results of a lipid panel are normal. The patient is admitted, started on intravenous hydration, and allowed nothing by mouth. An abdominal ultrasound study performed in the emergency department shows a normal gallbladder and common bile duct with poor visualization of the pancreas. Which of the following tests is most likely to reveal the etiology of this patient's condition?

A. Computed tomography (CT) of the abdomen
B. Endoscopic retrograde cholangiopancreatography (ERCP)
C. Urine drug screen
D. Gene testing for a mutation in the cationic trypsinogen gene (PRSS1)
E. Serum antinuclear antibody (ANA) level testing

530 Of the following statements, which is true regarding the performance of a lateral pancreaticojejunostomy for management of pain in a patient with chronic pancreatitis?

A. It carries a very high rate of surgical morbidity.
B. It is the procedure of choice for those with a normal-caliber pancreatic duct.

C. If relief of pain occurs, relief will probably last longer than if endoscopic therapy had been performed.
D. Surgical alterations will preclude endoscopic biliary access postoperatively.

531 A 38-year-old woman presents to the emergency department with a several-hour history of nausea and severe abdominal pain. The patient describes her pain as unrelenting midepigastric pain that radiates to the back. On examination, the patient is in the fetal position and reluctant to move. She is tachycardic and has a low-grade fever. Orthostatic hypotension is noted. Her amylase level is 1100 U/L and lipase level is 1900 U/L. Which of the following tests is most appropriate to assess the severity of her illness?

A. Abdominal radiography (imaging of the kidneys, ureters, and bladder [KUB])
B. Abdominal ultrasonography (US)
C. Computed tomography (CT)
D. Magnetic resonance imaging (MRI)
E. Endoscopic retrograde cholangiopancreatography (ERCP)

532 Which of the following statements is *most* accurate regarding the epidemiology of chronic pancreatitis?

A. Alcohol abuse accounts for two thirds of cases of chronic pancreatitis.
B. Chronic pancreatitis is seen equally in men and women.
C. The prevalence of alcoholic pancreatitis is 25 per 10,000 population.
D. There is limited geographical variation in the prevalence of chronic pancreatitis.

533 A 20-year-old man with cystic fibrosis has had large-volume, greasy stools for several years and weakness and poor coordination for 3 months. The weakness and poor coordination developed gradually and have worsened over the last 4 weeks. He denies any new medications, change in diet, or recent travel. On physical exam he appears thin but in no acute distress. His height is 5'8" and his weight is 130 pounds. The neurologic exam reveals mild ataxia, decreased vibratory sense, and bilateral hyporeflexia. What is the most likely nutritional deficiency present in this patient?

A. Vitamin A
B. Vitamin C
C. Vitamin D
D. Vitamin E
E. Zinc

534 Which of the following individuals is most likely to experience decreased pain from oral pancreatic enzymes supplementation?

A. A 34-year-old woman with early-onset idiopathic chronic pancreatitis

B. A 55-year-old woman with chronic calcific pancreatitis and pancreatic duct stones

C. A 61-year-old man with pancreatic pseudocyst and steatorrhea

D. A 71-year-old man with pancreatic cancer arising in the setting of chronic calcific pancreatitis

535 A 48-year-old woman with severe chronic renal insufficiency complains to her physician that she has nonspecific abdominal discomfort. Her serum amylase level is 4 times the upper limit of normal and her serum lipase level is twice the upper limit of normal. When interpreting these findings it is important to consider that:

A. Renal insufficiency does not affect the level of serum lipase

B. The amylase creatinine clearance ratio (ACCR) can distinguish elevations of amylase due to renal insufficiency from elevations due to other causes

C. There is no clear relationship between creatinine clearance and serum amylase levels

D. An elevated lipase level is only seen when there is disease of the pancreas

536 Oral administration of pancreatic enzymes has been advocated to manage pain related to chronic pancreatitis. Oral enzyme replacement acts by:

A. Decreasing acinar cell secretion of bicarbonate

B. Decreasing enterohepatic metabolism of substance P

C. Increasing destruction of CCK-releasing peptide

D. Increasing somatostatin production from islet D cells

537 An 18-year-old man who recently emigrated from India visits his physician. He has a history of periumbilical pain since age 6; the pain is intermittent and radiates to the back. The patient has noticed increasing weight loss and diarrhea during the last 5 months. He has no family history of similar complaints. He is noted to be of very lean build and to have gross pallor. Abdominal examination reveals localized rigidity in the epigastrium but no tenderness or distension.

His blood glucose level is 297 mg/dL and his amylase level is 560 IU/L. An x-ray of the abdomen shows a radiopaque shadow in the region of the pancreas and left kidney. On ERCP, a ductal obstruction is found and a subsequent CT scan shows marked dilatation of the pancreatic duct. The mostly likely diagnosis in this case is:

A. Hereditary pancreatitis

B. Tropical pancreatitis

C. Cystic fibrosis

D. Shwachman-Diamond syndrome

E. Gallstone pancreatitis

538 A 48-year-old man with chronic calcific pancreatitis complains of increasing postprandial midepigastric abdominal pain that is no longer relieved by standard doses of acetaminophen. He states that he has not experienced vomiting and his weight is stable. He denies fevers. He has not ingested alcohol for more than a year but he smokes one pack of cigarettes daily. He remains employed as a customer service agent. Which of the following medications would be *most* appropriate to manage this patient's his pain?

A. Amitriptyline

B. Gabapentin

C. Hydromorphone

D. Ketorolac

E. Tramadol

539 A 60-year-old man with mild underlying coronary artery disease is admitted to the hospital with acute pancreatitis. During the first 48 hours he is found to have six Ranson's criteria and Grey Turner's sign. His care in the intensive care unit should include:

A. Gentle fluid resuscitation

B. Swan-Ganz catheter insertion for monitoring intravascular volume without precipitating congestive heart failure

C. Correction of low serum calcium level

D. Broad-spectrum antibiotic therapy

E. Nasogastric suctioning

540 Trypsin:

A. Is an exopeptidase

B. Is produced by the action of trypsin on trypsinogen

C. Converts prolipase to lipase

D. Is produced by the action of enterokinase on trypsinogen

541 A 59-year-old man is admitted to the hospital with acute pancreatitis. One week following admission an abdominal CT demonstrates peripancreatic fat stranding and a 4-cm cyst in the head of the pancreas. He experiences respiratory failure, sepsis, and disseminated intravascular coagulation but after a 2-month stay he is discharged from the hospital. At the office follow-up visit 3 weeks later, he complains of ongoing abdominal pain of moderate severity. A CT scan shows no change in appearance of the

4-cm cyst in the head of the pancreas. The pancreatic duct and bile duct both appear normal. The correct next step is as follows:

A. Endoscopic cystogastrostomy should be performed to alleviate the patient's abdominal pain.
B. ERCP should be performed for further evaluation of the cyst.
C. EUS of the cyst should be performed to exclude malignancy.
D. The pseudocyst should not be treated because cysts of this size are unlikely to cause a complication.

542 A 46-year-old man presents to the emergency department with abdominal pain. He has no history of such episodes. His amylase and lipase levels are mildly elevated (twice the upper limit of normal) and CT reveals pancreatic calcification and dilation of the main pancreatic duct in the body and tail of the gland. When questioned, he admits to smoking a pack of cigarettes daily and drinking two glasses of Scotch on most evenings and up to six or seven on weekend nights.

The *best* information to provide this patient about alcoholic chronic pancreatitis is as follows:

A. Abstinence from alcohol will stop progression of the disease.
B. He is more likely to develop diabetes mellitus than malabsorption and steatorrhea as a complication of this disease.
C. His case is unusual in that the abnormalities identified on CT are more severe than would be expected given that this is his first episode of pain.
D. His tobacco use is unlikely to be contributing to his pancreatitis.
E. One third of heavy alcohol users develop chronic pancreatitis.

543 A 45-year-old man was admitted to the intensive care unit 10 days ago with severe gallstone pancreatitis. He has become tachycardic, there is fresh blood in his nasogastric aspirate, and his hemoglobin has decreased from 13.6 to 8.2 g/dL. Upper endoscopy reveals small esophageal and large gastric varices. In addition to pancreatitis, which of the following conditions is most likely to be present?

A. Chronic viral hepatitis
B. Alcohol abuse
C. Cavernous transformation of the portal vein
D. Splenic vein thrombosis
E. Hemosuccus pancreaticus

544 A 44-year-old man presents to the emergency department with severe midepigastric abdominal pain of 24 hours' duration. He states that one

day before the onset of his symptoms he had attended a party where he had consumed six beers. He states that he drinks three to six beers a few nights per week and has experienced postprandial midepigastric abdominal pain and diarrhea periodically for the past 4 months. On physical examination he has midepigastric tenderness but no other findings. He has elevated serum levels of amylase (1245 U/L; upper limit of normal is 132 U/L) and lipase (863 U/L; upper limit of normal is 52 U/L) and is admitted to the hospital. A Sudan stain of his stool reveals 3+ fecal fat.

MRI with MRCP is performed and shows evidence of acute peripancreatic inflammation as well as pancreas divisum with a normal-caliber pancreatic duct.

In explaining to the patient the significance of this finding, the *best* statement is as follows:

A. An ERCP with minor duct papillotomy should be performed to help improve the acute symptoms of pain.
B. An ERCP with minor duct stent placement should be performed to help improve the acute symptoms of pain.
C. Pancreas divisum is a sequela of chronic pancreatitis.
D. Pancreas divisum is unlikely to be a cause of his chronic pancreatitis.

545 The sequence of events that is postulated to lead to acute pancreatitis in most cases is as follows:

A. Acinar cell injury, expression of endothelial adhesion molecules, release of proinflammatory cytokines, release of anti-inflammatory cytokines, activation of hepatic Kupffer cells
B. Acinar cell injury, release of inflammatory mediators into the systemic circulation, translocation of bacteria into systemic circulation, systemic inflammatory response syndrome
C. Bile reflux into pancreatic duct, duct cell injury, increase in intraductal secretion of calcium and protein, increased vascular permeability, release of tumor necrosis factor
D. Increased acinar cell glutathione, acinar cell injury, release of anti-inflammatory mediators, recruitment and activation of macrophages, release of reactive oxygen metabolites

546 A 62-year-old woman with a 25-year history of type 1 diabetes mellitus visits the emergency department because of frequent nausea and vomiting for 3 months. She is admitted for intravenous hydration and evaluation of her problem. Diabetic gastroparesis is diagnosed, but all accepted medical treatments are unsuccessful in maintaining adequate nutritional intake. The decision is made to place a feeding tube and begin enteral feedings. Enteral feeding is expected to last for more than 6 months.

Which enteral feeding modality would be most appropriate in this patient?

A. Direct percutaneous jejunostomy (DPJ)
B. Nasogastric tube (NGT)
C. Nasojejunal tube (NJT)
D. Percutaneous endoscopic gastrojejunostomy (PEG/J)
E. Percutaneous endoscopic gastrostomy (PEG)

547 Idiopathic pancreatitis can be classified as "early-onset idiopathic pancreatitis" or "late-onset idiopathic pancreatitis." The two types of idiopathic pancreatitis are primarily differentiated by the patient's age at onset of the disease; however, they are also distinct in other ways. The statement that *best* describes the differences between early- and late-onset idiopathic pancreatitis is as follows:

A. Abdominal pain is common in early-onset idiopathic pancreatitis whereas pancreatic exocrine insufficiency is common in late-onset idiopathic pancreatitis.
B. Early-onset idiopathic pancreatitis has a female predominance whereas late-onset idiopathic pancreatitis has an even gender distribution.
C. Patients with early-onset idiopathic pancreatitis are less likely to have abnormalities in genes associated with pancreatitis than those with late-onset idiopathic pancreatitis.
D. Structural alterations to the pancreas are more readily identifiable in patients with early-onset idiopathic pancreatitis compared to those with late-onset idiopathic pancreatitis.

548 The estimated cumulative lifetime risk for patients with hereditary pancreatitis to develop pancreatic cancer is:

A. 5%
B. 10%
C. 20%
D. 40%
E. 60%

549 Which of the following is the *best* statement of how to perform a standard pancreatic hormone stimulation test?

A. A catheter is placed in the pancreatic duct to collect secretions.
B. Following cholecystokinin stimulation, pancreatic bicarbonate is measured.
C. Pancreatic secretions are collected over 2 hours.
D. Serum lipase is measured simultaneously with pancreatic secretions.

550 A 62-year-old man with a known history of dyslipidemia presents to the emergency department with acute pancreatitis. He has fever, tachypnea, diffuse abdominal tenderness, and oliguria. His white blood cell (WBC) count is 22,000/mL, glucose is 260 mg/dL, lactate dehydrogenase is 500 U/L, and PaO_2 is 82 mmHg. CT shows evidence of pancreatic necrosis and diffuse bilateral pulmonary infiltrates consistent with acute respiratory distress syndrome (ARDS). Which of the following is a likely contributor to this patient's respiratory decompensation?

A. Surfactant degradation by phospholipase A2
B. Infectious pneumonia
C. Elastase release from the injured pancreas
D. Increased intravascular fluid volume

551 A 40-year-old man suffers acute gallstone pancreatitis and is hospitalized for 1 week. Three weeks after discharge, CT shows a 9- × 12-cm pseudocyst adjacent to the stomach. The patient is tired but otherwise feels well. He is eating a low-fat diet without nausea or vomiting. His WBC count and levels of total bilirubin, aspartate aminotransferase (AST), alanine aminotransferase (ALT), amylase, and lipase are normal. His alkaline phosphatase level is minimally elevated. What is the recommended management in such a case?

A. Follow up clinically and radiographically only.
B. Perform endoscopic cystogastrostomy.
C. Wait 2 weeks to allow for formation of an adequate cyst wall and then proceed with surgical cystogastrostomy.
D. Perform percutaneous drainage during an interventional radiology procedure.
E. Administer octreotide (Sandostatin LAR) to decrease pancreatic secretions and promote resolution of pancreatitis.

552 Which one of the following tests is *most* likely to alter the plan for treating the patient described in question 522?

A. DEXA scan
B. Fecal elastase test
C. Fecal chymotrypsin test
D. Serum prealbumin concentration measurement
E. Serum vitamin B_{12} concentration measurement

553 In the diagnosis of acute pancreatitis, serum amylase:

A. Rises within 2 hours after the onset of symptoms
B. Has a half-life of 20 hours
C. Is primarily excreted by the kidneys

D. Remains elevated for approximately 7 to 10 days

E. May be normal in patients with severe pancreatitis

554 Which of the following is true regarding the histologic changes seen in chronic pancreatitis?

A. Intestinal metaplasia of ductal epithelium occurs late in the disease.

B. Islets of Langerhans are affected in the late stages of the disease.

C. Lobular neutrophilic infiltrate is a hallmark of chronic pancreatitis.

D. Transient fibrosis of the main pancreatic duct is common.

E. Histology readily identifies the cause of chronic pancreatitis.

555 The most common cause of hereditary pancreatitis is a mutation in the cationic trypsinogen gene (PRSS1). PRSS1 mutation causes pancreatitis by:

A. Altering the regulatory domains in trypsinogen controlled by calcium

B. Cleaving trypsinogen activation peptide (TAP)

C. Promoting cAMP activation of protein kinase A (PKA)

D. Stimulating the Golgi apparatus to produce excessive trypsinogen

556 The *most* significant limitation to establishing a screening diagnostic test for chronic pancreatitis is:

A. Diurnal variation in pancreatic secretions

B. Lack of a gold standard test

C. Lack of availability of effective pancreatic stimulant medications

D. Numerous causes of chronic pancreatitis

E. Variability in the clinical manifestations of disease

557 A 36-year-old man with a known history of Crohn's disease presents for evaluation of fatigue, decreased exercise tolerance, and dyspnea on exertion. He has predominantly distal ileal disease that required surgical resection 2 years earlier. His disease has been relatively quiescent since his surgery, and his recent treatment consists of mesalamine. CT and an upper gastrointestinal series with small-bowel follow through confirm the presence of disease in the terminal ileum. He denies any bright red blood per rectum, melena, or change in bowel habits. He appears comfortable, his temperature is 98.7°F, heart rate is 102 beats/minute, and blood pressure is 118/72 mmHg. A stool sample obtained by rectal examination is heme negative. His hemoglobin level is 9.2 g/dL.

Which of the following deficiencies is the most likely cause of this patient's anemia?

A. Vitamin B_{12} deficiency

B. Folic acid deficiency

C. Iron deficiency

D. Zinc deficiency

558 On admission, the patient described in question 531 had a WBC count of 22,000/mL, hemoglobin of 15.0 g/dL, total bilirubin of 3.2 mg/dL, alkaline phosphatase of 375 IU/L, AST of 130 IU/L, ALT of 170 IU/L, and PO_2 of 85 mmHg. In this patient, which of the following laboratory test results is most indicative of severe disease?

A. Alkaline phosphatase level

B. Amylase level

C. AST level

D. WBC count

E. Bilirubin level

559 The *primary* goal of endoscopic therapy for symptoms of chronic pancreatitis is to:

A. Alleviate pressure exerted by an inflamed duodenal papilla

B. Decrease pancreatic duct pressure

C. Decrease pancreatic secretion

D. Directly stimulate insulin release

E. Prevent episodes of pancreatic sepsis

560 A 46-year-old man seeks emergency care for a 12-hour history of severe midepigastric pain that radiates to the back and is associated with fever, nausea, vomiting, and light-headedness. He has a history of chronic low back pain for which he takes nonsteroidal antiinflammatory drugs (NSAIDs). His wife relates that he works as a mechanic and has one or two drinks on the weekends. He appears acutely ill, has orthostatic hypotension, decreased bowel sounds, and diffuse abdominal tenderness. Laboratory tests show leukocytosis, elevation of serum amylase, and mild elevations of liver enzymes. CT of the abdomen shows cholelithiasis and evidence of acute edematous pancreatitis. Which of the following is the most likely cause of this patient's signs and symptoms?

A. Alcohol abuse

B. Gallstones

C. Helminthic infection

D. Adverse effects of NSAID use

E. Pancreas divisum

561 A 45-year-old Asian woman is referred to a gastroenterologist for an upper endoscopy for surveillance of Barrett's esophagus. The patient has a 12-year history of heartburn that is well controlled with proton-pump inhibitors. She has no abnormalities on physical examination. On upper endoscopy an irregular, yellow mucosal nodule is seen in the duodenum. The nodule is biopsied; the pathologist reports it to be ectopic pancreatic tissue. The most appropriate next step in this patient's care is:

A. Endoscopic ultrasonography (EUS)
B. Surveillance esophagogastroduodenoscopy (EGD) in one year
C. CT of the abdomen
D. No further evaluation
E. Colonoscopy

562 The *main* limitation of EUS in diagnosing chronic pancreatitis is:

A. Difficulty in accurate identification of the pancreatic duct
B. Difficulty in imaging pancreatic calcifications
C. Inability to obtain tissue for histologic review
D. Lack of uniform diagnostic criteria to establish a diagnosis

563 The initial pathophysiologic event in acute pancreatitis is:

A. Intra-acinar cell conversion of trypsinogen to trypsin
B. Release of phospholipase A_2
C. Increased capillary permeability
D. Fat necrosis
E. Decrease in cell membrane protein GP2

564 The main mediator of meal-stimulated enzyme secretion from the pancreas is:

A. Secretin
B. VIP
C. Glucagon
D. CCK
E. Acetylcholine

565 Which of the following statements is correct with regard to the natural history of acute pancreatitis?

A. Forty percent of patients have "mild" pancreatitis.
B. Overall mortality may be as high as 25%.
C. Twenty percent of patients have "severe" pancreatitis.
D. Most patients suffering acute pancreatitis have persistent morphologic and functional changes after recovery.

566 CT of the abdomen of a 63-year-old woman shows pancreatic calcification and a dilated pancreatic duct but no hepatobiliary abnormality. The patient has a 25-year history of consuming four glasses of vodka daily. She does not complain of abdominal pain at present but

has had intermittent bouts in the past for which she has not sought medical care. She states that she has four bulky bowel movements daily. She has lost 5 pounds in the past 3 months, but otherwise feels well. The results of a complete blood count (CBC) and levels of electrolytes, bilirubin, ALT, AST, and lipase are normal.

Steatorrhea is suspected, based on findings of pancreatic exocrine dysfunction. Which of the following statements is most accurate in planning a 72-hour stool collection to evaluate for this condition?

A. A high-fat diet is required for at least 3 days prior to a 72-hour collection.
B. Mixing of the stool every 2 hours is required to prevent bacterial metabolism.
C. The most sensitive test is a 72-hour stool collection while the patient is on a diet that includes 50 g of fat per day.
D. The presence of an elevated fecal fat level determined by 72-hour collection is diagnostic for chronic pancreatitis.

567 After 6 months of pancreatic enzyme supplementation, the patient described in the previous question complains of urinary frequency. Urinalysis reveals glycosuria and multiple random fasting blood samples show elevated glucose levels. You correctly advise this patient that:

A. Diabetes due to chronic pancreatitis is difficult to manage because damaged islet cells are not producing insulin or somatostatin.
B. Diabetes occurs in patients with chronic pancreatitis when there are virtually no beta islet cells remaining.
C. Diabetes is uncommon in chronic pancreatitis; this patient's situation is unusual.
D. She should manage her diabetes similar to diabetics from other causes in order to prevent end-organ damage.

568 *SPINK1:*

A. Protects pancreatic acinar cells by inhibiting prematurely activated trypsin
B. Regulates bicarbonate conductance
C. Causes trypsin to be resistant to lysis by intracellular trypsin inhibitor
D. Increases concentrations of trypsinogen activation peptide

569 A 34-year-old white woman presents to her primary care doctor with complaints of a 4-month history of abdominal pain and episodes of vomiting. She is otherwise healthy. The results of routine laboratory tests, including measurements of amylase, lipase, and CA 19–9 levels, are normal. CT of the abdomen shows a 2-cm cyst in the pancreatic head. On the primary physician's recommendations, the patient is sent for an EUS, which shows a 2-cm smooth-walled anechoic cystic lesion in the pancreatic head without any debris, septations, or papillary projections. The pancreatic duct was seen to be dilated upstream from the cyst. What is the recommended next step for this patient?

A. Repeat EUS in 6 months.
B. Perform surgical resection of the cyst.
C. Perform CT-guided fine-needle aspiration of the cyst.
D. Test for a mutation in the cationic trypsinogen gene (PRSS1) to evaluate for congenital pancreatitis as a cause of the patient's cyst.
E. Perform MRI/MRCP to evaluate for pancreatic cyst.

570 A 31-year-old woman presents with a 4-hour history of severe abdominal pain. She is in acute distress, her blood pressure is 70/40 mmHg, and her heart rate is 130 beats per minute. Her abdomen is diffusely tender with no peritoneal signs and her stool tests negative for occult blood. Laboratory evaluation reveals a hematocrit of 20%, a serum amylase value twice the upper limit of normal, normal liver enzyme levels, and normal serum lipase level. The most likely diagnosis is:

A. Acute pancreatitis
B. Mesenteric ischemia
C. Perforated peptic ulcer
D. Ruptured ectopic pregnancy

571 A 12-year-old white boy with a previous history of cystic fibrosis confirmed by genetic testing and sweat chloride testing is brought to his pediatrician with a 2-month history of weight loss; foul-smelling, bulky bowel movements; and slow growth. Pancreatic insufficiency is diagnosed on the basis of clinical findings and the patient is prescribed an uncoated formulation of pancreatic lipase at a dose of 4000 units with each meal. Two weeks later, the patient's symptoms are essentially unchanged. The next best step would be:

A. Increase the dose to 8000 units of lipase with each meal
B. Add a proton pump inhibitor
C. Stop the pancreatic enzyme supplement and start metronidazole, 250 mg orally three times daily
D. Obtain a CT scan of the pancreas

572 Death in patients with severe pancreatitis:

A. Most often occurs in the first 24 hours
B. Is most often associated with hemorrhagic pancreatitis

C. Is frequently associated with infection
D. Is not influenced by patient age

573 A 41-year-old male with a history of ulcerative colitis is admitted to the hospital with abdominal pain and elevated pancreatic enzymes. After 6 days of bowel rest he has no improvement in symptoms and his pancreatic enzymes remain elevated. MRCP reveals pancreatic duct narrowing at the genu without an associated mass. A course of glucocorticoid therapy is being considered to confirm the suspicion of autoimmune pancreatitis. Which of the following statements is true regarding autoimmune pancreatitis?

A. An elevated serum IgG4 level is pathognomonic of autoimmune pancreatitis.
B. Autoimmune pancreatitis may progress to complete pancreatic failure over 2 to 3 months if left untreated.
C. In cases of autoimmune pancreatitis, clinical improvement in symptoms would be expected after 5 to 7 days of glucocorticoid therapy.
D. Glucocorticoid therapy is contraindicated in cases of autoimmune pancreatitis because it will induce severe hyperglycemia.

574 Which of the following is *most* accurate regarding the use of transabdominal ultrasound for establishing the diagnosis of chronic pancreatitis?

A. Advanced age results in changes of the pancreas that may confound the diagnosis.
B. The sensitivity of this test is approximately 30%.
C. Sound waves emitted by the probe may disrupt pancreatic duct stones, predisposing to acute pancreatitis.
D. Strictures of the pancreatic duct can be readily identified.

575 A 60-year-old woman is taken to the hospital following an automobile accident in which she suffered blunt trauma to the mid-abdomen when she was thrown against the steering wheel because she was not wearing a seatbelt. The most accurate test to diagnose pancreatic injury with pancreatic duct disruption is:

A. Endoscopic retrograde cholangiopancreatography
B. Elevated serum amylase level
C. Seeing fluid in the anterior pararenal space on CT scan
D. MRI with MRCP
E. The response to octreotide infusion

576 Which behavioral modification is most likely to benefit a patient with chronic pancreatitis?

A. Increasing daily activity level
B. Following a low-fat diet
C. Resuming alcohol use
D. Smoking cessation

577 Which of the following is most important in the treatment of malabsorptive steatorrhea?

A. Administration of at least 30,000 IU (90,000 USP) of lipase with each meal
B. Concomitant acid suppression with enzyme replacement
C. Consumption of a no-fat diet
D. Eating five small meals daily
E. Monitoring for fat-soluble vitamin deficiency

578 A 72-year-old white woman has been referred for evaluation of acute recurrent pancreatitis. She had been admitted to a district hospital through the emergency department four times in the previous 2 years for episodes of epigastric pain associated with nausea, vomiting, and markedly elevated serum lipase levels. In every episode, her transaminase levels had been elevated without an elevation of the alkaline phosphatase. At this evaluation, an abdominal sonogram shows dilation of the common bile duct and diffuse swelling of the pancreas but no stones in the gallbladder. On ERCP an anomalous pancreatobiliary ductal union is seen in association with diffuse dilation of the common bile duct and a diverticulum in the proximal (upstream) common bile duct. This patient is at increased risk for:

A. Sclerosing cholangitis
B. Colon cancer
C. Cholangiocarcinoma
D. Colon polyposis syndrome
E. Pancreatic neuroendocrine tumor

579 A patient with abdominal pain and elevation of the amylase and lipase levels undergoes an ERCP. On ERCP the patient is seen to have ectasia of the secondary radicals of the pancreatic duct without duct dilation or stricture. A pancreatic sphincterotomy is performed and the patient is prescribed narcotics and enzyme replacement therapy. Two months after ERCP she continues to have intolerable pain. The *most* appropriate intervention for this patient at this time is:

A. EUS-guided celiac axis ablation
B. Modified Puestow procedure
C. Repeat ERCP with planned stent placement
D. Subtotal pancreatectomy
E. Whipple procedure

580 An ERCP is performed and a stent is placed traversing a stricture of the pancreatic head in a woman with pancreatitis due to alcohol abuse. Her symptoms do not improve and the stent is removed. She returns to the office 2 weeks later complaining of new abdominal pain and dark urine and she appears jaundiced. Laboratory studies reveal a total bilirubin of 9.0 mg/dL with a direct fraction of 5.5 mg/dL. What would be the *most* appropriate next step?

A. Abdominal CT
B. Liver biopsy
C. Pancreaticobiliary EUS
D. Repeat ERCP
E. Measurement of serum haptoglobin level

581 Which of the following has been implicated in the pathophysiology of pain resulting from chronic pancreatitis?

A. Damage to the perineural sheaths of intrapancreatic neurons
B. Reduced pancreatic duct pressure in side branches of the main duct
C. Elevated pH in the pancreatic parenchyma in patients with chronic pancreatitis
D. Increased blood flow to regions of pancreatic inflammation
E. Stranding of the peripancreatic adipose tissues

582 Acinar cell protective mechanisms include all of the following *except:*

A. Presence of *SPINK1*
B. Sequestration of pancreatic enzymes within separate intracellular compartments
C. Presence of nonspecific anti proteases
D. High intracellular calcium concentration

583 A 52-year-old man with a history of alcohol abuse presents for evaluation of diarrhea that has lasted 4 weeks. In addition, he describes significant hair loss and impaired taste. On physical examination, a superficial scaling eruption is noted in the groin and around the mouth. What is the likely nutrient deficiency?

A. Vitamin A
B. Vitamin B_{12}
C. Vitamin C
D. Magnesium
E. Zinc

584 Which of the following statements is correct regarding diabetes mellitus due to pancreatic endocrine dysfunction?

A. Aggressive glucose control is advocated to prevent ketoacidosis.
B. Endocrine insufficiency uniformly precedes exocrine dysfunction.
C. Insulin requirements are higher than in type I diabetes.
D. Endocrine insufficiency is an independent predictor of mortality.

585 By definition an episode of pancreatitis is considered chronic pancreatitis if:

A. It is a recurrent episode
B. It occurs in conjunction with alcohol use
C. There are radiographic findings of ductal irregularity and parenchymal fibrosis
D. It is associated with steatorrhea
E. A pseudocyst is present

586 A 42-year-old man visits his primary care physician for a routine physical examination. He has no specific complaints and no specific medical history except for mild hypertension. He is 68 inches (173 cm) tall and weighs 220 pounds (100 kg).

What is this patient's body mass index (BMI) and weight classification?

A. 33.3/overweight
B. 33.3/obese
C. 33.3/super obese
D. 57.8/obese
E. 57.8/super obese

ANSWERS

497 **E.** (S&F, ch57)

Fecal elastase levels are low in patients with chronic pancreatitis. Other causes of abnormally low levels include malabsorptive conditions of the small intestine (Crohn's disease, celiac sprue) and those causing a dilute fecal stream (diabetic diarrhea). Primary sclerosing cholangitis will not alter fecal elastase levels. Jejunal diverticulosis results in overgrowth of bacteria in the small bowel, which may result in malabsorption.

498 **C.** (S&F, ch56)

Types I and V are the types of inherited hyperlipidemia most commonly associated with development of pancreatitis in adults. Type II hyperlipidemia is also associated with pancreatitis but to a lesser extent.

499 **D.** (S&F, ch58)

Refeeding syndrome is a common metabolic consequence of parenteral nutrition (PN). This syndrome results from sudden provision of a large number of calories, especially carbohydrates, to a malnourished patient. Upon PN infusion, the metabolism of these patients rapidly becomes anabolic. As a result, insulin production is increased, pushing potassium, phosphorus, and magnesium into intracellular compartments and thereby lowering the serum levels of these substances. Management of refeeding syndrome focuses on the close monitoring of electrolytes and adequate repletion as needed.

500 **E.** (S&F, ch53–55)

Of the systemic diseases listed, hemolytic uremic syndrome (HUS) is the most common cause of acute pancreatitis. Acute hemorrhagic colitis, which was first recognized in two separate outbreaks in Michigan and Oregon in 1982, has been associated mainly with a specific serotype of *E. coli*, O157:H7. This organism is estimated to be responsible for 0.6% to 2.4% of all cases of diarrhea and 15% to 36% of cases of hemorrhagic colitis in Canada, the United Kingdom, and the United States. The spectrum of disease associated with *E. coli* O157:H7 includes bloody diarrhea, which is seen in as many as 95% of patients, nonbloody diarrhea, hemolytic-uremic syndrome, acute renal insufficiency, and thrombotic thrombocytopenic purpura.

501 **C.** (S&F, ch56)

It is important to distinguish mild from acute pancreatitis, because severe pancreatitis is associated with high disease-related mortality. Several physiologic parameters and scoring systems have been developed to define severe pancreatitis. These include the presence of three or more Ranson's criteria, an APACHE II score of more than 8, a CRP level of more than 200 mg/dL, and hematocrit of more than 50%. Tachypnea is a physiologic consequence of severe pancreatitis, but alone it is insufficient for diagnosis.

502 **A.** (S&F, ch53–55)

Pancreas divisum occurs in approximately 7% of patients undergoing ERCP for diagnosis of nonpancreatic diseases. It occurs when the embryologic dorsal and ventral pancreases fail to fuse. Whether pancreas divisum is related to pancreatitis or abdominal pain is controversial. Pancreatitis in people with divisum develops in adulthood, not in childhood. On ERCP in a patient with pancreatic divisum, injection of contrast following cannulation of the ampulla of Vater will reveal a small pancreatic duct of Wirsung draining the pancreatic head, and cannulation of the minor ampulla will show filling of a separate, larger duct of Santorini draining the entire pancreatic body and tail.

503 **C.** (S&F, ch57)

The serum trypsinogen level is highly specific for chronic pancreatitis in late-stage disease when morphologic changes can be seen on imaging studies. In late-stage disease, abnormally low values of trypsinogen will be found. When pancreatic imaging is normal, as in early chronic pancreatitis, the serum trypsinogen level is often normal. The trypsinogen level may be falsely elevated when the pancreatic duct is obstructed, as in the case of cancer. The serum trypsinogen level is abnormal in patients with pancreatic steatorrhea, but the level will be normal when steatorrhea is due to other causes.

504 **D.** (S&F, ch58)

Energy requirements can be calculated using mathematical equations. Many different methods of estimating energy needs have been used over the years, including estimations based on body surface area, body weight, body height, and the age of the patient. The equations most commonly used for calculating energy need are the Harris-Benedict equations. The equations are as follows:

Men: Energy need (in kilocalories/24 hours)
$= 66 + (13.7 \times W) + (5 \times L) - (6.8 \times A)$

Women: Energy need (in kilocalories/24 hours)
$= 655 + (9.6 \times W) + (1.7 \times L) - (4.7 \times A)$

where W = weight in kilograms (kg), A = age in years, and L = height in centimeters (cm)

The energy need calculated using one of these equations is often supplemented by a "stress factor": The stress factors are 10% for mild disease, 25% for moderate disease, and 50% for severe disease.

As an example, the baseline caloric need of the patient in the question is 1858 kilocalories (kcal)/day, calculated using the Harris-Benedict equation for a man. Given the severity of the patient's condition, a stress factor of 0.5 (50%) should be used. Multiplying the baseline energy need by 0.5 and adding the result (929 kcal/day) to the baseline gives a total energy need for this patient of 2787 kcal/day.

505 **A.** (S&F, ch57)

A change in a patient's symptoms should prompt an evaluation for complications of chronic pancreatitis such as pseudocyst or obstruction of the pancreatic duct or bile duct. An abdominal

CT would identify these complications. Patients with a dilated pancreatic duct may benefit from endoscopic or surgical therapies. ERCP and EUS require sedation, which carries risks. Gastric emptying scintigraphy and small bowel x-ray would not be appropriate first-line examinations for evaluation of causes of pain.

506 **C.** (S&F, ch53–55)

507 **B.** (S&F, ch56)

The most common mechanism for drug-induced pancreatitis is a hypersensitivity reaction. Examples of drugs that act by this mechanism include 6 mercaptopurine, aminosalicylates, and metronidazole. Accumulation of a toxic metabolite and induction of hypertriglyceridemia are less common mechanisms for drug-induced pancreatitis. Alteration of acinar cell membrane permeability and alteration in trypsin inhibitor are not mechanisms of drug-induced pancreatitis.

508 **A.** (S&F, ch57)

Pancreatic endocrine dysfunction due to chronic pancreatitis may cause diabetes mellitus, however this mechanism accounts for only 1% of cases of diabetes. When chronic pancreatitis develops in a person with pre-existing diabetes, it is more likely to develop in patients with type 1 diabetes than in those not requiring insulin. Abnormalities of the pancreatic parenchyma and/or ducts may be seen in as many as 50% of diabetics, and the results of pancreatic function tests will be abnormal in a similar proportion of diabetic individuals. Pancreatic exocrine failure is rare in patients with diabetes.

509 **E.** (S&F, ch53–55)

Annular pancreas is a band of pancreatic tissue encircling the second part of the duodenum and is of ventral pancreas origin. Annular pancreas has a bimodal presentation, with peaks in neonates and in adults in the fourth and fifth decades. This entity is a common cause of duodenal obstruction in infants; in these cases, obstruction is usually due to growth of pancreatic tissue into the wall of the duodenum. In adults annular pancreas may present as duodenal stenosis, peptic ulceration, chronic pancreatitis, or as an incidental finding. The most common symptom in adults is upper abdominal pain. Biliary obstruction is a rare complication. Because pancreatic tissue often extends into the duodenal wall and because the annular tissue may contain a large pancreatic duct, symptomatic cases are best treated by surgical bypass rather than by surgical resection.

510 **B.** (S&F, ch53–55)

In contrast with other forms of pancreatic insufficiency, that due to cystic fibrosis is characterized by greater impairment of bicarbonate secretion within the duodenum and biliary tree. Lower levels of duodenal bicarbonate result in a more acidic duodenum (i.e., lower duodenal pH).

511 **E.** (S&F, ch57)

ERCP is considered the gold standard test for the diagnosis of chronic pancreatitis. Direct imaging of the pancreatic duct allows ready identification of dilation, stricture, and pseudocyst. MRI with MRCP is an excellent test for evaluation of the main pancreatic duct; however, the secondary branches are less easy to identify on MRI. Transpapillary biopsies are not routinely advocated to establish a diagnosis of chronic pancreatitis. ERCP cannot reliably determine if changes of the duct are due to aging or are a sequela of pancreatic inflammation.

512 **A.** (S&F, ch56)

There is no difference in the incidence of post-ERCP pancreatitis after studies performed with ionic contrast agents and those performed with nonionic contrast agents. Balloon sphincteroplasty poses a greater risk of post-ERCP pancreatitis than sphincterotomy. Randomized controlled trials show no difference in the incidence of post-ERCP pancreatitis in patients receiving gabexate versus patients not receiving gabexate. This patient has a 5% to 7% risk of developing post-ERCP pancreatitis and a 35% to 70% risk of developing asymptomatic hyperamylasemia.

513 **A.** (S&F, ch53–55)

Pancreatic abnormalities are present in approximately 85% to 90% of patients with cystic fibrosis. In the mild cases, there may be only accumulations of mucus in the small ducts, causing dilation of the exocrine glands. In advanced cases, usually seen in older children or adolescents, the ducts are totally plugged, as demonstrated in this slide, causing atrophy of the exocrine glands and progressive fibrosis.

514 **B.** (S&F, ch57)

The major mediator of hydrogen ion–stimulated bicarbonate and water secretion is secretin. The quantity of secretin released as well as the volume of pancreatic secretion is dependent on the load of titratable acid delivered to the duodenum. Secretin-induced bicarbonate secretion is augmented by CCK when both agents are infused to reproduce concentrations observed during a meal. CCK alone causes no bicarbonate secetion. The bicarbonate response to secretin is also dependent on cholinergic input because atropine partially inhibits the response stimulated by exogenous secretin. Thus, the complete meal-stimulated response results from a combination of mediators. The mediators of the enzyme secretory response from intestinal stimuli are both neural and humoral. Truncal vagotomy and atropine markedly inhibit the enzyme (and bicarbonate) responses to low intestinal loads of amino acids and fatty acids. These results suggest a vagovagal enteropancreatic reflex that mediates enzyme secretion and augments bicarbonate secretion stimulated by secretin.

515 **B.** (S&F, ch57)

Early-onset idiopathic chronic pancreatitis is characterized by the development of pancreatic pain at a young age, generally without evidence of pancreatic calcification or pancreatic duct abnormalities. Most individuals with early-onset disease only develop objective findings of calcification or evidence of endocrine or exocrine pancreatic dysfunction after they have had the condition for 20 years or longer.

516 **C.** (S&F, ch53–55)

Pancreatic secretory trypsin inhibitor (SPINK1) is a 56–amino-acid peptide that specifically inhibits trypsin by physically blocking its active site. SPINK1 is synthesized by pancreatic acinar cells along with trypsinogen, and it co-localizes with trypsinogen in the zymogen granules. SPINK1 is believed to act as the first line of defense against prematurely activated trypsinogen in the acinar cell. However, because of a 1:5 stoichiometric disequilibrium between SPINK1 and trypsinogen, SPINK1 is capable of inhibiting only about 20% of trypsin that may be formed. Thus, within the pancreas SPINK1 appears to have a limited role in the first-line defense against premature activation of trypsinogen.

517 **D.** (S&F, ch57)

The most sensitive tests for diagnosing chronic pancreatitis are hormonal tests of pancreatic function, (i.e., secretin or cholecystokinin stimulation tests). Imaging with ERP is the next most sensitive examination for diagnosis of this condition.

518 **E.** (S&F, ch57)

Steatorrhea occurs in those with chronic pancreatitis when gland function is reduced by 90% or more because at this point lipase secretion is inadequate for fat absorption. At this level of gland function, inadequate pancreatic bicarbonate production results in an acidic duodenal milieu, which causes precipitation of bile salts and deactivation of pancreatic lipase. Gastric motility is usually decreased in those with chronic pancreatitis.

519 **C.** (S&F, ch56)

Statistically the *most* common cause of acute pancreatitis in children is blunt trauma to the abdomen; the trauma often occurs in the setting of child abuse. The other causes of acute pancreatitis in children are less common.

520 **C.** (S&F, ch57)

Endoscopic therapy directed to the minor papilla in individuals with pancreas divisum is most successful in those with a dilated dorsal duct and ERCP can identify these individuals. Surgical therapies may offer improved outcomes compared to endoscopic therapies, but the incremental benefit is minimal. The greatest benefit of endoscopic therapy in these cases is that it may decrease the number of bouts of acute pancreatitis; however, chronic pain or pancreatic insufficiency do not generally respond to endoscopic intervention.

521 **D.** (S&F, ch53–55)

Vitamin deficiencies may develop as a consequence of fat maldigestion and malabsorption and therefore patients with cystic fibrosis are at risk. Nearly half of all newly diagnosed cystic fibrosis patients have a deficiency of vitamin A, D, and/or E. Chronic vitamin E deficiency is associated with hemolytic anemia (usually seen in infants); it may also cause neuroaxonal dystrophy with prominent neuromuscular symptoms, although these symptoms appear to be rare. Supplementation with pancreatic enzymes, a multivitamin preparation, and additional vitamin E usually leads to rapid normalization of serum albumin, retinol, and 25-hydroxyvitamin D levels. However, frequent monitoring of the trend in serum concentrations of fat-soluble vitamins is essential in children with cystic fibrosis because deficiencies, especially of vitamin E, may occur even during therapy.

522 **A.** (S&F, ch57)

Endoscopic therapy may be helpful in short-term management of pain in patients with chronic pancreatitis, but evidence for a long-term benefit is lacking. Immediate relief of pain occurs in 60% of individuals after placement of a stent to manage duct obstruction, this procedure has a complication rate of 20%. There is no reliable relationship between pancreatic duct pressure and response to therapy.

523 **C.** (S&F, ch56)

The presentation described (a poorly controlled obese diabetic with underlying hyperlipidemia) is classic for pancreatitis secondary to hypertriglyceridemia in adults. Other common predisposing factors for this condition are hypertriglyceridemia with concomitant alcohol abuse and drug- or diet-induced hypertriglyceridemia. When pancreatitis is due to hypertriglyceridemia, serum amylase may not be substantially elevated.

524 **D.** (S&F, ch57)

Autoimmune pancreatitis (AIP) is a rare cause of pancreatitis that is seen predominantly in middle-aged men. Other autoimmune diseases are seen in 50% or fewer of patients with AIP. It is typical to find single or multifocal strictures of the pancreatic duct. Typical histologic findings are a lymphocytic acinar infiltrate with fibrosis of the interlobular ducts.

525 **D.** (S&F, ch58)

Percutaneous endoscopic gastrostomy (PEG) was developed by Ponsky and Gauderer in the early 1980s. The procedure involves the percutaneous placement of a gastrostomy tube at a site chosen by endoscopic transillumination of the abdominal wall. Insertion of the PEG tube may be achieved by either the Sachs-Vine (push) or Ponsky (pull) technique, depending on the physician's preference. Prospective evaluations of PEG tube placement have found this procedure to be associated with few procedure-related complications

The most common complication is peristomal wound infection, which is usually treated for 7 days with an oral antibiotic, such as cephalexin, that has activity against skin-colonizing microorganisms.

Other complications are rare and include hematoma, peritonitis, gastric or colonic perforation, and fistulas—hepatogastric, gastrocolic, or colocutaneous.

526 **A.** (S&F, ch57)

Studies have demonstrated that the quality of life in patients with chronic pancreatitis is lower than that of the general population and that the strongest predictor of poor quality of life in these patients is ongoing alcohol use. Tobacco use also results in decreased quality of life, albeit to a lesser degree. The onset of pancreatic exocrine and endocrine insufficiency does not in itself strongly predict worsening health status. Diabetes, steatorrhea, and loss of income are also more common among individuals with chronic pancreatitis, but they are not the major causes of a poor quality of life in these patients.

527 **C.** (S&F, ch56)

Nutrition therapy should be instituted early in the course of treating severe acute pancreatitis. Although the standard of care had been total parenteral nutrition (TPN), several recent studies showed that the parenteral route is associated with more complications and no benefit (decrease) in length of stay when compared to the nasojejunal route. Nasojejunal feeding is therefore the preferred method for providing nutrition for patients with severe acute pancreatitis. If TPN is the selected route, however, there is no additional risk to providing intralipids via this route, although in this case serum triglyceride levels should be monitored.

528 **E.** (S&F, ch57)

Tropical pancreatitis is a disease commonly found in regions of India, Africa, and Southeast Asia. The overwhelming majority of cases are diagnosed in adolescents, particularly those in their early teens. The hallmarks of the disease are protein-calorie malnutrition, abdominal pain, and endocrine pancreatic insufficiency. On histologic examination, the pancreatic parenchyma will appear atrophic with dilation of the pancreatic duct and ductal lithiasis.

Although the patient in this case is the typical age and background for this diagnosis, there are many illnesses in addition to tropical pancreatitis that could present with the symptoms described. Mutations of the *SPINK1* gene are highly prevalent among those with tropical pancreatitis. This patient's elevated lipase is a nonspecific finding relative to the imaging findings. Betel nut use is associated with esophageal squamous cell carcinoma. Diets rich in cassava have been linked epidemiologically to tropical pancreatitis.

529 **D.** (S&F, ch53–55)

The disease of hereditary pancreatitis is an autosomal dominant disorder with high penetrance (80% of gene mutation carriers are affected) and variable expression. Hereditary pancreatitis was identified by studies over the past 50 years of several large kindreds with a high incidence of pancreatitis. These kindreds all proved to have an aberrant gene locus on chromosome 7. The disease gene was identified as the cationic trypsinogen gene (*PRSS1*). Several common mutations in the cationic trypsinogen gene are now known to be associated with hereditary pancreatitis. In addition, mutations in the *SPINK1/PSTI* gene have recently been associated with familial pancreatitis and with idiopathic chronic pancreatitis. Growing

experience with genetic testing reveals that family history alone is not an accurate predictor of detecting or excluding specific genes or mutations that predispose to pancreatitis. Thus, family history serves as an important clue to a genetic predisposition, but confirming a suspected diagnosis of hereditary pancreatitis requires genetic testing.

530 **C.** (S&F, ch57)

Lateral pancreaticojejunostomy (modified Peustow procedure) is the most widely performed surgery for patients with chronic pancreatitis. Technical success and relief of pain are both maximal in individuals with dilation of the pancreatic duct to more than 7 mm. Although surgery can be performed in patients with pancreatic ducts of normal caliber, surgery is unlikely to provide symptom relief in these cases. As is the case with all surgical therapies for chronic pancreatitis, the duration of effect after surgery is prolonged relative to the duration of effect after an endoscopic approach. Complications rarely occur with surgery because the procedure is relatively straightforward and the local vascular and biliary structures are not altered. Biliary access is readily obtained postoperatively because the duodenum and duodenal papillae are preserved.

531 **C.** (S&F, ch56)

Computed tomography (CT) is the modality of choice to assess the severity of acute pancreatitis and the presence of associated complications. More specifically, CT with dynamic intravenous contrast injection can determine the presence and extent of pancreatic necrosis, which remains the primary determinant of length of hospitalization and mortality. Although a KUB study can rule out other etiologies for abdominal pain, it does not directly show the pancreas. Transabdominal ultrasound is severely limited in usefulness by poor transmission of ultrasound waves through bowel gas that normally surrounds the pancreas. Compared to CT, MRI is not superior for delineating the pancreas in cases if acute pancreatitis and is both less available and more expensive. ERCP is contraindicated in patients with acute pancreatitis unless there is evidence of concurrent cholangitis.

532 **A.** (S&F, ch57)

The incidence of chronic pancreatitis in nonendemic areas is as high as 8/100,000 individuals, although there is significant regional variation, which indicates that environmental factors may play a role in the pathogenesis of this condition. Men are affected 3.5 times more often than women. The most common cause of chronic pancreatitis is alcohol abuse, which accounts for up to two thirds of cases.

533 **D.** (S&F, ch58)

Vitamin E comprises a group of eight compounds that are found in plants and known as tocols (saturated side chains) or tocotrienols (unsaturated side chains). Alpha-tocopherol provides 75% of the total vitamin E found in man. The largest store of vitamin E is found in adipose tissue. The principal function of vitamin E is to protect cell membranes from the effects of oxidation. The major routes of vitamin E excretion are the feces and the skin. Deficiency of vitamin E is rare and generally occurs in the context of severe fat-soluble vitamin malabsorption such as occurs in short-bowel syndrome, cystic fibrosis, pancreatic insufficiency, or advanced liver disease. Vitamin E deficiency can lead to neuromuscular dysfunction.

534 **A.** (S&F, ch57)

Pancreatic enzyme replacement appears to be most effective in women, those with idiopathic pancreatitis, and those without significant structural abnormalities (small duct disease). Those with readily identifiable morphologic changes or late-stage disease, as evidenced by pancreatic insufficiency, are less likely to benefit from this therapy.

535 **C.** (S&F, ch56)

There is no clear relationship between creatinine clearance and serum amylase levels. Individuals with impaired renal function may have serum amylase levels up to 5-fold greater than the upper limit of normal and serum lipase levels up to three times the upper limit of normal. On the other hand, 30% of patients with renal insufficiency maintain normal serum amylase levels. The amylase urinary-to-creatinine clearance ratio (ACCR) can only be used to diagnose macroamylasemia; it cannot be used to distinguish elevations of amylase due to renal insufficiency from elevations due to other causes. An elevated serum lipase level is not 100% specific for pancreatic disorders.

536 **C.** (S&F, ch57)

Cholecystokinin (CCK) release is stimulated by CCK-releasing peptide (CCK-RP), which is found in the proximal small bowel. CCK-RP undergoes constant degradation by luminal proteases. Patients with chronic pancreatitis are unable to digest protease adequately and therefore their CCK-RP levels rise. Pancreatic enzymes are thought to exert an analgesic effect by decreasing pancreatic stimulation. One mechanism by which this occurs is by decreasing CCK-mediated pancreatic stimulation. Oral replacement of pancreatic enzymes promotes digestion of CCK-RP, which lowers the CCK level, and in turn reduces pancreatic stimulation.

537 **B.** (S&F, ch53–55)

Tropical pancreatitis is the most common form of chronic pancreatitis in regions of India and Asia. The disease typically is diagnosed in young people, who usually present with abdominal pain, severe malnutrition, and exocrine or endocrine insufficiency. Clinically apparent steatorrhea is rarely seen because this population has a very low intake of dietary fat. Endocrine insufficiency is an inevitable consequence of tropical chronic pancreatitis and is often classified as a specific type of diabetes called fibrocalculous pancreatic diabetes. Pancreatic calculi develop in more than 90% of these patients. The pathophysiology of tropical pancreatitis is unknown. Protein-calorie malnutrition is present in the majority of these patients. Treatment for tropical pancreatitis is similar to treatment for other forms of chronic pancreatitis.

538 **E.** (S&F, ch57)

The goal of medical management of abdominal pain in patients with chronic pancreatitis is to afford adequate relief and avoid narcotic addiction and abuse. Optimally, therapy should begin with a non-narcotic analgesic such as acetaminophen; when this medication proves inadequate, the least-potent opioid should be prescribed. Tramadol would be the next choice amongst the options given. Hydromorphone is a potent narcotic. A tricyclic antidepressant such as amitriptyline may be used as adjuvant therapy; however, on its own it is inadequate for analgesia. Gabapentin has not been adequately studied to make recommendations for its use.

539 **B.** (S&F, ch56)

Mortality among patients with six Ranson's criteria is 60%. Grey Turner's sign is a manifestation of hemorrhagic pancreatitis. In most patients with underlying heart disease and severe acute pancreatitis, a Swan-Ganz catheter is recommended so that aggressive fluid resuscitation can be provided without inducing congestive heart failure. Fluid resuscitation in those with acute pancreatitis should almost never be "gentle." Hypocalcemia is often a manifestation of hypoalbuminemia, which does not need to be corrected, or of hypomagnesemia, which should be corrected. Nasogastric suctioning is recommended only in patients with intestinal ileus or intractable vomiting. The use of antibiotics in these cases is controversial; if employed, antibiotics should only be used when there is clinical evidence of infection or necrotizing disease.

540 **D.** (S&F, ch53–55)

Enterokinase, secreted by duodenal mucosal cells that activates trypsinogen.

541 **C.** (S&F, ch57)

Pseudocysts, which often complicate pancreatitis, are difficult to manage. Although most lesions resolve spontaneously, intervention is advocated for pseudocysts that are enlarging, causing enteral on pancreatic duct obstruction, or are infected. Intervention is more often necessary for cysts larger than 6 cm; however, size in itself is not an indication for intervention. When a patient's symptoms are stable and there is no pancreaticobiliary duct dilation, endoscopic decompression of a cyst is unlikely to provide significant relief. ERCP should generally be avoided to prevent possible introduction of infectious organisms into the cyst. A minority of pancreatic cysts have malignant potential; these are the cysts that are not sequelae of pancreatitis but may be its cause, or cysts found incidentally when pancreatitis occurs due to another cause.

One should not presume that a pancreatic cyst found during a bout of pancreatitis is a result of the inflammation. Pancreatic cysts may be congenital or neoplastic. To further evaluate such a cyst, EUS should be performed. The presence of septations or of mural nodules raises the suspicion for neoplasia. Fine-needle aspiration of the cyst may identify mucin or dysplastic epithelium, and fluid analysis can differentiate benign lesions from malignancy or those with malignant potential.

542 **D.** (S&F, ch57)

Alcoholic chronic pancreatitis occurs in a minority of patients with heavy alcohol use: Although estimates vary, chronic pancreatitis will develop in fewer than 15% of heavy drinkers. Tobacco use has been associated with an increased risk of chronic pancreatitis and increased severity of disease in alcohol users. Clinical presentations of alcoholic chronic pancreatitis vary from no clinical symptoms in patients whose pancreatitis is first suspected from abnormal findings on an imaging study, to acute bouts of pain, to exocrine and endocrine insufficiency. It would not be unusual for a patient with alcoholic chronic pancreatitis to present in the manner described in this scenario.

Studies of the natural history of alcoholic chronic pancreatitis demonstrate that exocrine insufficiency is somewhat more common and occurs earlier in the disease process than endocrine failure. These complications of pancreatic insufficiency may be slowed by cessation of alcohol ingestion, but unfortunately the disease often continues to progress even during abstinence.

543 **D.** (S&F, ch56)

Acute pancreatitis may result in splenic vein thrombosis due to the peripancreatic inflammation. Splenic vein thrombosis, in turn, leads to gastric varices and the potential for gastrointestinal hemorrhage. Cavernous transformation of the portal vein may develop in cases of chronic portal vein thrombosis, but not within 10 days from the onset of acute pancreatitis. Hemosuccus pancreaticus is bleeding from the pancreatic duct into the duodenum. It is often secondary to erosion of a pseudocyst or pseudoaneurysm into the peripancreatic vasculature. It is a rare cause of gastrointestinal hemorrhage related to pancreatitis. In this patient there is no basis to suspect viral hepatitis or alcohol abuse.

544 **D.** (S&F, ch57)

Although this patient may have pancreas divisum, his pancreatitis is more likely to be due to alcohol use than divisum. This patient has symptoms of both acute pancreatitis (pain) and exocrine pancreatic insufficiency. Pancreas divisum is associated more strongly with acute recurrent pancreatitis than with chronic pancreatitis and pancreatic insufficiency. Thus the alcohol consumption is implicated rather than the divisum as the cause of pancreatitis in this case. Pancreas divisum is identified in 4% to 11% of the general population; a minority of those with divisum develop pancreatitis. An ERCP to manage this patient's acute symptoms would not be an appropriate intervention.

545 **A.** (S&F, ch56)

The sequence in answer **A** is correct.

546 **A.** (S&F, ch58)

The preferred method of meeting the nutritional needs of this patient with severe gastroparesis is to give enteral feedings via the jejunum. Enteral feeding using the stomach would be contraindicated given the severity of this patient's gastroparesis. This would eliminate answer choices **A** and **C**. Nasoenteric tube placement is the most common method of enteral access; however, nasoenteric tubes more readily become occluded or dislodged, leading to interruption of feedings and disruption of medication regimens. Therefore, nasoenteric tubes should only be used in patients who are expected to require either nasogastric or nasojejunal access for less than 1 month.

A PEG/J tube allows for both gastric decompression and jejunal feeding and should be used in patients who will need jejunal feedings for more than one month, but less than 6 months, because the jejunal feeding tube may become occluded or displaced if left in place longer than 6 months. A retrospective study by Fan et al compared the number of physician re-interventions required to manage J-tube complications in a group of patients who received PEG/J tubes compared with another group of patients who received DPJ tubes. The patients with DPJ tubes had significantly fewer re-interventions. DPJ tube placement should be performed in patients who will require long-term jejunal feedings (more than 6 months) or in whom gastric access for decompression or medication instillation is not necessary.

547 A. (S&F, ch57)

Early-onset idiopathic pancreatitis is characterized as a disease of pancreatic abdominal pain without morphologic features of chronic pancreatitis. Patients rarely present with exocrine or endocrine insufficiency and only develop these complications after decades of disease. Genetic abnormalities are found in a significant proportion of patients, although the specifics of the genetic contribution in this subgroup with chronic pancreatitis have yet to be worked out. In contrast, late-onset idiopathic pancreatitis usually presents with exocrine and endocrine dysfunction and less commonly presents with pain. The overwhelming majority of patients with late-onset idiopathic pancreatitis will have pancreatic calcification, which may be present at the time of diagnosis. The gender distribution is about equal in both early-onset and late-onset idiopathic pancreatitis.

548 D. (S&F, ch53–55)

The reason for the high incidence of pancreatic cancer in patients with hereditary pancreatitis is unknown. The recurrent damage to the pancreas caused by unregulated trypsinogen activation and subsequent inflammation appears to provide an environment that promotes oncogenesis. The *PRSS1* gene does not appear to play a role in the development of pancreatic cancer in this population.

549 C. (S&F, ch57)

The pancreatic hormone stimulation test is performed by placing a tube into the third portion of the duodenum under fluoroscopic guidance, administering a secretagogue, and measuring the resultant pancreatic secretion. With cholecystokinin stimulation, pancreatic lipase secretion is measured; with secretin stimulation, bicarbonate secretion is measured. Collection requires 2 hours. The test is generally performed in specialized laboratories that have established reference values so that test results can be clearly interpreted as normal or abnormal. Another test that can be performed is the intraductal secretin test. For this test, a catheter is placed within the pancreatic duct and output is measured over 15 minutes. However, this test does not add any useful diagnostic information to that obtained from the pancreatic hormone stimulation test, and the intraductal secretin test alone is likely to be less accurate for diagnostic purposes than the pancreatic hormone stimulation test.

550 A. (S&F, ch56)

The injured pancreas releases many systemically active substances. The release of phospholipase A2 into the systemic circulation results in degradation of surfactant and contributes to the development of adult respiratory distress syndrome (ARDS).

Infectious pneumonia is a rare complication of acute pancreatitis. Elastase is also released by the injured pancreas, but this enzyme primarily affects blood vessels. Patients with acute pancreatitis suffer from decreased intravascular fluid volume.

551 A. (S&F, ch56)

Regardless of size, an asymptomatic pseudocyst does not require treatment. Therefore none of the procedural interventions listed (answers **B**, **C**, or **D**) should be entertained. In addition, there is no evidence that Sandostatin LAR is beneficial in a patient with a pancreatic pseudocyst. Periodic clinical and radiographic assessment is the recommended strategy for managing an asymptomatic pseudocyst.

552 A. (S&F, ch57)

This patient has findings consistent with chronic pancreatitis secondary to alcohol abuse, and tests of pancreatic function such as a fecal chymotrypsin test or fecal elastase test are unlikely to offer any additional useful information. Vitamin B_{12} deficiency is rare, so testing for a deficiency is unlikely to alter the treatment plan. In contrast, osteopenia is increasingly being recognized in patients with chronic pancreatitis and its presence would warrant consideration of calcium and vitamin D supplementation and addition of a bisphosphonate to the patient's medication regimen.

553 **E.** (S&F, ch56)

The serum amylase level is not 100% sensitive for diagnosis of acute pancreatitis; in fact, the amylase level may be normal or minimally elevated in patients with fatal pancreatitis, mild-to-moderate pancreatitis, or an attack superimposed on chronic pancreatitis. Serum amylase rises within 6 to 12 hours of the onset of an acute attack, has a half-life of 10 hours, and remains elevated for 3 to 5 days. It is likely that only 25% of serum amylase is removed by the kidneys, although all routes of excretion have not been elucidated.

554 **B.** (S&F, ch57)

The histologic features of chronic pancreatitis include progressive fibrosis of the lobules and ductal structures. The islet cells are affected in the later stages of disease. Regions of fibrosis are interspersed with cellular infiltrates of plasma cells, lymphocytes, and macrophages. Although infiltrating neutrophils may be seen in histologic sections from patients with chronic pancreatitis, this is a feature of acute pancreatic inflammation, which can occur superimposed on chronic disease, rather than being a hallmark of chronic pancreatitis. Changes of the pancreatic duct in cases of chronic pancreatitis include eosinophilic plugging, calcification, and intraductal stone formation, fibrosis of the duct with resultant stricture formation, obstruction, and proximal dilation. This course of events is progressive and not a transient or intermittent process.

The changes seen in chronic pancreatitis are not unique to the cause of the condition. Although some authorities propose that there are patterns of inflammation and fibrosis that are more specific to a given cause of inflammation, it is universally accepted that there is overlap in the histologic changes that occur with diseases of various etiologies.

555 **A.** (S&F, ch53–55)

Hereditary pancreatitis is a syndrome of recurrent acute pancreatitis that develops in an individual from a family in which the pancreatitis phenotype appears to be inherited through a disease-causing gene mutation expressed in an autosomal dominant pattern. The most common cause is a mutation in the cationic trypsinogen gene (*PRSS1*) that appears to cause a gain-of-function through altering the regulatory domains in trypsinogen usually controlled by calcium. In two large studies, 19% and 35% of affected patients from families with hereditary pancreatitis had no identifiable *PRSS1* mutations, suggesting that other genes or factors may be responsible for the high risk of pancreatitis.

556 **B.** (S&F, ch57)

Lack of a gold standard is the primary limiting factor in establishing a test that is adequately sensitive and specific to serve as a screening test for chronic pancreatitis. Histologic evidence of chronic inflammation is regional and thus false-negative results of histologic evaluations are common. Detectable anatomic alterations such as pancreatic duct stricture often only occur late in the course of the disease, if at all. Thus the performance characteristics of many diagnostic tests cannot be defined.

557 **A.** (S&F, ch58)

Vitamin B_{12} belongs to a group of compounds called corrinoids, which contain a cobalt atom in the center of four pyrrole rings with various side-chain attachments. Cyanocobalamin is the most common, commercially available form. Animal products are the only source of vitamin B_{12} for humans. Ingested cobalamin is liberated from proteins in the stomach by the action of pepsin and becomes bound to factors known as R-binders. In the small intestine, pancreatic enzymes cleave vitamin B_{12} from R-binders and facilitate the attachment of vitamin B_{12} to intrinsic factor (IF). After vitamin B_{12} has bound to IF receptors in the distal ileum, the IF-B_{12} complex disassociates and the vitamin B_{12} molecule is absorbed and transported by specific proteins to the liver. Vitamin B_{12} is excreted in the bile. Although a vegan diet does not provide the minimal recommended daily allowance of vitamin B_{12}, most cases of vitamin B_{12} deficiency result not from dietary deficiency but from factors related to digestion and absorption such as intrinsic factor deficiency, bacterial overgrowth, pancreatic insufficiency, or impaired absorption of vitamin B_{12} because of distal ileal disease or loss. Deficiency usually presents as a megaloblastic anemia or peripheral neuropathy.

558 **D.** (S&F, ch56)

Ranson's criteria have been found to be reliable indicators of disease severity and prognosis. Ranson's criteria include five variables evaluated at admission: Patient age older than 55 years, WBC count more than 16,000/mL, blood glucose level more than 200 mg/dL, LDH more than 350, and AST more than 250 IU/L; and five criteria determined at 48 hours after admission: Hematocrit decreased by more than 10% from admission, BUN increase of more than 5 mg/dL from admission, calcium level of less than 8 mg/dL, PO_2 less than 60 mmHg, and base deficit greater than 4. Amylase and lipase levels are not good predictors of disease severity or prognosis.

559 **B.** (S&F, ch57)

The primary role of endoscopic management of chronic pancreatitis is to decrease pancreatic ductal pressures. Thus, patients with evidence of a stricture in the head of the pancreas with proximal dilation are most likely to benefit from an endoscopic intervention.

560 **B.** (S&F, ch56)

When gallstones are present and the results of liver function tests are abnormal, gallstone pancreatitis is the most likely diagnosis. Although alcohol is a common cause of acute pancreatitis, it is not as common a cause as gallstones, and when alcohol causes acute pancreatitis, it most often is heavy alcohol use. The other listed causes are far less common and unlikely to be the cause of pancreatitis in this case.

561 **D.** (S&F, ch53–55)

Heterotopic, ectopic, or aberrant pancreatic tissue, or pancreatic rest, is defined as the presence of pancreatic tissue that lacks anatomic and vascular continuity with the main body of the pancreas. Focal expression of human pancreatic cells outside of the pancreatic gland is relatively common, as indicated by their identification on histologic examination of 1% to 14% of various series of autopsy cases. It is rarely of clinical significance. Heterotopic pancreatic tissue is usually seen in the stomach, duodenum, and jejunum. Heterotopic pancreatic tissue usually appears as discrete, firm, yellow submucosal nodules between 2 and 4 cm in diameter. The management of heterotopic pancreatic tissue has been controversial because it is usually of no clinical significance. When complications occur, surgical excision is curative. Surgical excision should be considered if there is doubt regarding the diagnosis or if the lesion is large.

562 **D.** (S&F, ch57)

EUS provides detailed images of the pancreatic parenchyma and duct. Abnormalities such as pseudocysts, duct dilation, and calcification are readily seen. Studies of EUS for the diagnosis of chronic pancreatitis have not resulted in a uniform set of diagnostic criteria, thus limiting the utility of this procedure. Tissue sampling may be performed at the time of EUS but the added benefit of this has not been documented in a rigorous manner.

563 **A.** (S&F, ch56)

The initial step in the pathogenesis of acute pancreatitis is the conversion of trypsinogen to trypsin within acinar cells in sufficient quantities to overwhelm normal mechanisms to remove active trypsin. Release of phospholipase A_2, increased capillary permeability, and fat necrosis are subsequent steps in this disease process. A decrease in the cell membrane protein GP2 is one postulated mechanism for direct alcohol-induced acinar cell cytotoxicity in the development of chronic pancreatitis.

564 **D.** (S&F, ch53–55)

CCK is the major humoral mediator of meal-stimulated pancreatic enzyme secretion. The circulating concentration of CCK increases with a meal. Experiments using highly specific CCK receptor antagonists have demonstrated that pancreatic enzyme secretion with a meal is largely mediated by CCK. CCK is released from the upper small intestinal mucosa by digestion products of fat and protein and, to a small extent, by starch digestion products. Experimental data suggest that CCK activates afferent neurons in the duodenal mucosa. These afferent neurons mediate an enteropancreatic reflex that causes pancreatic enzyme secretion.

565 **C.** (S&F, ch56)

About 80% of pancreatitis attacks are mild, and normal pancreatic morphology and function are the rule after recovery. The remaining 20% of patients suffer severe pancreatitis that is accompanied by pancreatic necrosis and organ failure. For this latter group, the disease-related mortality is 25% to 35%, but the overall mortality of pancreatitis is 2% to 10%.

566 **A.** (S&F, ch57)

A 72-hour fecal fat study is the most sensitive and specific test for determining pancreatic exocrine dysfunction. The patient must consume a diet that includes 100 g of fat per day for 3 days before the start of the 72-hour collection period. This test offers no diagnostic information regarding the etiology of steatorrhea; it only confirms the presence of excess fecal fat.

567 **D.** (S&F, ch57)

Diabetes mellitus develops in the majority of patients who have had chronic pancreatitis for many years. Pancreatic diabetes results from decrease in both the number and function of beta islet cells. Insulin secretion can be demonstrated in those with pancreatic endocrine insufficiency due to chronic pancreatitis. In addition to the loss of function of beta islet cells, glucagon-producing alpha cells are damaged as well, which makes management of diabetes particularly troublesome in this population. Patients with diabetes due to chronic pancreatitis should be monitored as closely for complications such as nephropathy and retinopathy as those with diabetes not due to chronic pancreatitis.

568 A. (S&F, ch56)

SPINK1 protects the pancreatic acinar cell by inhibiting premature activation of trypsin. Mutation of the *SPINK1* gene results in pancreatitis by limiting the activity of this protein. Heterozygous mutations of the *CFTR* gene change bicarbonate conductance and mutations to the trypsin gene cause hereditary pancreatitis by making trypsin resistant to lysis. Trypsinogen activation peptide is a marker for acute pancreatitis.

569 B. (S&F, ch53–55)

Congenital cysts of the pancreas are rare and are distinguished from pseudocysts by the presence of an epithelial lining. It is believed that these cysts are caused by anomalous development of the pancreatic ductal system in which sequestered segments of a primitive ductal system give rise to microscopic or macroscopic cystic lesions. Clinical presentations can include an asymptomatic mass, abdominal distension, vomiting, and jaundice due to biliary obstruction. Symptomatic pancreatic cysts should be surgically removed whenever possible.

570 D. (S&F, ch56)

All the conditions listed may result in an elevated serum amylase. In this young woman, the most likely cause of abrupt onset of abdominal pain, shock, and severe anemia is a ruptured ectopic pregnancy.

571 B. (S&F, ch53–55)

Fat and protein maldigestion with fecal losses are the primary manifestations of pancreatic involvement in cystic fibrosis. Numerous pancreatic enzyme preparations are available commercially, but enzyme activity varies considerably from one product to another, and reduced activity of lipase remains a problem for some patients. The use of histamine H_2-receptor blockers or proton pump inhibitors along with uncoated or enteric-coated pancreatic enzyme supplements should also be considered in patients with cystic fibrosis. Enteric-coated enzyme microspheres are now the preferred form of replacement because they protect the digestive enzymes from destruction by gastric acid (pH less than 4) and are effective in treating steatorrhea. Initial therapy for pancreatic exocrine insufficiency in patients with cystic fibrosis includes pancreatic enzyme replacement at doses ranging from 500 to 2000 units of lipase activity per kilogram of body weight per meal, given just before a meal and with snacks.

572 C. (S&F, ch56)

In patients with severe acute pancreatitis, overall mortality is 25% to 35%. Death tends to occur either within the first 48 hours of symptom onset or after the second week of disease, in which case the major cause of death is pancreatic infection in association with multisystem organ failure. Patients who are older and have concurrent illnesses have a substantially higher risk of death due to pancreatitis than younger patients. Hemorrhagic pancreatitis is not an independent risk factor for death from pancreatitis.

573 B. (S&F, ch57)

The diagnosis of autoimmune pancreatitis can be difficult to confirm. Clinical and laboratory findings supportive of the diagnosis include elevated immunoglobulins, in particular elevated IgG4, although this feature alone is not diagnostic. When autoimmune pancreatitis is suspected, a therapeutic trial of glucocorticoids is appropriate because pancreatic insufficiency may develop over months. Glucocorticoid-induced hyperglycemia can generally be managed with medications. One would expect to observe clinical improvement within 2 to 4 weeks.

574 A. (S&F, ch57)

Transabdominal ultrasound is 50% to 60% sensitive for a diagnosis of chronic pancreatitis. Ultrasound may demonstrate features of late-stage disease and allow for identification of complications such as pseudocyst or calcifications, but the results are often nondiagnostic in those with early chronic pancreatitis. Ultrasound does not delineate duct anatomy or allow for identification of strictures. Additionally, there is a spectrum of normal findings and age-related changes of the pancreas that overlap with subtle findings of chronic pancreatitis, thereby decreasing the utility of the test.

575 A. (S&F, ch56)

After blunt trauma to the abdomen the most reliable way to diagnose and treat a pancreatic duct disruption is ERCP. Serum amylase may be elevated secondary to pancreatic contusion or injury to other intra-abdominal organs. Pancreatic or peripancreatic inflammatory changes may suggest pancreatic duct disruption but these changes are not diagnostic. A CT scan may also appear normal. MRI with MRCP is not significantly better than CT for the diagnosis of pancreatic duct disruption.

576 **D.** (S&F, ch57)

Studies have demonstrated that ongoing tobacco use by patient with chronic pancreatitis is associated with increased abdominal pain and a decrement in quality of life. A low-fat diet may result in decreased pain, although greater benefit can be expected from smoking cessation. Increasing exercise would not be expected to decrease pain and resumption of alcohol use would be contraindicated.

577 **B.** (S&F, ch53–55)

The administration of adequate pancreatic enzyme in the dose of 30,000 IU of lipase with each meal is the most important principle in the management of steatorrhea. Often, adjuvant measures include the use of a proton pump inhibitor, enteric-coated preparations, and eating multiple small meals. A no-fat diet should be avoided to prevent fat-soluble vitamin deficiency. Periodic monitoring for fat-soluble vitamin deficiency should be performed.

578 **C.** (S&F, ch53–55)

Anomalous pancreaticobiliary union is a congenital malformation of the confluence of the pancreatic and bile ducts. A common channel for the bile and pancreatic fluid is formed by the absence of a septum between the ducts. This malunion is associated with pancreatitis, choledochal cysts, and proliferative abnormalities that can manifest in adults. Choledochal cysts are frequently associated with this abnormality (in 94% and 100% of cases in two series). Malunions were seen in the following percentages in adults with the following diseases: gallbladder cancer, 62.5%; gallbladder adenomyomatosis, 50.0%; common bile duct cancer, 33.3%; and pancreatitis, 13.4%. Considering the cancer risk of a dilated bile duct associated with a pancreaticobiliary malunion, it may be advisable to perform cholecystectomy, resection of the bile duct, and hepaticojejunostomy. Diverting the bile duct from the pancreatic duct by choledochal cyst excision prevents the recurrence of pancreatitis in most cases.

579 **A.** (S&F, ch57)

This patient has evidence of chronic pancreatitis; however, she does not have a dilated pancreatic duct, and therefore further endoscopic or surgical interventions are unlikely to be helpful. Neurolysis of the celiac nerve plexus would be the most appropriate of the choices presented.

580 **A.** (S&F, ch57)

The time period over which jaundice may develop in patients with pancreatitis due to alcohol is broad. Ongoing alcohol use may precipitate acute alcoholic hepatitis and a superimposed viral hepatitis is always a possibility. Biliary complications of chronic pancreatitis, including both benign and malignant causes of obstruction, may occur. Benign etiologies include benign inflammatory stricture and obstructing pseudocyst. The most appropriate plan would be to repeat cross-sectional imaging and if no anatomic cause of biliary obstruction is found, to consider alternative diagnoses.

581 **A.** (S&F, ch57)

Tissue ischemia and acidosis, reduced pancreatic blood flow, and neuronal changes have been implicated in the pathogenesis of abdominal pain secondary to chronic pancreatitis. There is an increase in the number and diameter of intrapancreatic neurons, and damage to the perineural sheaths has been well documented.

582 **D.** (S&F, ch56)

Pancreatic secretory trypsin inhibitor (SPINK1) binds and inactivates about 20% of trypsin. Other mechanisms involve mesotrypsin, enzyme Y, trypsin itself, and nonspecific proteases such as alpha$_2$-antitrypsin and alpha$_2$-macroglobulin. Additional protective mechanisms are the sequestration of pancreatic enzymes within intracellular compartments of the acinar cell during synthesis and transport and the separation of digestive enzymes from lysosomal hydrolases such as cathepsin B as they pass through the Golgi apparatus. Low intracellular concentrations of calcium prevent further autoactivation of trypsin.

583 **E.** (S&F, ch58)

Zinc deficiency can result in a characteristic skin rash (acrodermatitis), poor wound healing, impaired or abnormal taste, glucose intolerance, alopecia, depression, and diarrhea.

584 **D.** (S&F, ch57)

Individuals with diabetes mellitus resulting from pancreatic endocrine insufficiency have an increased risk of disease-related mortality compared to those without pancreatic diabetes. Management of glucose levels is difficult in these patients and tight glucose control should be avoided because disordered glucagon homeostasis may result in profound hypoglycemia. Diabetic ketoacidosis is rare.

585 **C.** (S&F, ch56)

Chronic pancreatitis is a persistent or progressive disorder in which changes in pancreatic structure and function usually precede symptoms and always persist even after the precipitating cause of pancreatitis has been corrected. The only way to confirm that an attack of pancreatitis represents chronic pancreatitis is to demonstrate characteristics consistent with chronic pancreatitis, including ductal irregularity and parenchymal fibrosis. Acute pancreatitis may recur, particularly in those who use alcohol. Pseudocysts can be seen in patients with either acute or chronic pancreatitis.

586 **B.** (S&F, ch58)

There has recently been an emphasis on evaluating a patient's weight and body habitus using the body mass index (BMI), defined as weight/height^2 in kg/m^2. BMI numbers help to categorize patients as underweight, ideal weight, overweight, obese, or super obese, as shown in the following list:

BMI	Category
<18	Underweight
18–26.5	Ideal weight
26.5–30	Overweight
30–40	Obese
>40	Super obese

QUESTIONS

587 A 44-year-old chef questions the safety of a wild mushroom he has harvested. The fungus is identified as *Amanita phylloides*. Which of the following preparation methods will render this mushroom safe to eat?

A. Broiling (500°F)
B. Dehydrating
C. Freeze-drying
D. Frying (350°F)
E. None of the above

588 A 2-year-old infant is admitted to the hospital with severe drug-induced hepatotoxicity. Which of the following agents is most likely to be implicated?

A. Diclofenac
B. Isoniazid
C. Nitrofurantoin
D. Phenytoin
E. Valproic acid

589 Which is the most appropriate treatment for secondary bacterial peritonitis?

A. Four weeks of intravenous (IV) cephalosporin/antianaerobic drug
B. IV cephalosporin/anti-anaerobic drug; duration determined by response
C. Surgical intervention; 2 weeks IV cephalosporin/antianaerobic drug
D. Surgical intervention; 4 weeks IV cephalosporin/antianaerobic drug
E. Surgical intervention; perioperative IV cephalosporin/antianaerobic drug

590 A gastroenterology consult was called for a 68-year-old man who was brought to the emergency department. He was found unconscious in his home, where he had suffered a non-hemorrhagic stroke. His liver test results are abnormal. On exam, he is intubated, anicteric, has no stigmata of chronic liver disease, and no abnormalities on abdominal examination. His laboratory test results are as follows:

Serum bilirubin:
   Total   1.4 mg/dL
   Direct   0.3 mg/dL

Serum alkaline phosphatase: 84 U/L

Serum aminotransaminase:
   Aspartate (AST)   1570 U/L
   Arginine (ALT)   128 U/L

Which is the most likely diagnosis?

A. Acetaminophen overdose
B. Acute alcoholic hepatitis
C. Ischemic hepatitis
D. Mesenteric vasculitis
E. Rhabdomyolysis

591 A 55-year-old woman presents with a 6-week history of fatigue and dull right upper quadrant discomfort followed by a 4-week history of jaundice. She is perimenopausal and has had frequent urinary tract infections, which have been treated with antibiotics. She has an elevated direct bilirubin level, minimally elevated alkaline phosphatase, aminotransaminase levels 10 times normal, and normal albumin. Her antinuclear antibody titer is 1:40. Which of the following is the most likely cause of her drug-induced hepatic injury?

A. Amoxicillin
B. Cephalexin
C. Ciprofloxacin
D. Nitrofurantoin
E. Trimethoprim/sulfamethoxazole

592 Which of the following is the best initial approach to treat systemic hypertension following liver transplantation?

A. Angiotensin-converting enzyme inhibitor
B. Diltiazem
C. Nifedipine
D. Reduction in doses of immunosuppressant medications

593 A man with hemochromatosis has his only male child tested for this disease. His child's hemochromatosis genotype is found to be compound heterozygote (C282Y/H63D). Which of the following courses of action is most appropriate to recommend?

A. Immediate institution of weekly phlebotomy to prevent iron overload
B. Liver biopsy
C. No subsequent testing for iron
D. Referral for transplant evaluation
E. Yearly measurement of ferritin level and phlebotomy when the level is elevated

594 A 48-year-old woman has a 1-year history of abnormal results of serum tests, which show a pattern of hepatocellular injury. Her medical history is notable for type II diabetes mellitus and hypertriglyceridemia. Serum tests for possible liver pathogens are negative. Ultrasonography reveals increased hepatic echogenicity. The most likely finding on histologic evaluation of a biopsy specimen is:

A. Interface hepatitis with lymphocytoplasmic infiltrate
B. Nonsuppurative destructive cholangitis
C. Periodic acid–Schiff (PAS)–positive diastase-resistant periportal globules
D. Perisinusoidal fibrosis and Mallory's hyaline
E. Portal lymphoid aggregates with germinal centers

595 A 31-year-old woman becomes infected with hepatitis B virus. The infection is self-limited, with full recovery after a period of jaundice. This patient's risk of chronic HBV infection is:

A. 5%
B. 15%
C. 50%

D. 75%
E. 90%

596 A patient has abnormal aminotransaminase levels and suspected nonalcoholic fatty liver disease (NAFLD), based on negative results of serum tests for liver pathogens or other infectious agents and imaging studies to evaluate for other liver diseases. What is the best rationale for performing a percutaneous liver biopsy in this patient?

A. To exclude occult iron overload disorders
B. To counsel the patient on possible risk for future complications
C. To establish the diagnosis
D. To identify the most appropriate pharmacotherapeutic approach

597 After a 3-day fast, which of the following is the primary source of glucose supplied to the brain?

A. Beta oxidation of fatty acids
B. Hepatic gluconeogenesis
C. Hepatic glycogen
D. Muscle glycogen

598 A 24-year-old woman is admitted to the intensive care unit following intentional acetaminophen overdose. She is intubated, unresponsive, mildly hypotensive, and has no stigmata of chronic liver disease. She is most likely to die of:

A. Cerebral herniation
B. Coagulopathy with bleeding
C. Hemodynamic collapse
D. Liver synthetic failure
E. Renal failure

599 A 50-year-old Asian man presents with cirrhosis due to hepatitis B virus, complicated by ascites that has been controlled with diuretics, and a 2.5-cm hepatocellular carcinoma. His alanine aminotransferase level is three times the upper limit of normal. A test for hepatitis B surface antigen is positive, the hepatitis B e antigen test is negative, and the hepatitis B viral DNA level is 5 million copies/mL. It is decided that the patient would benefit from liver transplantation. Which therapy would be most likely to minimize the risk of recurrence of hepatitis B after liver transplantation?

A. Adefovir, administered orally
B. Chemoembolization of the tumor
C. Immediate listing for liver transplantation
D. Pegylated interferon combined with oral lamivudine

600 A 42-year-old woman presents for management of chronic hepatitis C virus (HCV) after being refused as a blood donor. Her risk factor for HCV infection is a brief period of intravenous drug use while in her teens. She has no symptoms, the results of her physical examination are unremarkable, her serum ALT level was normal on two occasions, and she is found to have an HCV RNA (genotype 1a) level of 430,000 IU/mL. Which of the following is most helpful in estimating her prognosis?

A. ALT level
B. Duration of HCV infection
C. HCV genotype
D. HCV viral load
E. Results of a liver biopsy

601 An 83-year-old man presents to the emergency department with abdominal pain and hypotension. An 8-cm vascular mass, actively bleeding, is seen in the right lobe of the liver on angiography. Exploratory laparotomy is performed to control the bleeding and biopsy the mass. The results of histologic evaluation of the biopsy specimen are consistent with angiosarcoma. Which occupational exposure is likely to have contributed to development of this patient's cancer?

A. Asbestos
B. Pesticides
C. Petroleum
D. Plastics

602 A consult is called for a 25-year-old woman who has presented to the emergency department with a 1-month history of abdominal pain and distention. On physical exam she is found to have tender hepatomegaly and ascites, but no asterixis. Her medications include acetaminophen, albuterol inhalers, and oral contraceptives. Which is the most likely diagnosis?

A. Acetaminophen-induced liver failure
B. Acute hepatitis B virus infection
C. Alpha-1 antitrypsin deficiency
D. Budd-Chiari syndrome
E. Hemochromatosis

603 A 57-year-old homeless man with a long history of tobacco and intravenous drug abuse is evaluated for new-onset ascites. He has not seen a physician for 25 years and is taking no medications. On physical exam he is thin, with temporal atrophy and muscle wasting in the upper extremities. He has needle track marks on his arms, moderate ascites, and ankle edema. Ascites fluid analysis shows a leukocyte count of 1000/μL (35% polymorphonuclear leukocytes, 65% lymphocytes) and serum ascites albumin gradient of 1.0 g/dL; a Gram-stained slide shows no bacteria, and culture results are pending. What is the most likely diagnosis?

A. Cardiac ascites
B. Cirrhosis
C. Peritoneal carcinomatosis
D. Spontaneous bacterial peritonitis
E. Tuberculous peritonitis

604 A 35-year-old liver transplant recipient with hepatitis C virus infection who is in her third postoperative year presents with hypertension and renal insufficiency. What is the most likely cause of her problems?

A. Calcineurin inhibitor–induced nephrotoxicity
B. Immunosuppression-related renal cell cancer
C. New-onset diabetes mellitus
D. Recurrent hepatitis C virus infection complicated by membranoproliferative renal disease

605 A 26-year-old woman presents with abnormal serum aminotransaminase levels and the clinical triad of pharyngitis, fever, and lymphadenopathy. Which of the following is the most likely cause of her signs and symptoms?

A. Epstein-Barr virus (EBV) infection
B. Hepatitis G virus (GBV-C) infection
C. Hepatitis A virus infection
D. Herpes simplex virus (HSV) infection
E. Transfusion-transmitted virus (TTV)

606 A patient has a new diagnosis of autoimmune hepatitis confirmed by liver biopsy. The first choice for single-drug therapy for this patient would be:

A. Cyclosporine
B. Mesalamine
C. Prednisone
D. Tacrolimus
E. Ursodiol

607 Which of the following is a predictor of fibrosis in nonalcoholic fatty liver disease (NAFLD)?

A. Patient age younger than 50 years
B. AST/ALT less than 1
C. Female gender
D. New onset of liver test abnormalities
E. Triglycerides = 1.7 mmol/L

608 A 50-year-old woman presents with persistently elevated serum aminotransaminase levels and a body mass index (BMI) of 40 kg/m². Serologic tests are negative for autoimmune, infectious, or metabolic diseases. Ultrasonography demonstrates a fatty liver and evaluation of a biopsy specimen shows steatosis, lobular inflammation, and fibrosis. Which feature of this patient's presentation raises the possibility of progression to advanced liver disease?

A. Elevated serum transaminase levels
B. Her gender and age
C. Inflammation and fibrosis on biopsy
D. High BMI (obesity)
E. Steatosis on biopsy

609 A 40-year-old man presents to his primary care doctor with complaints of polydipsia, polyuria, arthralgias, abdominal pain, and impotence. His brother, who had diabetes mellitus, died recently of heart failure. On physical examination the patient has tan-appearing skin with spider angiomas on his chest and back and he has abdominal ascites. The most likely cause of this man's cirrhosis is:

A. Alcohol
B. Autoimmune hepatitis
C. Hemochromatosis
D. Hepatitis C virus infection
E. Nonalcoholic fatty liver disease

610 A 41-year-old woman chronically infected with hepatitis C virus, genotype 1a, 580,000 IU/mL, whose liver biopsy showed stage 2, grade 1 disease has been receiving peginterferon alfa-2b, 150 mcg subcutaneously per week, and ribavirin, 600 mg orally twice daily. After 12 weeks of therapy she has had no adverse effects of therapy, her absolute neutrophil count is 800/mL, her hemoglobin level is 10.8 g/dL, her platelet count is 127,000/mL, and her HCV RNA level is 25,000 IU/mL. Which of the following is the most appropriate next step in this patient's care?

A. Add erythropoietin, 40,000 IU/week, to her medication regimen
B. Continue current therapy for 12 weeks, then recheck HCV RNA level
C. Decrease ribavirin to 400 mg twice daily
D. Discontinue therapy
E. Increase peginterferon to 180 mcg/week

611 A 43-year-old man with decompensated cirrhosis secondary to hepatitis C virus infection is being evaluated for liver transplantation. Pretransplant testing reveals that the patient is infected with GBV-C (hepatitis G virus). GBV-C virus poses risk of which of the following complications for this patient?

A. Fulminant hepatic failure
B. Increased hepatitis C viral load
C. Increased post-transplant mortality
D. New onset of pancytopenia
E. No clinically significant complications

612 A 65-year-old woman is noted to have jaundice 2 days following uncomplicated abdominal hysterectomy. The surgery and postoperative course were uneventful, without documented episodes of hemodynamic instability, and her surgical incision has no signs of infection. She has an elevated indirect bilirubin level and her serum ALT is 1.5 times the upper limit of normal, but the results of a complete blood count (CBC) with differential are normal. Which of the following is the most likely diagnosis?

A. Analgesic-induced hepatotoxicity
B. Anesthetic-induced hepatotoxicity
C. Hemolytic anemia
D. Ischemic hepatitis
E. Postoperative cholestasis

613 The characteristic histologic findings in autoimmune hepatitis include:

A. Florid bile duct lesion, granulomas, ductopenia
B. Ground-glass appearance of hepatocytes
C. Interface hepatitis, plasmacytic infiltration, rosette formation
D. Microvesicular fat and Mallory's hyaline bodies
E. Piecemeal necrosis, lymphocytic infiltration

614 A liver biopsy specimen obtained from a patient with newly diagnosed primary biliary cirrhosis would most likely show:

A. Florid bile duct lesion
B. Ground-glass appearance of hepatocytes
C. Microvesicular fat
D. Obliterative fibrosis cholangitis
E. Piecemeal necrosis

615 A 60-year-old man who has recently emigrated from Brazil is evaluated for fever and lymphocyte-predominant ascites. Tuberculous peritonitis is suspected. What is the most appropriate next step in diagnosis?

A. Test ascitic fluid for adenosine deaminase.
B. Culture ascitic fluid for mycobacteria.
C. Perform blind peritoneal biopsy.
D. Perform laparoscopy with histologic examination of a biopsy specimen and culture of a fluid sample.

616 A 45-year-old man with hepatitis C cirrhosis is hospitalized with refractory ascites, oliguria, and failure to thrive. On physical exam he looks chronically ill and has noticeable ascites, but he has no fever, jaundice, peripheral edema, or encephalopathy. His blood urea nitrogen (BUN) and creatinine levels have increased over the last 6 weeks from 18 mg/dL and 1.5 mg/dL to 20 mg/dL and 1.8 mg/dL, respectively. The results of routine blood and urine cultures are negative; a sample of ascitic fluid shows a white blood cell (WBC) count of 200/mL with 40% neutrophils. A sample of nasogastric lavage fluid tests negative for blood. What is the best next step in managing this patient?

A. Start antibiotic therapy for spontaneous bacterial peritonitis.
B. Perform esophagogastroduodenoscopy.
C. Increase the dose of his current diuretic medication.
D. Administer intravenous fluids for intravascular volume expansion.
E. Insert a transvenous intrahepatic portosystemic shunt.

617 A 63-year-old man from mainland China presents with right upper quadrant abdominal pain and jaundice. Computed tomography (CT) of the abdomen reveals a 6-cm enhancing mass in the left hepatic lobe. The results of examining a biopsy specimen of the mass are diagnostic for hepatocellular carcinoma. What is the likelihood that his serum alpha-fetoprotein level will be in excess of 500 ng/mL?

A. 10%
B. 50%
C. 75%
D. 100%

618 A 62-year-old rancher presents with abdominal fullness and a palpable liver. A CBC of a peripheral smear shows 33% eosinophils. Ultrasonography reveals a 10-cm hepatic cyst with internal septations. Serologic testing for hydatidosis is positive. Which of the following is appropriate for management of this patient's condition?

A. Albendazole, 10 mg/kg for 28 days
B. Liver transplantation
C. Percutaneous aspiration-injection-re-aspiration (PAIR)
D. Percutaneous drainage
E. Surgical resection

619 A 48-year-old man with poorly compensated hepatitis C–induced cirrhosis undergoes magnetic resonance imaging (MRI) and a 3-cm hepatocellular carcinoma is seen in the right lobe. There is a thrombus in the right portal vein. Which of the following is the most appropriate approach to treatment of this patient?

A. Chemoembolization followed by transplantation
B. Liver transplantation
C. Local ablative therapy with radiofrequency ablation or ethanol injection
D. Surgical resection

620 A 38-year-old woman undergoes abdominal ultrasound because of a bout of right upper quadrant pain, and a mass is seen. She is otherwise well. Her only medication is oral contraceptives. MRI shows a brightly enhancing 6-cm mass in the periphery of the right lobe of the liver. The mass has a "spoke-wheel appearance" but no central scar. Which of the following is most appropriate for managing this patient's condition?

A. Arterial embolization
B. Exploratory laparoscopy
C. Radiologic percutaneous biopsy
D. Repeat MRI in 6 months
E. Surgical resection

621 The most common cause of acute liver failure worldwide is:

A. Acetaminophen
B. Autoimmune hepatitis
C. Budd-Chiari syndrome
D. Hepatitis A virus infection
E. Hepatitis B virus infection

622 A 51-year-old man with hepatitis B–related cirrhosis is noted to have a platelet count of 86,000/mL. Which of the following statements is true regarding platelet abnormalities in patients with cirrhosis?

A. Platelet count is inversely related to clinical outcome.
B. Splenic sequestration due to splenomegaly is the major cause of thrombocytopenia.
C. Thrombocytopenia is more common in patients with chronic hepatitis B virus infection than in those with chronic hepatitis C virus infection.
D. Thrombocytopenia usually responds well to administration of thrombopoietin.

623 A 45-year-old man with HCV-related cirrhosis is hospitalized with a 2-day history of fever and abdominal discomfort. His temperature is 39°C, he has abdominal distention with shifting dullness, and a small, reducible umbilical hernia is noted. Laboratory test results show a sodium level of 130 mEq/dL, albumin of 2.5 g/dL, ALT of 75 U/L, and hemoglobin of 9.0 g/dL. Ascitic fluid has an albumin level of 1.0 g/dL and a polymorphonuclear (PMN) leukocyte count of 500/μL. Which of the following is the most appropriate next step in managing this patient?

A. Administration of ampicillin plus an aminoglycoside
B. Large-volume paracentesis
C. Surgery to correct the umbilical hernia
D. Administration of a third-generation cephalosporin
E. Placement of a transjugular intrahepatic portosystemic shunt (TIPS)

624 A 37-year-old woman with splenic vein thrombosis presents with brisk hematemesis. The patient is hemodynamically stable. She is given transfusion products to bring hemoglobin into the normal range, started on octreotide, and sent for endoscopy. At endoscopy, a large pool of blood is seen in the fundus, and inferior to this pool are large bleeding gastric varices. Which of the following is the most appropriate next step in managing this patient's condition?

A. Balloon tamponade
B. Endoscopic band ligation
C. Endoscopic sclerotherapy
D. Epinephrine injection
E. TIPS placement

625 A 36-year-old woman presents to the emergency department with brisk gastrointestinal hemorrhage. Following volume resuscitation and achievement of hemodynamic stability she undergoes esophagogastroduodenoscopy (EGD). Bleeding esophageal varices are noted; hemostasis is achieved using band ligation. Which of the following is the best way to estimate this patient's portal venous pressure?

A. Measure portal pressure directly.
B. Measure variceal pressure endoscopically.
C. Determine the hepatic vein pressure gradient.
D. Measure splenic pulp pressure.

626 A 43-year-old woman known to have advanced primary biliary cirrhosis presents with new onset of weight loss, greasy stools, and easy bruising. Stool studies show the presence of fecal fat. The best course of management for this patient would be:

A. Colonoscopy with random biopsies
B. Esophagogastroduodenoscopy (EGD) with duodenal biopsy
C. Fat-soluble vitamin replacement
D. Lactase replacement
E. Pancreatic enzyme replacement

627 A patient has been newly diagnosed with decompensated autoimmune hepatitis manifested by new onset of ascites and encephalopathy. She is started on diuretic therapy and lactulose. The next best step in management is:

A. Azathioprine
B. Cyclosporine
C. Steroids and transplant evaluation
D. Tacrolimus
E. Transplant evaluation only

628 A 64-year-old man presents with increasing abdominal girth and peripheral edema. He is a Vietnam veteran who lives in a small hamlet supplied by well water. He admits to consumption of home-distilled alcoholic beverages. His serum-ascites albumin gradient is 2.0, but liver biopsy reveals mild, nonspecific periportal inflammation without fibrosis. Which of the following is the most likely cause of ascites in this case?

A. Agent Orange
B. Arsenic
C. Paraquat
D. Polychlorinated biphenyls (PCBs)

629 A 35-year-old man develops cholestasis and hepatocellular inflammation following treatment with an aminopenicillin. Which of the following techniques is most specific for a diagnosis of drug-induced hepatotoxicity?

A. Drug rechallenge
B. In vitro testing
C. Liver biopsy
D. Peripheral eosinophil count
E. Skin biopsy

630 Spontaneous hepatitis B e surface antigen (HBeAg) seroconversion is seen in approximately what percent annually of patients chronically infected with hepatitis B virus?

A. 10% per year
B. 25% per year
C. 50% per year
D. 75% per year

631 A 6-week-old infant is brought for evaluation of lethargy and seizures. Hepatomegaly and lactic acidosis are present. Which of the following tests is the best to establish the diagnosis of glycogen storage disease, type I?

A. Abdominal CT with contrast
B. Fasting serum glucose measurement
C. Glucagon response test
D. Liver biopsy

632 A 57-year-old woman is referred for evaluation of persistently elevated serum levels of liver enzymes. Her medical history is notable for chronic atrial fibrillation, hypertension, and diabetes mellitus. Her medication regimen includes nifedipine, warfarin, and metformin. She has had no exposures to hepatotropic viruses, nor does she drink alcohol. Her laboratory test results are as follows:

Serum bilirubin:

Total	0.6 mg/dL
Direct	0.1 mg/dL

Alkaline phosphatase: 78 U/L

Gamma-glutamyl transpeptidase: 250 U/L

Serum aminotransaminases:

AST	23 U/L
ALT	16 U/L

Which of the following is the most appropriate next step in management for this patient?

A. Perform abdominal ultrasound.
B. Perform endoscopic retrograde cholangiopancreatography.
C. Obtain a liver biopsy.
D. Perform no further testing because none is required.
E. Measure her serum 5'-nucleotidase level.

633 Hepar lobatum (coarse lobulations of the liver) develops as a result of:

A. Congenital anomalies
B. Extensive fibrosis
C. Obliterative lesions in the vessels
D. Regenerative nodules

634 Which of the following is thought to be the principal mechanism of liver fibrosis in individuals with alcohol-related liver disease?

A. Alcohol-mediated free radical injury
B. Chronic intrahepatic cholestasis
C. Increase in matrix degradation
D. Increase in stellate cell activation

635 A 55-year-old man with cirrhosis and a history of hepatic encephalopathy is admitted to the hospital for the third time this month with tense ascites. At each previous admission, he underwent therapeutic paracentesis with removal of 2 to 3 L of fluid. He has been following a 2-gram sodium/day diet and taking furosemide 160 mg and spironolactone 400 mg daily for diuresis. His urine sodium concentration is low, confirming that he has been compliant with his low-sodium diet. His serum sodium and potassium levels are 125 mEq/L and 4.2 mEq/L, respectively. Which of the following is the most appropriate initial approach to managing this patient's ascites?

A. Administer intravenous (IV) furosemide.
B. Remove all ascites fluid possible and add amiloride to his medication regimen.
C. Remove all ascites fluid possible and start IV albumin replacement.
D. Remove up to 5 L of ascites fluid and increase the dosages of both diuretics.
E. Place a TIPS.

636 A 42-year-old woman with cryptogenic cirrhosis notes progressive exertional dyspnea, despite being fully compliant with a salt-restricted diet and a high-dose diuretic medication regimen. Pulse oximetry shows an oxygen saturation of 92% while sitting and 88% when standing. The results of her cardiac and pulmonary system examinations are normal, she has minimal ascites and trace ankle edema, and her weight

has been stable over the past several months. Which of the following is the most likely diagnosis in this case?

A. Hepatopulmonary syndrome
B. Portopulmonary hypertension
C. Sarcoidosis
D. Hepatic hydrothorax

637 A 45-year-old man with chronic back pain was prescribed acetaminophen with oxycodone for pain control. His typical alcohol intake is three beers daily with dinner. He presents to the emergency department of a community hospital with new-onset jaundice, nausea, and renal failure. On exam he is noted to be oriented but has asterixis. N-acetylcysteine has been started. The next step in treating this patient would be to:

A. Admit to a medical-surgical unit and observe
B. Begin antibiotic therapy
C. Discharge to home with close follow-up
D. Perform liver biopsy
E. Refer to a transplant center

638 A 56-year-old immigrant from India presents with variceal hemorrhage. His condition is stabilized and he undergoes serologic, radiologic, and histologic evaluations. Tests for markers for hepatotrophic viruses are negative and serum aminotransaminase levels and measures of hepatic protein synthesis function are normal. On ultrasound the liver appears normal and the hepatic veins, portal vein, and superior mesenteric vein appear patent. Histologic evaluation of a liver biopsy specimen shows no fibrosis and minimal, nonspecific portal inflammation. Which of the following is the most appropriate way to manage this patient's condition?

A. Perform coil embolization of portal collaterals.
B. Evaluate for liver transplantation.
C. Prescribe a long-acting somatostatin analogue.
D. Insert a mesocaval shunt.

639 Which of the following groups of diseases are most likely to be associated with type I autoimmune hepatitis (AIH):

A. Autoimmune thyroiditis, dermatomyositis, Crohn's disease
B. Autoimmune thyroiditis, Grave's disease, chronic ulcerative colitis
C. Autoimmune thyroiditis, Grave's disease, Crohn's disease
D. Diabetes mellitus, Grave's disease, chronic ulcerative colitis
E. Diabetes mellitus, Grave's disease, chronic Crohn's disease

640 A cardiologist expresses concern about increased risk for cardiovascular disease in a patient with primary biliary cirrhosis who has been found to have an abnormal low-density lipoprotein (LDL) level. Which of the following is the most appropriate recommendation to address the abnormal LDL level?

A. Prescribe an exercise regimen.
B. Prescribe a low-fat diet.
C. Prescribe a niacin supplement.
D. No intervention is necessary.
E. Order a stress test.

641 A 25-year-old intravenous drug user presents to the emergency department with jaundice, fever, hypotension, elevated transaminase levels, and an elevated international normalization ratio (INR). Determining the level of which of the following factors may help to distinguish sepsis from acute liver failure?

A. Factor II
B. Factor V
C. Factor VII
D. Factor VIII
E. Factor IX

642 A 65-year-old woman with cirrhosis due to autoimmune hepatitis presents with encephalopathy and ascites. The ascites persists despite dietary salt restriction and a diuretic regimen. She has no co-morbid illnesses and lives with her extended family. What is the most reasonable next step in this patient's care?

A. Prescribe high-dose diuretic therapy and nonabsorbable antibiotic therapy.
B. Evaluate for liver transplantation.
C. Insert a splenorenal shunt.
D. Place a transjugular portosystemic shunt.

643 A 65-year-old man presents with increasing abdominal girth. He is found to have a 6-cm enhancing mass in the left hepatic lobe with associated portal vein thrombosis. Which of the following is most likely to have caused this patient's liver cancer?

A. Aflatoxin
B. Copper
C. HBV infection
D. Iron

644 A 28-year-old man presents with asymptomatic elevation of serum aminotransaminase levels. Serologic evaluation reveals the presence of anti-HCV antibodies. From an epidemiologic perspective, which is the most likely source of viral transmission?

A. Blood transfusion
B. Intravenous drug use

C. Occupational needle-stick injury
D. Perinatal transmission
E. Sex with an HCV-infected partner

645 A 33-year-old man presents for evaluation of chronic HCV infection discovered during a life insurance physical examination. His risk factor for HCV infection was a blood transfusion following a motor vehicle accident at the age of 9 years. His wife of 7 years tests negative for anti-HCV antibody and wishes to become pregnant. Which of the following recommendations is most appropriate?

A. Avoid breast-feeding the baby.
B. Plan delivery of the baby by cesarean section.
C. Administer HCV immune globulin to the infant at the time of delivery.
D. Test the infant for HCV after the age of 12 months.
E. Use Latex condoms.

646 A 6-year-old child develops jaundice, rash, myalgias, eosinophilia, and severe elevations in serum aminotransaminase levels following surgery to repair an umbilical hernia. Which anesthetic agent was most likely used for his surgery?

A. Desflurane
B. Enflurane
C. Isoflurane
D. Methoxyflurane
E. Sevoflurane

647 A 42-year-old woman with cirrhosis secondary to alcohol use and HCV infection is hospitalized with a 3-day history of abdominal pain and fever. Her prehospitalization medication regimen included spironolactone, furosemide, and nadolol. Her temperature is 39.5°C, her blood pressure is 100/65 mmHg, and she has palmar erythema, moderate ascites, and no signs of hepatic encephalopathy. Laboratory tests show a white blood cell count of 6000/µL, hemoglobin of 8.0 g/dL, platelets of 85,000/µL, albumin of 2.6 g/dL, total bilirubin of 2.2 mg/dL, ALT of 90 U/L, and INR of 2.5. Spontaneous bacterial peritonitis (SBP) is suspected. What is the most appropriate next step in management of this patient's condition?

A. Treat SBP empirically and perform paracentesis when the INR falls to below 1.5.
B. Administer fresh frozen plasma, and then perform paracentesis.
C. Perform paracentesis now.
D. Administer vitamin K subcutaneously and then perform paracentesis.

648 A 65-year-old man from India is visiting the United States. In India he is a farmer and sells vegetables for a living. When his family meets him, they note that he has jaundice and take him to the emergency department. A chest x-ray shows an infiltrate and laboratory tests show eosinophilia, a total bilirubin of 4.2 mg/dL, direct bilirubin of 2.8 mg/dL, and alkaline phosphatase of 541 U/L. Endoscopic retrograde cholangiopancreatography (ERCP) is performed and the cause of his signs and symptoms is both diagnosed and treated during the procedure. The most likely cause of this patient's biliary obstruction is:

A. Ascariasis
B. Cholangiocarcinoma
C. Choledocholithiasis
D. Metastatic colon cancer
E. Sarcoidosis

649 A 75-year-old woman with congestive heart failure and respiratory failure suffers cardiopulmonary arrest but is successfully resuscitated within 3 minutes. The next morning she has markedly elevated liver function enzymes (AST is 12,000 U/L and ALT is 9,000 U/L). Her INR is also elevated at 2.4. The most appropriate treatment for this patient would be:

A. Anticoagulation therapy
B. Administration of hepatitis B immunoglobulin (HBIG) and initiation of lamivudine therapy
C. Administration of N-acetylcysteine
D. A course of prednisone
E. Provision of supportive care and treatment of her underlying conditions

650 A 23-year-old woman is brought to the emergency department with rhabdomyolysis, hypotension, hyperpyrexia, disseminated intravascular coagulation, and renal failure. Serum aminotransaminase levels are in excess of 1000 U/L. Ingestion of which substance is most likely responsible for this patient's condition?

A. Cocaine
B. Ecstasy (3,4-methylenedioxymethamphetamine)
C. Heroin
D. Methamphetamine
E. Phencyclidine ("Angel dust")

651 Which of the following criteria are used in predicting the need for liver transplantation in cases of acute liver failure secondary to acetaminophen toxicity?

A. Platelet count, lactate level, hemoglobin level, creatinine level, presence of encephalopathy
B. Platelet count, lactate level, INR, creatinine level, presence of encephalopathy
C. pH, lactate level, INR, bilirubin level, albumin level

D. pH, lactate level, INR, creatinine level, presence of encephalopathy
E. pH, lactate level, INR, creatinine level, transaminase levels

652 A 55-year-old man with a history of HCV-related cirrhosis undergoes orthotopic liver transplantation. The surgery is uneventful, the patient is extubated on day 2, and he is discharged from the hospital on day 8. Two months later the patient develops jaundice associated with elevated alkaline phosphatase and mildly increased serum aminotransaminase levels. Ultrasound shows that hepatic vessels are patent and a cholangiogram reveals a normal biliary anastomosis. Liver biopsy reveals profound cholestasis, minimal chronic portal inflammatory infiltrates, and extensive portal-portal fibrous bridging. Which of the following is the most accurate prediction of this patient's clinical course?

A. Development of cirrhosis within 5 years
B. Graft failure and death within 6 months
C. Resolution of laboratory test abnormalities over 6 months
D. Retransplantation within 1 year

653 A 24-year-old woman in her third trimester of pregnancy returns from an 8-week business trip in the Middle East. She seeks medical attention after developing flu-like symptoms followed by dark urine, jaundice, and clay-colored stools. Right upper quadrant ultrasound shows a nondilated biliary tree. She denies a history of intravenous drug use and has not been sexually active for the past 2 months. She has immunoglobulin G (IgG) antibodies to HAV. Which of the following is the most likely diagnosis in this case?

A. Acute hepatitis A virus infection
B. Acute hepatitis B virus infection
C. Acute hepatitis C virus infection
D. Acute hepatitis D virus infection
E. Acute hepatitis E virus infection

654 A 72-year-old Asian man with chronic *Clonorchis sinensis* infection has had multiple admissions to the hospital with fever, right upper quadrant pain, tender hepatomegaly, and eosinophilia. At this admission he presented with weight loss and a palpable abdominal mass. Which of the following is the most likely diagnosis at this time?

A. Cholangiocarcinoma
B. Gallbladder cancer
C. Gastric cancer
D. Hepatocellular carcinoma
E. Pancreatic cancer

655 A 65-year-old woman with a known history of pancreatic cancer presents with variceal bleeding. She does not have any history of liver disease, and on abdominal CT performed 1 month earlier to stage pancreatic cancer, the liver appeared normal. The results of liver function tests are normal. Doppler ultrasound confirms that the most likely cause of variceal bleeding is:

A. Budd-Chiari syndrome
B. Hepatitis C virus infection
C. Metastatic pancreatic cancer
D. Portal vein thrombosis
E. Sarcoidosis

656 Which of the following is true regarding the hepatic arteries?

A. Arterial ligation is usually well tolerated in persons with normal liver function.
B. The common hepatic artery usually arises from the superior mesenteric artery.
C. The cystic arteries usually arise from the celiac artery.
D. The hepatic artery supplies 70% of the blood flow to the hepatic parenchyma.

657 A 45-year-old homosexual man with a new diagnosis of acute HAV infection asks if any precautions should be taken to prevent transmission of HAV to his sexual partner. Which of the following answers is best?

A. The partner should receive HAV serum immunoglobulin alone for prophylaxis.
B. The partner should receive HAV serum immunoglobulin and start immunization against HAV.
C. The partner should receive HAV vaccine alone.
D. No prophylaxis is necessary.

658 A 35-year-old man with a 2-year history of abnormal results of serum tests of liver function is found to have steatohepatitis and evaluation of a liver biopsy specimen shows fibrosis. Which of the following agents has been shown in clinical trials to lead to improvement in the histologic findings in cases of NAFLD?

A. Insulin
B. Leptin
C. Pioglitazone
D. Ursodiol
E. Vitamin E

659 Pentoxifylline, a nonselective phosphodiesterase inhibitor, may be an alternative to glucocorticoids in the treatment of acute alcoholic hepatitis. In which of the following circumstances is pentoxifylline more appropriate than glucocorticoids?

A. Ascites and spontaneous bacterial peritonitis
B. Mild jaundice and encephalopathy, with active infection
C. Severe jaundice, coagulopathy, and encephalopathy
D. Severe jaundice, encephalopathy, and hepatorenal syndrome

660 A 60-year-old man with a history of alcohol-induced cirrhosis presents 3 months after liver transplantation with jaundice and an alkaline phosphatase level that is three times the upper limit of normal. A Doppler ultrasound shows normal arterial flow, no masses, and no bile duct dilatation. A liver biopsy shows bile duct proliferation and no rejection. What test should be performed next?

A. Abdominal computed tomography (CT) with intravenous contrast
B. Cytomegalovirus (CMV) culture
C. Endoscopic retrograde cholangiopancreatography
D. Hepatic arteriogram

661 A 37-year-old man undergoes a bone marrow transplant and is treated with several chemotherapeutic agents, including dacarbazine. One month later, he presents with painful hepatomegaly, weight gain, ascites, and mild hyperbilirubinemia. He undergoes liver biopsy and histologic evaluation of the biopsy specimen shows sinusoidal dilatation and severe hepatic congestion. Inflammation is notably absent. Which is the most likely diagnosis?

A. Budd-Chiari syndrome
B. Congestive heart failure
C. Drug toxicity
D. Graft versus host disease
E. Veno-occlusive disease

662 A 22-year-old man with a history of cystic fibrosis is referred for evaluation of constant, achy right upper quadrant discomfort. Ultrasonography shows notable nodularity of the liver and evidence of portal hypertension. Histologic examination of a needle biopsy specimen is likely to show which of the following?

A. Inflammatory changes, bile duct proliferation
B. PAS-positive, diastase-resistant periportal globules
C. Steatosis, hepatocyte ballooning, Mallory's hyaline bodies
D. Widespread staining with Prussian blue

663 A 16-year-old high school student is brought to the emergency room by his mother because over the past 24 hours he has become lethargic and is slurring his speech. He has a 3-day history of jaundice and bleeding gums. His family has noticed that over the past few months, he has become withdrawn and irritable and started to have problems with homework. Laboratory tests show that his hemoglobin level is 8.6 g/dL, total bilirubin is 22.3 mg/dL, direct bilirubin is 8.4 mg/dL, AST is 890 U/L, ALT is 984 U/L, alkaline phosphatase is 104 U/L, and prothrombin time is 16.4 seconds. Which of the following is the most appropriate course of treatment for this patient?

A. Admit to hospital and order CT of the head.
B. Admit to the intensive care unit (ICU) and initiate transplantation evaluation.
C. Initiate penicillamine therapy for Wilson disease.
D. Start intravenous fluids and check the serum alcohol level.
E. Administer IV fluids, test blood samples for abnormal hepatic function indicators or pathogens, and discharge to home.

664 A 12-year-old boy is seen in consultation for growth retardation, episodic irritability, lethargy, and refusal to eat animal protein such as milk, eggs, and meat. Which of the following abnormalities is most characteristic of ornithine transcarbamylase (OTC) deficiency?

A. Elevated plasma ammonia
B. Elevated plasma citrulline
C. Metabolic acidosis
D. Serum aminotransaminase levels less than 1000 U/L

665 A 33-year-old woman attends a holiday party on a cruise ship. She has some alcoholic drinks and eats freely from the buffet table. Two weeks later she presents with diarrhea, fever, myalgias, and periorbital edema. A CBC shows leukocytosis and eosinophilia. A muscle biopsy is diagnostic, and she is treated promptly with albendazole. The food that was most likely the source of the pathogen causing her infection was:

A. Canned fruit
B. Cream pie
C. Pork
D. Potato salad
E. Refried rice

666 Classic histologic findings of alcoholic hepatitis include which of the following?

A. Hepatocellular necrosis, bridging fibrosis, steatosis
B. Hepatocyte ballooning, Mallory's hyaline bodies, neutrophilic infiltrate
C. Regenerative nodule formation with Mallory's hyaline bodies
D. Steatosis with chronic inflammatory infiltrate

667 The currently recommended medical therapy for primary biliary cirrhosis is:

A. Chlorambucil
B. Cyclosporine
C. Glucocorticoids
D. Ursodeoxycholic acid

668 A 40-year-old man with alcoholic cirrhosis presents with increasing abdominal girth, ankle edema, and a 20-pound weight gain over the past 3 months. On physical exam he is found to have scleral icterus and moderate ascites. Laboratory test findings included the following: sodium 130 mEq/L, potassium 3.6 mEq/L, creatinine 1.0 mg/dL, albumin 3.0 g/dL, total bilirubin 2.7 mg/dL, ALT 75 U/L, and AST 62 U/L. Ascitic fluid analysis showed an albumin level of 1.2 g/dL and neutrophil count of 180/μL. In addition to a salt-restricted diet, which of the following is recommended to manage his ascites?

A. Diuretic therapy with a loop diuretic
B. Diuretic therapy with a loop diuretic and spironolactone
C. Fluid restriction
D. Serial large-volume paracentesis
E. Transjugular intrahepatic portosystemic shunt

669 A 28-year-old female healthcare worker presents following an accidental self-puncture with an 18-gauge hollow-bore needle that had been used to withdraw blood from an HCV-infected patient. At the time of presentation she tests negative for anti-HCV antibodies, HCV RNA is detectable at a level of 5690 IU/mL, and serum transaminase levels are normal. Which of the following choices is most appropriate for management of this case?

A. Administer HCV immune globulin, 1.5 mL intramuscularly.
B. Start interferon therapy, 3 million units subcutaneously t.i.w. for 24 weeks.
C. No further evaluation is necessary.
D. Start peginterferon, 180 μg/week, and ribavirin, 600 mg orally twice a day, for 48 weeks.
E. Recheck for viremia at 3 months.

670 Infections with transfusion-transmitted virus (TT virus; TTV) and SEN virus have which of the following characteristics in common?

A. Adverse effect on treatment for chronic HCV infection
B. Association with increased mortality
C. Both parenteral and fecal-oral transmission
D. Progression to chronic infection
E. Progression to end-stage liver disease

671 A 56-year-old woman is hospitalized for management of a toxic level of theophylline. While interviewing the patient, it is discovered that she takes a variety of herbal preparations. Which of the following is most likely to have contributed to her high theophylline level?

A. Dandelion root
B. Ginkgo biloba
C. Milk thistle
D. Saw palmetto
E. St. John's wort

672 A 65-year-old woman with a history of primary biliary cirrhosis (Child-Pugh class B, Model for End-stage Liver Disease [MELD] score of 12) presents with upper gastrointestinal hemorrhage. After she has been resuscitated she undergoes EGD, which reveals bleeding esophageal varices. Hemostasis is achieved using band ligation, but rebleeding occurs 6 hours later. On repeat EGD the bands placed previously are in place but there is brisk bleeding. More bands are applied and they control bleeding briefly, but rebleeding occurs again later that day. Which of the following is the most appropriate therapy for this patient at this time?

A. Distal splenorenal shunt
B. Endoscopic sclerotherapy
C. Repeat band ligation
D. Sengstaken-Blakemore tube placement
E. TIPS insertion

673 Which of the following is positively associated with sustained virologic response as a result of treatment for HCV infection?

A. African-American ethnicity
B. Body mass index of greater than 30
C. Biopsy-proven bridging fibrosis or cirrhosis
D. HCV genotype 2
E. Presence of steatosis on biopsy

674 A 66-year-old man with a history of ischemic heart disease undergoes liver function testing and the results indicate a combination of cholestatic and hepatocellular disease. Ultrasonography shows no abnormality. Liver biopsy reveals steatosis, portal acute and chronic inflammatory infiltrates, and central hyaline sclerosis. Which drug is most likely to have caused this patient's condition?

A. Amiodarone
B. Androgenic steroids
C. Methotrexate
D. Phenytoin
E. Pioglitazone

675 A 64-year-old man has a TIPS placed to manage ascites refractory to other treatments, and after shunt placement his portosystemic gradient decreases, from 18 mmHg to 10 mmHg. However, although he maintains his diuretic medication regimen and sodium-restricted diet, he continues to require high-volume paracentesis every 2 weeks. Which of the following is the most accurate method to assess TIPS patency?

A. Doppler ultrasound
B. Liver/spleen scan
C. MRI with gadolinium contrast
D. Serum ascites albumin gradient
E. TIPS venogram

676 Which of the following has been shown to increase the risk of hepatorenal syndrome in patients with cirrhosis and ascites?

A. Higher Child-Pugh class
B. Cirrhosis attributable to alcohol
C. Cirrhosis attributable to hepatitis C virus infection
D. Hyponatremia
E. Large liver size

677 Immediately following orthotopic liver transplantation, which constellation of findings most strongly indicates poor graft function?

A. Electrolyte imbalance and renal failure
B. Liver enzyme levels 10 times the upper limit of normal on the first postoperative day
C. Non–anion gap acidosis
D. Poor bile production and impaired cognition

678 Which of the following changes occurs in the sinusoids with the development of cirrhosis?

A. Passage of macromolecules across the sinusoidal walls is increased.
B. Subendothelial material becomes scanty.
C. The endothelial fenestrations increase in size and number.
D. Disse's spaces become widened with collagen.

679 A 55-year-old man presents with a variceal hemorrhage. After his condition has been stabilized he is referred to a liver transplant center, where a blood sample is analyzed to determine the cause of his cirrhosis. Which of the following genotypes would make the diagnosis of hereditary hemochromatosis most likely?

A. C282Y/C282Y
B. C282Y/wt
C. H63D/H63D
D. H63D/wt
E. wt/wt

680 A 42-year-old woman presents with a 3-week history of progressive fatigue, right upper quadrant discomfort, nausea, and jaundice. Her serum ALT level is 10 times the upper limit of normal. Presence of which of the following in a blood sample is most indicative of acute hepatitis B infection?

A. Anti-HBc IgG
B. Anti-HBc IgM
C. Anti-HBs
D. HBsAg

681 A 56-year-old man with hemophilia and AIDS presents to the emergency department with multiple red papular skin lesions, fever, hypotension, and elevated transaminase levels. On history, his only exposure to infectious agents was while cat-sitting recently for his uncle. The organism most likely causing this patient's condition is:

A. *Actinomyces* sp.
B. *Bartonella henselae*
C. *Listeria monocytogenes*
D. *Staphylococcus aureus*
E. *Yersinia* sp.

682 Which structure is involved in the transport to hepatocyte cytoplasm of mRNAs synthesized in hepatocyte nuclei?

A. Endoplasmic reticulum
B. Golgi complex
C. Lysosome
D. Nuclear pore complex
E. Peroxisome

683 A 45-year-old man is referred for evaluation of abnormal liver test results. He has a past medical history of dyslipidemia and hypertension. Physical examination reveals central obesity and a smooth, palpable liver edge. His serum aminotransaminase levels are twice the upper limit of normal with maintained hepatic synthetic function. Which of the following procedures is best able to differentiate between steatosis and steatohepatitis?

A. Computed tomography
B. Liver biopsy
C. Magnetic resonance imaging
D. Positron emission tomography
E. Ultrasonography

684 Match the liver cell type with its function:

1. Bile duct epithelial cell
2. Hepatic sinusoidal endothelial cell
3. Hepatic stellate cell
4. Kupffer cell

A. Activated to become myofibroblasts
B. Mediates uptake of conjugated bile salts
C. Removes particulate and foreign substances from portal blood
D. Selective barrier between blood and hepatocytes

685 An 18-year-old intravenous drug user who is known to be infected with HIV is admitted to the medical intensive care unit with jaundice, asterixis, confusion, and markedly elevated transaminase levels. A review of his medication list reveals that he was recently prescribed acyclovir by his primary care physician. Based on the histologic appearance of a liver biopsy specimen (see figure), the most likely diagnosis is:

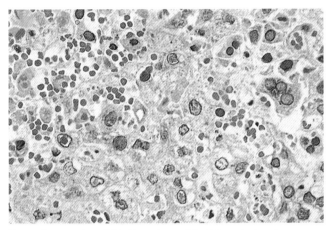

Figure for question **685**. (From Lucas SB: Other viral and infectious diseases and HIV-related liver disease. In MacSween RNM, Burt AD, Portmann BC, et al [eds]: Pathology of the Liver, 4th ed. London, Churchill Livingstone, 2001, p 366.)

A. Acyclovir toxicity
B. Hepatitis A virus infection
C. Hepatitis B virus infection
D. Herpes simplex virus infection
E. Tylenol toxicity

686 A 63-year-old man with HCV-related cirrhosis is noted on CT to have a patent periumbilical vein. Considering the mechanisms involved in portal hypertension, which of the following is likely to be present?

A. Decreased cardiac output
B. Increased mean arterial pressure
C. Peripheral vasoconstriction
D. Splanchnic vasodilation

687 A 23-year-old woman without known liver disease presents with increasing abdominal girth and right upper quadrant abdominal pain. A 10-cm mass is found in the right lobe of the liver. What is histologic evaluation of the mass likely to show?

A. Hepatocellular carcinoma, fibrolamellar histology
B. Hepatocellular carcinoma, standard histology
C. Lymphoma
D. Metastatic adenocarcinoma

688 Which of the following inflammatory conditions is most likely to lead to a pyogenic liver abscess?

A. Cholangitis/cholecystitis
B. Diverticulitis
C. Endocarditis
D. Inflammatory bowel disease
E. Perforated appendix

689 A 15-year-old boy with Wilson's disease has been taking penicillamine for 2 years. He had been feeling well until recently when he noticed weight gain, increasing abdominal girth, and peripheral edema. Urinalysis shows 3+ protein. What course of treatment is recommended?

A. Continue penicillamine; test for diabetes.
B. Discontinue penicillamine; re-challenge once symptoms resolve.
C. Continue penicillamine; start furosemide 40 mg orally each day.
D. Discontinue penicillamine; start trientine.
E. Decrease the dose of penicillamine; add zinc.

690 A 31-year-old woman with chronic HCV infection is pregnant and asks about the risk of transmitting HCV infection to her newborn. The most accurate estimate is:

A. 5%
B. 20%
C. 50%
D. 80%
E. 95%

691 A 43-year-old factory worker is brought to the emergency department with nausea, vomiting, diarrhea, and jaundice. Laboratory tests reveal direct hyperbilirubinemia, serum transaminase levels of 20 times the upper limits of normal, and evidence of renal failure. A liver biopsy shows significant steatosis but there is no evidence of zone 3 necrosis. This patient's condition is most likely due to which of the following?

A. Acetaminophen
B. *Amanita phylloides*
C. Carbon tetrachloride
D. Phosphorus

692 A 23-year-old white woman in whom acute hepatitis A virus infection was diagnosed approximately 1 month ago complains of continued jaundice and new symptoms of dark urine and fatigue. She denies fever or abdominal pain. Her laboratory test results are positive for

HAV IgM, negative for HBsAg, and negative for HCV antibody. A right upper quadrant ultrasound shows a normal biliary tree and no gallstones. The best course of action at this time is:

A. Begin broad-spectrum antibiotics.
B. Continue symptomatic care.
C. Schedule emergency ERCP.
D. Schedule MRCP of the abdomen and pelvis.

693 A 67-year-old man is found to have significantly abnormal liver function test results following surgery to repair an abdominal aortic aneurysm. During the surgery, he had received 6 units of packed red blood cells and an additional 2 units of his own blood salvaged through the "cell saver" device. He is still intubated and sedated but hemodynamically stable. His urine output is less than 20 mL/hour. The results of serologic tests are most likely to support a diagnosis of:

A. Acute biliary obstruction
B. Acute viral hepatitis
C. Autoimmune hepatitis
D. Drug hepatotoxicity
E. Ischemic hepatitis

694 A drug in phase II trials caused elevations of ALT to more than eight times the upper limit of normal in 2 of 2500 subjects who received the drug. According to "Hy's rule," this finding during the trial indicates that during the marketing phase, one case of acute liver failure would be expected per every:

A. 2500 persons receiving the drug
B. 12,500 persons receiving the drug
C. 50,000 persons receiving the drug
D. 100,000 persons receiving the drug
E. 1,000,000 persons receiving the drug

695 A 54-year-old man with a history of end-stage liver disease secondary to alpha-1-antitrypsin deficiency presents with upper gastrointestinal hemorrhage. Volume resuscitation and intravenous octreotide are started. On upper endoscopy, active bleeding in the esophagus impedes visibility. This condition should be managed by?

A. Band ligation of the esophagus every 2 cm in a spiral pattern
B. Circumferential band ligation of the lower esophagus
C. Endoscopic sclerotherapy
D. Withdrawal of the endoscope and esophageal balloon tamponade
E. Withdrawal of the endoscope and immediate placement of a TIPS

696 A 46-year-old man is brought to the emergency department with fever and sharp, diffuse abdominal pain. On physical exam he appears to be in moderate distress. His temperature is 39°C, pulse is 90 beats/minute, and blood pressure is 110/78 mmHg. His abdomen is distended and diffusely tender without rebound or guarding. An abdominal ultrasound reveals a large amount of ascites fluid and paracentesis is performed. Which of the following results for total protein, glucose, and lactic dehydrogenase (LDH) is consistent with a diagnosis of secondary bacterial peritonitis?

A. Total protein 0.6 g/dL, glucose 120 mg/dL, LDH 300 U/L
B. Total protein 0.6 g/dL, glucose 20 mg/dL, LDH 100 U/L
C. Total protein 1.0 g/dL, glucose 100 mg/dL, LDH 150 U/L
D. Total protein 2.0 g/dL, glucose 100 mg/dL, LDH 150 U/L
E. Total protein 2.0 g/dL, glucose 20 mg/dL, LDH 300 U/L

697 The best medical treatment for schistosomiasis is:

A. Albendazole
B. Chloroquine
C. Mebendazole
D. Metronidazole
E. Praziquantel

698 Which of the following is the most appropriate treatment for nonalcoholic fatty liver disease?

A. Antioxidant drug therapy
B. Bariatric surgery for morbid obesity
C. Iron reduction therapy
D. Treatment of the underlying disorder

699 A 49-year-old woman presents with increasing abdominal girth and painful hepatomegaly. The hepatic venous system appears to be patent, but a liver biopsy specimen shows evidence of hepatic veno-occlusive disease. Which of the following herbal therapies has most likely caused liver disease in this case?

A. Chaparral *(Larrea tridentata)*
B. Comfrey *(Symphytum officinale)*
C. Germander *(Teucrium chamaedrys)*
D. Kava kava *(Piper methysticum)*
E. Pennyroyal *(Hedeoma pulegioides)*

700 A 57-year-old man with chronic ulcerative colitis complains of several weeks of lassitude, low-grade fever, and right upper quadrant abdominal discomfort and more recent onset of jaundice. On examination he is found to have mild temporal wasting, scleral icterus, and tenderness in the right upper quadrant without rebound. Ultrasonography reveals a misshapen liver but there is no ductal dilatation. Which of the

following is the most likely cause of this patient's symptoms?

A. Cholangiocarcinoma
B. Choledochocele
C. Gallbladder carcinoma
D. Hepatic adenoma
E. Hepatocellular carcinoma

701 Which of the following cutaneous porphyrias is most likely to present with severe Coombs-negative hemolytic anemia?

A. Congenital erythropoietic porphyria
B. Erythropoietic protoporphyria
C. Hepatoerythropoietic porphyria
D. Porphyria cutanea tarda

702 A 30-year-old patient with Wilson disease has been stable on penicillamine therapy for many years. She now reports that she is pregnant. Which of the following courses of action is recommended?

A. Do not change her medication.
B. Discontinue penicillamine; do not start any new medications.
C. Inform her that penicillamine is not associated with birth defects.
D. Discontinue penicillamine; start oral zinc.
E. Discontinue penicillamine; start trientine.

703 A 65-year-old woman has had pruritus, fever, and weight loss for 3 weeks. She does not have icterus but there is bilateral temporal wasting and a palpable, smooth liver edge. Her bilirubin level and aminotransaminase levels are normal but alkaline phosphatase is four times the upper limit of normal and the level of gamma glutamyltransferase is elevated. Ultrasonography shows an echogenic liver without ductal dilatation. On the basis of these findings, which of the following is the most likely diagnosis?

A. Extrahepatic biliary obstruction
B. Granulomatous hepatitis
C. Nonalcoholic fatty liver disease
D. Paget's disease of bone
E. Renal cell carcinoma

704 A 63-year-old woman with a 30-year history of chronic HCV infection presents with leg swelling and purpura consisting of round, 1- to 3-mm palpable lesions that coalesce to form plaques in some areas. Which of the following is the most important to test for?

A. Anti-glomerular basement membrane antibody
B. Antineutrophil cytoplasmic antibody
C. Anti-nuclear antibody
D. Rheumatoid factor
E. Serum cryoglobulin

705 A 28-year-old Hispanic man presents with a 2-week history of abdominal pain, fever, malaise, and myalgias. He is found to have a fluid-filled abscess in his liver. The radiologist who aspirated the fluid for diagnostic purposes describes the aspirate as reddish brown and pasty. Trophozoites are identified on microscopic examination. This patient most likely has an infection caused by:

A. *Bacteroides fragilis*
B. *Echinococcus* sp.
C. *Entamoeba histolytica*
D. *Escherichia coli*
E. *Strongyloides* sp.

706 A 30-year-old woman is diagnosed with acute HEV infection. This condition is most likely to progress to:

A. Resolution; this is an acute, self-limited disease
B. Chronic hepatitis
C. Fulminant hepatic failure
D. Cirrhosis
E. Hepatocellular cancer

707 A 44-year-old American man has active upper gastrointestinal hemorrhage, scleral icterus, gynecomastia, spider angiomata, and splenomegaly. Which of the following medications should be prescribed first?

A. Nitroglycerine
B. Octreotide
C. Propranolol
D. Terlipressin
E. Losartin

708 A 57-year-old immigrant from Pakistan is found to have acute hepatitis with antibody against hepatitis E virus. How did he most likely become infected?

A. Blood transfusion
B. Consumption of contaminated drinking water
C. Consumption of raw pork
D. Exposure to an infected child
E. Sexual transmission

709 Which of the following agents is the most likely to cause hepatotoxicity?

A. Amoxicillin/clavulanic acid
B. Ibuprofen
C. Isoniazid
D. Tamoxifen
E. Troglitazone

710 Women have greater susceptibility than men to the injurious effects of alcohol on the liver. Risk factors that predispose to this heightened susceptibility in women include which of the following?

A. Increased endotoxemia and lipid peroxidation
B. Lower body mass index
C. Less gastric mucosal secretion of alcohol dehydrogenase
D. Slower alcohol metabolism

711 In which of the following patients with elevated liver enzymes would a diagnosis of nonalcoholic fatty liver disease be most likely, excluding other causes?

A. A 40-year-old female patient with insulin resistance
B. A 55-year-old male patient with hypertension
C. A 65-year-old male patient who consumes 15 grams of alcohol per day
D. A 70-year-old female patient with a BMI of 28

712 A 63-year-old woman with alcohol-related cirrhosis, Child-Pugh class A, has been abstinent from alcohol for 10 years. She presents with variceal hemorrhage, which is controlled by band ligation. She is started on a beta blocker medication that provides adequate reduction in heart rate, but rebleeding occurs 4 weeks later. Band ligation is repeated and an oral nitrate is added to her medication regimen. At this time, her hepatic venous pressure gradient (HVPG) is less than 12 mmHg. Three days later, variceal bleeding recurs. The most appropriate action at this time is?

A. Place a distal splenorenal shunt
B. Perform esophageal balloon tamponade
C. Increase her dose of beta blockers
D. Place a TIPS

713 A 43-year-old woman has the following laboratory test results:

Serum bilirubin:
Total	4.4 mg/dL
Direct	0.4 mg/dL

Serum alkaline phosphatase: 110 U/L

Serum aminotransaminase:
AST	23 U/L
ALT	26 U/L

The most likely diagnosis is:

A. Chronic hepatitis C virus infection
B. Dubin-Johnson syndrome
C. Hemolytic anemia
D. Primary biliary cirrhosis
E. Primary sclerosing cholangitis

714 A 36-year-old woman has recurrent bouts of severe abdominal pain that have defied diagnosis. No abnormalities have been discovered by radiologic or endoscopic procedures. Finally, serum and fecal porphyrin tests are ordered. The results indicate a diagnosis of:

A. Erythropoietic protoporphyria
B. Hepatoerythropoietic porphyria
C. Porphyria cutanea tarda
D. Variegate coproporphyria

715 A right upper quadrant ultrasound in a patient with echinococcosis would most likely show:

A. A central scar with a thickened wall
B. An enhancing dominant lesion with multiple satellite lesions
C. Hypodense cysts with an air-fluid level
D. A single isodense, nonseptated cyst
E. Ring-like calcifications, intracystic septations, and daughter cysts

716 Which of the following is most infective?

A. HBV
B. HCV
C. HIV

717 A 25-year-old Chinese woman presents for a routine evaluation. The results of a test for hepatitis B virus surface antigen are positive despite normal results of liver function tests. How did this patient most likely acquire chronic HBV infection?

A. Horizontal transmission
B. Parenteral transmission
C. Sexual transmission
D. Vertical transmission

718 Which of the following is synthesized primarily outside the liver?

A. Apolipoproteins
B. Fatty acids
C. 3-Hydroxy-3-methyl-glutaryl-coenzyme A (HMG-CoA) reductase
D. Lipoprotein lipase

719 Which hepatic structure allows a difference in concentration of solutes between the cytoplasm and bile canaliculus?

A. Anchoring junction
B. Gap junction
C. Lipid rafts
D. Tight junction

720 A 37-year-old woman presents with blisters and scarring on the backs of both hands. Porphyria cutanea tarda is diagnosed. Which of the following is most appropriate for management of this condition?

A. Chloroquine
B. Fasting during an outbreak
C. Hematin infusion
D. Phlebotomy
E. Ultraviolet (UV) light therapy

721 A 31-year-old woman with chronic hepatitis B virus infection becomes pregnant. A test for hepatitis e antigen is positive. Which is the most accurate estimate of the risk of HBV infection in her newborn child?

A. 5%
B. 15%
C. 50%
D. 75%
E. 90%

722 The progression of alcohol-related liver disease is most profoundly influenced by coexistent:

A. Advanced age
B. Chronic hepatitis C virus infection
C. Diabetes mellitus and insulin sensitivity
D. Obesity and smoking

723 Which of the following two 20-year-old men (patient A or patient B) exposed to HBV is more likely to become a chronic carrier of HBV?

A. Patient A, whose mother has chronic HBV
B. Patient B, who acquired HBV via intravenous drug use at the age of 15

724 A 17-year-old woman has abnormal serum aminotransaminase levels and evaluation of a liver biopsy specimen shows the presence of PAS-positive, diastase-resistant periportal globules. Serologic evaluation is likely to show the presence of which of the following protease inhibitor (Pi) genotypes (allelic representations)?

A. PiMM
B. PiMZ
C. PiSS
D. PiSZ
E. PiZZ

725 A 31-year-old woman with chronic hepatitis B virus infection becomes pregnant. Her serum tests negative for hepatitis e antigen. Which of the following is the most accurate estimate of the risk of HBV infection in her newborn child?

A. 5%
B. 15%
C. 50%
D. 75%
E. 90%

726 Alcoholic liver disease develops in women after a shorter duration of alcohol use, and with lower daily intake of alcohol, than in men. Which of the following quantities and duration of alcohol use puts patients at risk for alcohol-induced cirrhosis?

A. 10 grams per day in women; more than 40 grams per day in men, for at least 20 years
B. 20 to 40 grams per day in women; 40 to 80 grams per day in men, for at least 10 years
C. 20 to 40 grams per day in women; 40 to 80 grams per day in men, for more than 20 years
D. 40 to 60 grams per day in women; 80 to 100 grams per day in men, for at least 10 years

727 Which of the following is the most accurate estimate of the duration of chronic HBV infection seen prior to the development of hepatocellular carcinoma?

A. 2 years
B. 5 years
C. 10 years
D. 25 years

728 Which of the following is true regarding the surface anatomy of the liver?

A. At the porta hepatis, the portal vein is anterior to the hepatic artery.
B. The caudate lobe of the liver is posterior to the transverse fissure.
C. The falciform ligament contains the obliterated umbilical artery.
D. All surfaces of the liver lie within the peritoneum.

729 Drug-mediated hepatotoxicity that results in formation of intracellular collagen is likely related to activation of which hepatic cell type?

A. Endothelial cells
B. Hepatocytes
C. Kupffer cells
D. Stellate cells

730 A 34-year-old woman presents for further evaluation of abdominal pain and abnormal liver test results. Her primary care physician sends the results of upper endoscopy, which were normal, and right upper quadrant ultrasound, which showed cholelithiasis without gallbladder wall thickening, pericholecystic fluid, or ductal dilatation. Her laboratory test results show an albumin level of 4.0 g/dL, bilirubin 1.0 mg/dL, alkaline phosphatase 320 U/L, AST 65 U/L, ALT 72 U/L, antimitochondrial antibody (AMA) 1 : 2560, antinuclear antibody (ANA) 1 : 20, HCV antibody negative, antibody to hepatitis B virus core antigen (anti-HBc) negative, hepatitis B virus surface antigen (HBsAg) negative, and antibody to hepatitis B virus surface antigen (anti-HBs) positive. Which is the most likely diagnosis?

A. Autoimmune hepatitis
B. Cholelithiasis
C. Hepatitis B virus infection
D. Hepatitis C virus infection
E. Primary biliary cirrhosis

731 A 46-year-old man taking isoniazid prophylactically is noted to have increased serum levels of aminotransaminases and bilirubin. Which of the following courses of action will be most effective?

A. Start cholestyramine.
B. Discontinue isoniazid.
C. Start glucocorticoids.
D. Start N-acetylcysteine.
E. Start ursodeoxycholic acid.

732 A 67-year-old man presents to the hospital with variceal hemorrhage. In deciding how to control the hemorrhage, the endoscopist should be aware of which of the following possible complications of sclerotherapy that is not seen with band ligation?

A. Elevation of hepatic venous pressure gradient
B. Esophageal perforation
C. Esophageal stricture
D. Esophageal ulceration

733 A 44-year-old woman with HCV cirrhosis and ascites reports at a routine follow-up visit that she feels good and has been following her sodium-restricted (2 grams/day) diet and her diuretic regimen of spironolactone 200 mg daily and furosemide 80 mg daily. The only significant finding on her physical exam is that she has gained 8 pounds since her last visit. A blood sample analyzed the same day as the visit shows a sodium level of 128 mEq/dL, potassium of 3.9 mEq/dL, and creatinine of 0.7 mg/dL, and a urine sample shows a sodium/potassium ratio of 0.8. What should be done to address this patient's weight gain?

A. Admit for intravenous administration of furosemide.
B. Further restrict sodium intake to 500 mg/day.
C. Educate the patient about how to follow a low-sodium diet.
D. Increase her dosage of spironolactone.
E. Increase her dosages of spironolactone and furosemide.

734 Hepatitis C virus infection recurs following liver transplantation in all patients who have HCV infection prior to transplantation. Graft failure due to hepatitis C virus infection may occur following transplantation. Most rapid progression to graft failure is seen in patients with:

A. Biochemical and histologic evidence of cholestasis
B. Concurrent rejection
C. A high pretransplantation viral load
D. Histologic evidence of hepatitis and fibrosis

735 A 62-year-old man with alcoholic cirrhosis has become progressively lethargic over the past few days. On physical exam he is somnolent but oriented and able to follow commands. He has asterixis and sluggish reflexes but no fever, jaundice, or ascites. Which of the following statements regarding ammonia (NH$_3$) measurements and hepatic encephalopathy (HE) is *true*?

A. The blood level of NH$_3$ is more accurately measured in a sample of arterial than in a sample of venous blood.
B. A normal serum NH$_3$ level excludes the diagnosis of HE.
C. Serial measurement of NH$_3$ levels are indicated to assess response to treatment.
D. The serum NH$_3$ level correlates poorly with the severity of HE.

736 A 55-year-old woman with HCV-induced cirrhosis is noted on screening EGD to have 4- to 5-mm esophageal varices but no stigmata of recent hemorrhage. In addition, she has no clinical signs or symptoms of blood loss. Which of the following is the most appropriate course of action for this patient?

A. Perform band ligation of the esophageal varices.
B. Administer octreotide intravenously.
C. Begin nonselective beta blocker therapy.
D. Begin oral nitrate therapy.
E. Perform sclerotherapy of varices.

737 Which of the following HCV genotypes has increased in incidence since 1995?

A. Genotype 1a
B. Genotype 1b
C. Genotype 2
D. Genotype 4

738 A 55-year-old woman presents with fatigue and persistently abnormal aminotransaminase levels. The results of a right upper quadrant ultrasound are normal. She has no abdominal pain, weight loss, or diarrhea. Blood tests for evidence of viral infection are negative. She was recently diagnosed with Grave's disease. Her laboratory tests show an ANA titer of 1:260, ferritin level of 200 ng/mL, alpha-1 anti-trypsin phenotype of MM, normal ceruloplasmin level, and test for AMA negative. Which of the following serologic tests would confirm the diagnosis?

A. Anti-Ro, Anti-La
B. Anti-smooth muscle antibody
C. Double-stranded DNA
D. HFE genotype
E. Liver/kidney microsome type 1 antibody

739 A 55-year-old man presents with new onset of increasing abdominal girth that is found to be due to ascites. The ascites fluid has a protein level of 2.6 g/dL and an albumin level of 2.1 g/dL. A simultaneously obtained serum sample has an albumin level of 3.4 g/dL. Which of the following is the most likely cause of ascites in this case?

A. Bowel obstruction
B. Cardiac disease
C. Nephrotic syndrome
D. Pancreatic disease
E. Peritoneal carcinomatosis

740 A 41-year-old woman undergoing ultrasound for infertility evaluation is noted to have a 3-cm hyperechoic mass in the left lobe of her liver. She is otherwise well and has no risk factors for or physical examination findings consistent with chronic liver disease. Liver function tests and serum alpha-fetoprotein are normal. Which is the most appropriate next step in care of this patient?

A. Hepatic artery embolization
B. Contrast-enhanced MRI
C. No further treatment or testing
D. Radiologic-guided biopsy of the mass
E. Surgical resection of the mass

741 Which of the following patients with acute alcoholic hepatitis would be most appropriately treated with glucocorticoids to reduce short-term mortality?

A. A 40-year-old man with jaundice, encephalopathy, severe coagulopathy, and renal failure
B. A 40-year-old woman with jaundice and encephalopathy but with no evidence of infection, renal failure, or gastrointestinal bleeding
C. A 60-year-old man with mild jaundice but with no coagulopathy, infection, renal failure, or encephalopathy
D. None; glucocorticoids have not been shown to reduce short-term mortality in patients with alcoholic hepatitis

742 Worldwide, the highest rate of reported disease due to hepatitis A virus infection is among:

A. Children 5 to 14 years old
B. Healthy adults 18 to 65 years old
C. Homosexual men of any age
D. Intravenous drug users of any age

743 Treating bleeding disorders due to cirrhosis with desmopressin leads to:

A. Decreased bleeding time by increased mobilization of platelets from the spleen
B. Decreased bleeding time by increasing factor VIII and von Willebrand's factor
C. Decreased partial thromboplastin time by increasing factor VIII and von Willebrand's factor
D. Decreased prothrombin time by increasing factor VII

744 A 55-year-old man with a history of alcohol-induced cirrhosis has been abstinent form alcohol for 3 years. He has been vaccinated against hepatitis A and hepatitis B, has twice yearly alpha fetoprotein determinations and regular cross-sectional images of the liver. Which of the following is most important in determining his prognosis?

A. Hepatic venous pressure gradient
B. Liver size on CT or MRI
C. Serum albumin level
D. Size of esophageal varices

ANSWERS

587 **E.** (S&F, ch84)

There are approximately 100 poisonous varieties of mushrooms among the more than 5000 known species of mushrooms, and more than 8000 mushroom poisonings were reported in the United States in 2001. More than 90% of cases of fatal poisonings are caused by *Amanita phylloides* ("death cap") or *A. verna* ("destroying angel"), which are found in the Pacific northwest and eastern parts of the country. A fatal outcome can follow ingestion of a single 50-g (2-oz) mushroom; the toxin is one of the most potent and lethal in nature. Alpha amatoxin is thermostable, can resist drying for years, and is not inactivated by cooking. Rapidly absorbed via the gastrointestinal tract, the amatoxin reaches hepatocytes via the enterohepatic circulation and inhibits production of mRNA and protein synthesis, leading in turn to cell necrosis.

588 **E.** (S&F, ch83)

Valproic acid has been associated with severe hepatotoxicity. Children are most at risk, particularly those younger than 3 years old. Cases in adults have been described rarely. Concomitant administration of other antiepileptic drugs is another predisposing factor, with the frequency of liver injury increasing in proportion to the number of agents ingested. The frequency of valproic acid hepatotoxicity varies from 1 per 500 high-risk persons exposed to 1 per 37,000 low-risk persons. Another risk factor is a family history of mitochondrial enzyme deficiencies (particularly those in the urea cycle or involved in long-chain fatty acid transport), Reye's syndrome, or a sibling affected by valproate hepatotoxicity.

589 **C.** (S&F, ch88)

The appropriate therapy for secondary bacterial peritonitis is surgical intervention plus approximately 2 weeks of intravenous (IV) administration of a cephalosporin (e.g., cefotaxime, 2 grams every 8 hours) plus an antibiotic with activity against anaerobic organisms (e.g., metronidazole).

590 **E.** (S&F, ch70)

It is important to note that ALT is relatively liver-specific, whereas AST is found in skeletal and cardiac muscle, kidney, brain, pancreas, and blood cells, in addition to hepatocytes. Therefore, the suspicion that an isolated elevation in AST is due to a liver condition should be confirmed by measuring the level of ALT, and an isolated or disproportionate elevation of the AST concentration should prompt a search for an extrahepatic source, in particular myocardial or skeletal muscle injury. For example, vigorous physical activity, such as long-distance running or weight lifting, may increase the serum AST level several fold. However, in rare cases, elevation of both AST and ALT may be due to muscle disease or injury (e.g., muscular dystrophy, myositis).

591 **D.** (S&F, ch83)

Nitrofurantoin, a synthetic furan-based compound, is a urinary antiseptic with a range of uncommon adverse effects. Liver test results are often noted to be abnormal during the first few weeks of drug administration but the abnormalities are of doubtful importance. The range of liver disease associated with nitrofurantoin includes acute hepatitis, in some cases with features of cholestasis; hepatic granulomas; chronic hepatitis with autoimmune phenomena; acute liver failure; and cirrhosis. Causality has been proven by drug rechallenge. There is no relationship between dose of nitrofurantoin and severity or type of adverse effects on the liver; cases of liver disease have even been described after ingestion of milk from a nitrofurantoin-treated cow. The frequency of nitrofurantoin hepatic injury ranges from 0.3 to 3 cases per 100,000 exposed persons, and it increases with age, particularly after age 64 years. Two thirds of acute cases occur in women, and the female:male gender ratio for chronic hepatitis due to nitrofurantoin is 8:1.

592 **C.** (S&F, ch92)

Angiotensin-converting enzyme inhibitors may exacerbate hyperkalemia, to which the liver transplant recipient may be predisposed as a side effects of calcineurin-inhibitor therapy. Diltiazem may interfere with calcineurin-inhibitor drug metabolism, leading to increased levels of calcineurin-inhibitor drugs. A reduction in the doses of immunosuppressant drugs administered after transplantation usually does not significantly affect hypertension, so dosage reduction should not be regarded as an appropriate initial approach to treating systemic hypertension after liver transplantation.

593 **E.** (S&F, ch71)

Once a proband with HFE-related HH has been identified and therapy initiated, there is still a responsibility to the patient's family. If the spouse of a patient who is homozygotic for C282Y is heterozygotic for C282Y, there is a 50% chance that their offspring will be homozygous for C282Y. Despite concerns about discrimination arising from genetic testing, HFE mutation analysis in children can eliminate the need for subsequent serum iron testing if the child is found *not* to have a genotype of C282Y/C282Y or C282Y/H63D, although children who are C282Y homozygotes or compound heterozygotes should have serum ferritin levels measured yearly and undergo phlebotomy if the ferritin level is elevated.

594 **D.** (S&F, ch82)

Choice **A** lists typical findings in cases of autoimmune hepatitis, choice **B** lists findings in cases of primary biliary cirrhosis, choice **C** lists findings in cases of alpha-1-antitrypsin deficiency, and choice **E** lists typical findings in cases of chronic hepatitis C virus infection. This patient is most likely, given her demographic profile, to have NAFLD. Choice **D** lists typical findings in cases of NAFLD.

595 **A.** (S&F, ch75)

The risk of chronicity after acute HBV infection is low in immunocompetent adults. The risk of chronic infection is greatly increased in patients in whom it is difficult to recognize and eradicate

viral infection (e.g., patients on chronic hemodialysis, those on immunosuppressant therapy following solid organ transplantation, and those receiving cancer chemotherapy). Patients with concomitant HIV infection are also at significant risk of developing chronic infection (20% to 30% of such patients continue to test positive for HBsAg after resolution of the acute infection). The risk of chronicity in patients who acquire the infection as neonates is extremely high (up to 90%), presumably because neonates have an immature immune system; it has been proposed that the fetal immune system becomes tolerant of HBV as a result of exposure in utero to viral proteins transmitted transplacentally. Children younger than age 6 years have a lower yet nevertheless significant risk of chronic infection (approximately 30%).

596 **B.** (S&F, ch82)

There is no need for further testing to establish the diagnosis, and no pharmacologic intervention is effective in cases of nonalcoholic fatty liver disease (NAFLD). In these cases, biopsy is performed to stage the disease and help establish a prognosis.

597 **B.** (S&F, ch69)

The liver is the main storage site for glycogen to supply glucose-dependent organs in the body (erythrocytes, retina, and renal medulla) and the brain, a preferential user of glucose. By gluconeogenesis, the liver is able to produce up to 240 mg of glucose a day, which is approximately twice the metabolic needs of the retina, red blood cells, and brain. The liver can store as much as a 2-day supply of glucose in the form of glycogen, before gluconeogenesis occurs using either the glucose itself or the glucose precursor lactate.

598 **A.** (S&F, ch83)

Encephalopathy is a defining criterion for acute liver failure. The severity of encephalopathy can range from subtle changes in affect, insomnia, and difficulties with concentration (stage 1); to drowsiness, disorientation, and confusion (stage 2); to marked somnolence and incoherence (stage 3); to frank coma (stage 4). The pathophysiologic mechanisms underlying encephalopathy associated with acute liver failure (ALF) are multifactorial. Many features of ALF, including hypoglycemia, sepsis, hypoxemia, occult seizures, and cerebral edema, can contribute to neurologic abnormalities. Notably, neurologic conditions are the reason for excluding approximately 25% of patients with ALF from liver transplantation and for the deaths of more than 20% of patients who have undergone liver transplantation.

599 **A.** (S&F, ch92)

Administration of a nucleoside/nucleotide analogue in combination with hepatitis B immune globulin has improved the outcome of liver transplantation in patients with liver disease due to hepatitis B virus infection. When this regimen is not followed, recurrent HBV infection is the rule and the graft is often lost as a result. Interferons are contraindicated in patients with decompensated HBV infection, because in these patients interferons can lead to elevations in aminotransaminase levels, loss of hepatocellular mass, and acute worsening of hepatic synthetic function.

600 **E.** (S&F, ch76)

The best test is liver biopsy because, although the prognostic implications of specific histologic findings are not clear, mild inflammation and negligible fibrosis are associated with a low risk of progression to cirrhosis. In contrast, severe inflammatory activity, necrosis, and advanced fibrosis are likely to lead to cirrhosis with time. Measurement of serum HCV RNA levels (viral load) may be useful in assessing the effectiveness of antiviral therapy and in evaluating the likelihood of a treatment response, but not in estimating overall prognosis.

601 **D.** (S&F, ch84)

In the past, exposure to vinyl chloride monomer (VCM) occurred in polymerization plants where vinyl chloride was heated to form polyvinyl chloride (PVC) in the manufacture of plastics. VCM is carcinogenic. Angiosarcoma develops after a mean latency of 25 years after exposure; the risk is related to the duration and extent of contact. Ingestion of alcohol concurrent with exposure appears to enhance the hepatocarcinogenicity of VCM in rodents and possibly in man, by inducing CYP2E1, which converts VCM to a toxic or carcinogenic metabolite (e.g., 2-chloroethylene oxide). A history of vinyl chloride exposure was found in 15% to 25% of all individuals in whom hepatic angiosarcoma was reported in the late 1970s, and strict controls on occupational exposure to vinyl chloride, instituted in 1974, have resulted in a marked decrease in the frequency of angiosarcoma.

602 **D.** (S&F, ch80)

Budd-Chiari syndrome is characterized by hepatic venous outflow obstruction. Classic Budd-Chiari syndrome is due to thrombosis of one or more hepatic veins at their opening into the inferior vena cava, which results in hepatomegaly, pain, ascites, and impaired hepatic function. Oral contraceptive use increases the risk of Budd-Chiari syndrome by more than 2-fold.

603 **E.** (S&F, ch88)

This patient has a serum-ascites albumin gradient (SAAG) of less than 1.1, which is not consistent with choices **A**, **B**, or **D**. Also the predominance of mononuclear cells in the differential count provides a clue to the diagnosis of tuberculous peritonitis or peritoneal carcinomatosis. There is nothing in the history or physical examination to suggest malignancy.

604 **A.** (S&F, ch92)

Renal toxicity is in an unfortunate and very common adverse effect of using a calcineurin-inhibitor drug for immunosuppression.

605 **A.** (S&F, ch78)

Epstein-Barr virus (EBV) infection is common and has a wide range of clinical presentations. Most affected infants or children are asymptomatic or have mild, nonspecific complaints, whereas adolescents and adults typically present with the triad of pharyngitis, fever, and lymphadenopathy. Although usually subclinical, liver abnormalities are nearly universal in patients with EBV mononucleosis and range from mild, self-limited elevations in levels of serum aminotransaminases to, rarely, fulminant and even fatal hepatitis.

606 **C.** (S&F, ch85)

Preferred treatment regimens for autoimmune hepatitis (AIH) include combination therapy and single-drug therapy. Prednisone alone or at lower doses but in combination with azathioprine induces clinical, biochemical, and histologic remission in 65% of patients within 3 years. The average treatment duration is 22 months. Single-drug therapy often consists of prednisone at a starting dose of 60 mg/day for 1 week, followed by slowly tapering doses. Combination therapy consists of prednisone at a starting dose of 30 mg/ day for 1 week, followed by slowly tapering doses of prednisone with concomitant administration of azathioprine, starting at 50 mg/day.

607 **E.** (S&F, ch82)

A variety of noninvasive scoring methods have been developed to predict the likelihood that NAFLD will progress. Risk factors for progression include older age, presence of diabetes mellitus, AST/ALT greater than 1, BMI > 28 kg/m^2, and triglycerides > 1.7 mmol/L.

608 **C.** (S&F, ch82)

Findings of inflammation and fibrosis on evaluation of a liver biopsy specimen is the only factor found in reproducible studies to be associated with progression of NAFLD to advanced disease.

609 **C.** (S&F, ch71)

Most patients with symptomatic hemochromatosis are between 40 and 50 years of age at the time of diagnosis. Although the defective gene is equally distributed between men and women, men have predominated in most clinical series. When patients present with symptoms, the most common symptoms are weakness, lethargy, arthralgias, abdominal pain, loss of libido, and impotence. Physical findings include hepatomegaly, splenomegaly, ascites, edema, and jaundice. Diabetes is typically not seen in the absence of cirrhosis. The bronze or slate gray skin pigmentation of hereditary hemochromatosis is often a subtle finding. Cardiomyopathy, atrial and ventricular dysrhythmias, and congestive heart failure can occur.

610 **D.** (S&F, ch76)

After 12 weeks (3 months) of treatment for HCV infection, it is useful to measure the HCV RNA level. If, as in this case, there has been less than a 2-log reduction in viral load, it is highly unlikely that the patient will have a sustained response to antiviral therapy and therapy should be discontinued.

611 **D.** (S&F, ch78)

GBV-C (hepatitis G virus) is a positive-strand RNA virus. GBV-C is found worldwide and is present in about 20% of HCV-infected persons. GBV-C infection does not appear to cause liver disease or any other disorder. In addition it does not appear to modulate the course or response to treatment of chronic HCV or HBV infection. GBV-C infection also does not affect the outcome of liver transplantation: Although liver transplant recipients have high rates of GBV-C infection, the outcome of transplantation is unaffected by current or past infection by GBV-C.

612 **E.** (S&F, ch84)

Between 25% and 75% of patients undergoing surgery experience postoperative hepatic dysfunction, ranging from mild elevations in serum levels of liver enzymes to hepatic failure. Drugs that may cause hepatoxicity in this setting include antibiotics (e.g., erythromycin, amoxicillin-clavulanate, and sulfamethoxazole-trimethoprim) and the halogenated anesthetics; most produce injury by causing a hypersensitivity reaction that becomes evident within 1 to 2 weeks of administration. Postoperative cholestasis is characterized by a short-latency elevation in the level of indirect bilirubin, lack of rash or eosinophilia, and assured recovery.

613 **C.** (S&F, ch85)

A histologic hallmark of autoimmune hepatitis (AIH) is interface hepatitis, which is characterized by disruption of the portal tract by a lymphoplasmacytic infiltrate. Typically, lobular hepatitis (mononuclear inflammatory cells line the sinusoidal spaces) coexists with interface hepatitis and it may be pronounced during an acute onset or during relapse after treatment withdrawal. Overall, histologic features are similar between symptomatic and asymptomatic patients, and both groups respond well to administration of glucocorticoid agents.

614 **A.** (S&F, ch86)

The initial lesion found on liver biopsy of a patient with primary biliary cirrhosis (PBC) is damage to epithelial cells in the small bile ducts. The most important and only diagnostic clue in many cases is ductopenia (defined as the absence of interlobular bile ducts in more than 50% of the portal tract). The florid duct lesion, in which the epithelium of the interlobular and segmental bile ducts degenerates segmentally with formation of poorly defined, noncaseating, epithelioid granulomas, is nearly diagnostic of PBC, although this lesion is found in a relatively small proportion of patients, mainly those with early-stage disease. According to the two most popular histologic staging systems (those proposed by Ludwig and Scheuer), disease is classified into four stages. Both systems describe pathologic changes beginning initially in the portal areas surrounding the bile ducts and culminating in cirrhosis.

615 **D.** (S&F, ch88)

Whereas mycobacterial culture of ascitic fluid with optimal processing has a sensitivity rate of approximately 50%, laparoscopy with histologic evaluation and culture of peritoneal biopsy specimens has a sensitivity rate of approximately 100% in detecting tuberculous peritonitis. In the United States, where more than 50% of patients with tuberculous peritonitis have underlying cirrhosis, the adenosine deaminase level has been found to be too insensitive for the diagnosis of tuberculous peritonitis.

616 **D.** (S&F, ch89)

Worsening renal function in a patient with cirrhosis and ascites can be the harbinger of hepatorenal syndrome. However, this diagnosis can only be made based on signs and symptoms in patients with normal intravascular volume. Therefore, intravenous administration of fluids for volume expansion should always be attempted.

617 C. (S&F, ch91)

Mild elevations in alpha-fetoprotein (AFP) level are common and nonspecific, but in adults, levels of 500 ng/mL or more are strongly suggestive of the diagnosis of hepatocellular carcinoma (HCC). At a cut-off of 500 ng/mL, the test has a predictive accuracy of approximately 75%. A progressively rising AFP level, even if the cut-off level has not yet been reached, is also highly suggestive of HCC.

618 E. (S&F, ch91)

Surgical resection is the most frequently recommended treatment for hydatid cysts. With larger cysts, great care must be taken to avoid spillage of the cyst contents into the peritoneal cavity. PAIR is safe and effective in treating cysts less than 5 cm in diameter. Aspiration alone is insufficient treatment and carries the risk of spillage of cyst contents into the peritoneum. Liver transplantation is sometimes indicated to treat echinococcal cysts, but not hydatid cysts.

619 C. (S&F, ch92)

Hepatocellular carcinoma with extension to the portal vein is not considered an indication for liver transplantation given the very high risk of recurrence. Chemoembolization is relatively contraindicated due to the portal vein thrombosis. Local ablative therapies would be most appropriate in this case.

620 E. (S&F, ch91)

The lesion in question is an hepatic adenoma, a benign tumor, but one that may rupture, especially if, as in this case, it is located peripherally. Surgical resection is the recommended treatment for such tumors, whenever feasible. Arterial embolization should be reserved for lesions not amenable to surgical resection. Biopsy results will add little to decisions regarding diagnosis or treatment. Because of the risk of rupture and reports of malignant transformation, observation by repeat imaging is not an appropriate way to manage these tumors.

621 A. (S&F, ch90)

The U.S. Acute Liver Failure Study Group identified the leading causes of acute liver failure

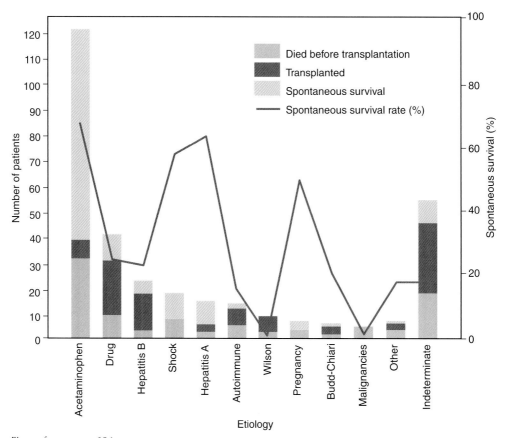

Figure for answer **621**

to be acetaminophen (39%) and idiosyncratic drug reactions (13%), based on a study of 308 adults conducted between 1998 and 2001 (see figure).

622 **A.** (S&F, ch89)

Cirrhosis is associated with both quantitative and qualitative abnormalities in platelets. Approximately 40% of patients with cirrhosis have bleeding times of longer than 10 minutes and platelet counts less than 100,000/mL. The severity of the thrombocytopenia is in direct proportion to the Child-Pugh class, and platelet counts of less than 50,000/mL are common. There is no consensus on the role of thrombopoietin; there is evidence for both decreased production of thrombopoietin and decreased sensitivity of the bone marrow to thrombopoietin. Defining the precise role of thrombopoietin is of great interest because thrombopoietin could be an alternative for treatment in some cirrhotic patients with thrombocytopenia. The key point is that lower platelet counts, regardless of the cause, generally predict a poorer clinical outcome in patients with cirrhosis.

623 **D.** (S&F, ch88)

This patient has spontaneous bacterial peritonitis (SBP), and cefotaxime, a third-generation cephalosporin, has been shown in a controlled trial to be superior to ampicillin plus tobramycin for the treatment of SBP. Thus, cefotaxime or a similar third-generation cephalosporin is the treatment of choice for suspected SBP. Elective surgical treatment of the hernia should be considered in patients with ascites. Ascites should be minimized preoperatively to reduce the risk of hernia recurrence. There is no indication for TIPS placement or large-volume paracentesis in this patient.

624 **E.** (S&F, ch87)

The preferred endoscopic therapy for gastric variceal bleeding is injection of polymers of cyanoacrylate, but these tissue adhesives are not currently available in the United States. Most patients with bleeding gastric varices that are not appropriate for or that do not respond to endoscopic and pharmacologic treatment will require TIPS, which has a success rate of more than 90% for control of gastric variceal bleeding, equivalent to its success rate for controlling esophageal variceal bleeding.

625 **C.** (S&F, ch87)

Use of the hepatic vein pressure gradient (HVPG) has been proposed for the following three indications: (1) monitoring of portal pressure in patients on pharmacotherapy for prevention of variceal bleeding; (2) assessing the risk for hepatic resection in patients with cirrhosis; and (3) delineation of the etiology of portal hypertension (that is, presinusoidal, sinusoidal, or postsinusoidal), usually in combination with concomitant venography, right-sided heart pressure measurements, and transjugular liver biopsy.

Splenic pulp pressure is an indirect method of measuring portal pressure and involves puncture of the splenic pulp with a needle catheter. Because of potential risks of splenic puncture, however, the procedure is now rarely used. Direct portal pressure measurements are carried out when the HVPG cannot be measured, such as in patients with Budd-Chiari syndrome with occluded hepatic veins in whom a surgical portosystemic shunt is being contemplated, or in patients with intrahepatic, presinusoidal causes of portal hypertension, such as idiopathic portal hypertension (in which case HVPG may be normal). Variceal pressure can be measured by inserting into the varices a needle connected to a fluid-filled catheter that is in turn connected to a pressure transducer; use of this method is not justified unless variceal pressure measurement can be followed by variceal injection sclerotherapy. Because variceal sclerotherapy has fallen out of favor, measuring variceal pressure by variceal puncture is seldom carried out except in research protocols.

626 **C.** (S&F, ch86)

Many patients with advanced primary biliary cirrhosis (PBC) have fat-soluble vitamin deficiency and should receive fat-soluble vitamin replacement therapy. Fat-soluble vitamin deficiency is almost always caused by malabsorption resulting from decreased amounts of bile salts in the intestinal lumen.

627 **C.** (S&F, ch85)

The presence of ascites or hepatic encephalopathy in patients with established autoimmune hepatitis (AIH) is indicative of a poor prognosis, but there is a chance that AIH may resolve completely with glucocorticoid therapy. In addition, liver transplantation is effective in the treatment of decompensated AIH. Decompensated patients with multilobular necrosis on histologic examination who have at least one laboratory parameter that fails to normalize or hyperbilirubinemia that does not improve after 2 weeks of treatment are at high risk of early mortality unless they undergo liver transplantation. Thus, the recommendation in this case is for glucorticoid therapy and evaluation for liver transplantation.

628 **B.** (S&F, ch84)

Agent Orange (2.4-dichlorophenoxyacetic acid), the defoliant widely used in Vietnam, has been reported to cause acute hepatitis after chronic exposure. Inorganic arsenic can be found in contaminated ground and well water and homemade alcohol. Doses of more than 3 grams can cause death in 1 to 3 days. Syndromes resembling hepatic veno-occlusive disease and noncirrhotic portal hypertension can develop with long-term exposure. Ingestion of or dermal exposure to dichloride-dimethyldipyridium (Paraquat) has been implicated in several instances of hepatotoxicity as a result of attempted suicide and homicide. Death results from a combination of renal, respiratory, cardiac, and hepatic failure; mortality rates are as high as 70%, and death often occurs within the first 48 hours.

Polychlorinated biphenyls (PCBs) are used in the manufacture of electrical transformers, condensers, capacitors, insulating materials for electrical cables, and industrial fluids. Liver damage appears as early as 7 weeks after ongoing exposure and is accompanied by anorexia, nausea, and edema of the face and hands. Acne-like skin lesions (chloracne) usually precede hepatic injury. Once jaundice appears, death occurs within 2 weeks in fulminant cases, or after 1 to 3 months in subacute cases. Cirrhosis develops in some persons who survive the acute injury.

629 **A.** (S&F, ch83)

The diagnosis of drug-induced hepatotoxicity requires clinical suspicion, a careful drug history, consideration of the temporal relationships between drug ingestion and liver disease, and exclusion of other disorders. The objective weighing of evidence for and against individual agents ("causality assessment") is a probabilistic method of arriving at a diagnosis. Several clinical scales have been described to identify and weigh various factors, and although use of these scales provides only a modest advantage in arriving at a diagnosis, they serve as a framework for identifying factors to be considered in cases of suspected hepatic adverse drug reactions and for improving the consistency of diagnosis. In some cases, a liver biopsy may be indicated to exclude other diseases and to provide further clues to the etiology of liver disease. In the future, in vitro tests may provide confirmatory evidence for the pathogenic role of particular drugs, but drug rechallenge remains the gold standard for confirming a diagnosis of drug-induced liver disease. Purposeful rechallenge is unsafe and not recommended.

630 **A.** (S&F, ch75)

Spontaneous HBeAg seroconversion is seen in only about 10% annually of patients with chronic hepatitis B virus infection. Early changes in serum markers in patients with HBV infection that progresses to chronicity are similar to those in patients with acute HBV infection that resolves. However, with chronic infection, HBsAg, HBeAg, and HBV DNA remain positive for 6 months or longer. After the acute phase of infection, serum ALT levels fall but often remain persistently abnormal (between 50 and 200 U/L). IgM anti-HBc titers typically fall to undetectable levels after 6 months but may become detectable again during reactivation of infection. Detectable levels of IgG anti-HBc persist indefinitely. HBV DNA is detectable by hybridization assays during the acute and chronic phases of disease. With time, there may be a spontaneous decrease in levels of HBV DNA and HBeAg, frequently in association with a flare of serum ALT levels and seroconversion to anti-HBe positivity. Spontaneous loss of reactivity to HBsAg is rare. Anti-HBs may be detected simultaneously with HBsAg in serum in fewer than 10% of cases. In some cases of chronic infection, active viral replication (HBV DNA positivity) occurs in the absence of HBeAg.

631 **D.** (S&F, ch73)

In patients with glycogen storage disease (GSD), the hepatic glycogen concentration is elevated and the most accurate test for making this diagnosis is direct analysis of enzyme activity in a fresh, rather than frozen, sample of liver tissue. Evaluation in fresh liver tissue is important to avoid disruption of microsomal G6Pase activity. Fasting glucose and lactate levels, a glucagon response test, or response to fructose or galactose administration may support the diagnosis but are not definitive; in fact, patients with GSD type I will not show the rise in serum glucose concentration expected after administration of these substances.

632 **D.** (S&F, ch70)

Hepatic gamma glutamyl transpeptidase (GGTP) is derived from hepatocytes and biliary epithelia but, like alkaline phosphatase (AP), GGTP is found in many extrahepatic tissues, including the kidney, spleen, pancreas, heart, lung, and brain. GGTP is a microsomal enzyme and is therefore inducible by alcohol and drugs, including most anticonvulsant medications and warfarin. In the case described, the elevation in

GGTP concentration is likely due to warfarin, and no further testing is indicated.

633 C. (S&F, ch68)

Coarse lobulations of the liver (hepar lobatum) are the result of obliterative lesions in large and medium-sized vessels, typically after invasion by neoplasms or in cases of syphilis.

634 D. (S&F, ch81)

A central event in the development of alcoholic liver fibrosis is activation of hepatic stellate cells. Stellate cells reside in Disse's space between hepatocytes and sinusoidal endothelia. In a normal liver, there is a stable population of stellate cells that play an important role in hepatic vitamin A storage. When liver injury occurs, however, whether by alcohol abuse or by other toxic or infectious insults, stellate cells alter their phenotype to become proliferative, myofibroblast-like cells. Activated stellate cells are the principal collagen-producing cells of the liver. They are responsible for the perisinusoidal fibrosis that is characteristic of alcoholic liver disease.

635 C. (S&F, ch88)

Therapeutic paracentesis is the accepted first-line therapy for patients with tense ascites. Because this patient has recurrent ascites despite maximal doses of diuretics, removal of all ascites fluid possible is indicated. In addition, albumin replacement with large-volume paracentesis has been shown to decrease mortality and renal failure. TIPS placement is a second-line choice because it is associated with an increased risk of hepatic encephalopathy.

636 A. (S&F, ch89)

Patients with cirrhosis are at increased risk for specific abnormalities of pulmonary mechanics, hemodynamics, and ventilation-perfusion matching that can adversely affect both quality of life and longevity. Two of the most common pulmonary manifestations of cirrhosis are alterations in lung mechanics caused by the presence of ascites and intrapulmonary shunting and abnormal gas exchange, which together comprise the hepatopulmonary syndrome.

637 E. (S&F, ch90)

Acute liver failure is defined as the rapid development of hepatocellular dysfunction (i.e., coagulopathy) and mental status changes (i.e., encephalopathy). The reported incidence of acute liver failure due to acetaminophen overdose has been rising recently. In many of these "therapeutic misadventures," patients ingested over-the-counter products containing acetaminophen along with prescription narcotic-acetaminophen congeners. Chronic heavy ethanol consumption may lower the threshold for acetaminophen toxicity in some patients via induction of cytochrome P450 enzyme activity. Only liver transplantation has been effective in treating patients with irreversible liver failure. Unfortunately, many patients with irreversible acute liver failure do not undergo transplantation because of late referral, contraindications, or lack of donor livers. Therefore, patients in acute liver failure should be evaluated for liver transplantation as soon as possible and, if no contraindications are identified, placed on a liver transplant waiting list.

638 D. (S&F, ch87)

This patient has idiopathic portal hypertension, which generally does not progress to end-stage liver disease. Ascites is uncommon and liver transplantation is rarely required in these patients. The dominant clinical features of idiopathic portal hypertension are variceal bleeding and a markedly enlarged spleen. Liver synthetic function is usually normal, although mild elevation in alkaline phosphatase may be seen. The hepatic venous pressure gradient is usually normal in patients with idiopathic portal hypertension, indicating that the site of increased resistance is presinusoidal. Surgical shunts are well tolerated in these patients, although hepatic encephalopathy may be seen when these patients are followed up long-term.

639 B. (S&F, ch85)

It has been reported that 41% of patients with autoimmune hepatitis (AIH) had concurrent extrahepatic immunologic diseases, the most common of which were autoimmune thyroiditis (in 12%), Grave's disease (in 6%), and chronic ulcerative colitis (in 6%). Rheumatoid arthritis, pernicious anemia, systemic sclerosis, Coomb's-positive hemolytic anemia, autoimmune thrombocytic purpura, symptomatic cryoglobulinemia, leukocytoclastic vasculitis, nephritis, erythema nodosum, systemic lupus erythematosus, and fibrosis alveolitis also occurred but each in fewer than 1% of those with AIH. Cholangiography is warranted in all patients who have concurrent chronic ulcerative colitis, to exclude primary sclerosing cholangitis.

640 D. (S&F, ch86)

Lipid abnormalities are found in up to 85% of patients with primary biliary cirrhosis (PBC). High-density lipoprotein (HDL) cholesterol levels are usually most prominently elevated in the early stages of PBC. As the disease progresses, HDL cholesterol levels decrease and low-density lipoprotein (LDL) cholesterol levels increase. However, the risk of atherosclerosis in these patients with PBC and hyperlipidemia does not appear to be increased.

641 **D.** (S&F, ch90)

The diagnosis of acute liver failure is made clinically on the basis of physical examination findings and laboratory test results. Infrequently, acute liver failure may be confused with other clinical entities that manifest as jaundice, coagulopathy, and encephalopathy; these include sepsis, a systemic disorder with liver and brain effects (lupus erythematosus, thrombotic thrombocytopenic purpura), and acute decompensation in a patient with chronic liver disease. In particular, sepsis and acute liver failure have similar hemodynamic profiles and severe sepsis is frequently associated with changes in mental status. In this situation, jaundice and coagulopathy may result from intrahepatic cholestasis and disseminated intravascular coagulation, respectively. Measurement of factor VIII levels may be helpful in differentiating sepsis (low factor VIII level) from acute liver failure (factor VIII level generally not reduced).

642 **B.** (S&F, ch92)

The development of ascites secondary to chronic liver disease is associated with a 50% 2-year survival and should prompt evaluation for liver transplantation.

643 **C.** (S&F, ch75)

Patients with chronic liver disease, particularly those with established cirrhosis, are at increased risk of developing hepatocellular carcinoma (HCC). The risk of developing HCC is increased 10- to 390-fold in patients with chronic HBV infection compared with those who are HBsAg-negative, and the risk is greater in those who acquired HBV infection perinatally rather than in adulthood. In regions where HBV is endemic, HCC is the leading cause of cancer-related deaths. Despite this strong epidemiologic link between HBV infection and HCC, and despite active research in this area for more than a decade, the mechanism by which HBV causes malignant transformation has not been elucidated.

644 **B.** (S&F, ch76)

The modes of transmission of HCV infection can be divided into percutaneous (blood transfusion and needle-stick inoculation) and nonpercutaneous (sexual contact, perinatal exposure). The latter mode may represent occult percutaneous exposure. Overall, receiving blood from unscreened donors and injection drug use are the two best-documented risk factors for HCV infection. Indeed, in initial studies, HCV was shown to be the etiologic agent in more than 85% of cases of post-transfusion non-A, non-B hepatitis. After the introduction of anti-HCV screening of blood donors in 1991, transfusion-related cases of HCV infection declined significantly, and non–transfusion-related cases came to account for a higher proportion of cases. Currently, among patients presenting with acute and chronic HCV infection, injection drug use is the most common risk factor identified and is present in 40% or more of patients.

645 **D.** (S&F, ch76)

Because antibodies to HCV (anti-HCV) can be acquired passively by the infant, recent studies have utilized polymerase chain reaction (PCR) amplification of HCV RNA to test for HCV infection in the infant. Testing of the infant for anti-HCV before 12 months is not recommended. If the mother were infected, the relative risk for HCV transmission with vaginal or caesarean delivery is a matter of controversy. The risk posed to the infant from breast-feeding when the mother tests positive for antibodies to HCV is believed to be negligible.

646 **D.** (S&F, ch84)

The anesthetic agent that most often causes hepatotoxicity is halothane, which is now rarely used. The likelihood that individual haloalkane anesthetics will cause liver injury appears to be related to the extent to which they are metabolized by hepatic CYP enzymes; the rate of metabolism is 20% to 30% for halothane, more than 30% for methoxyflurane, 2% for enflurane, 1% for sevoflurane, and 0.2% or less for isoflurane and desflurane, which are newer agents.

647 **C.** (S&F, ch88)

Early detection of spontaneous bacterial peritonitis (SBP), before symptoms of infection occur, may reduce mortality. Therefore, ascitic fluid should be sampled in all patients with ascites who are admitted to the hospital, especially if infection is suspected. Coagulopathy is a contraindication to paracentesis only in cases of clinically evident fibrinolysis or disseminated intravascular coagulation; no coagulation parameter limitations (e.g., INR values) to performing paracentesis have been identified. Giving fresh-frozen plasma or vitamin K routinely before paracentesis in patients with cirrhosis and coagulopathy is not supported by data.

648 **A.** (S&F, ch79)

Ascaris lumbricoides infection is present in at least 1 billion persons worldwide; it is most common among the poor. Humans are infected by ingesting embryonated eggs, usually in raw vegetables. The eggs hatch in the small intestine, and the larvae penetrate the mucosa, enter the portal circulation, and reach the liver, pulmonary artery, and lungs, where they grow in the alveolar spaces. From the alveolar spaces, they are regurgitated and swallowed and become mature adults in the intestine 2 to 3 months after ingestion, whereupon the cycle repeats itself. Symptoms generally occur in persons with a large worm burden; most infected persons are asymptomatic. Cough, fever, dyspnea, wheezing, substernal chest discomfort, and hepatomegaly may occur in the first 2 weeks. Chest radiography may show an infiltrate and eosinophilia may be present. Endoscopic retrograde cholangiopancreatography (ERCP) is both diagnostic and therapeutic for ascariasis.

649 **E.** (S&F, ch80)

The primary cause of ischemic hepatitis is tissue hypoxia, which may result from hypoperfusion secondary to cardiac failure, systemic hypoxemia from respiratory failure, or increased oxygen requirements from sepsis. Among all cases of extreme AST elevation (above 3000 U/L), ischemic hepatitis accounts for about one half. Most cases of ischemic hepatitis are transient and self-limited. The overall prognosis is primarily dependent on the severity of the underlying predisposing condition, not the severity of the liver disease. Treatment for ischemic hepatitis is nonspecific and directed at improving cardiac output and systemic oxygenation.

650 **A.** (S&F, ch84)

Cocaine is a dose-dependent hepatotoxin. Acute cocaine intoxication affects the liver in 60% of patients and many affected persons have markedly elevated serum ALT levels (more than 1000 U/L). Associated features include rhabdomyolysis, hypotension, hyperpyrexia, disseminated intravascular coagulation, and renal failure.

Ecstasy (3,4-methylenedioxymethamphetamine) is a euphorigenic and psychedelic amphetamine derivative that can lead to hepatic necrosis as part of a heat-stroke-like syndrome that occurs as a result of exhaustive dancing in hot nightclubs ("raves"). Phencyclidine ("angel dust") is another stimulant that can lead to hepatic injury as part of a syndrome of malignant hyperthermia that

produces zone 3 hepatic necrosis, congestion, and collapse, with high serum AST and ALT levels similar to those seen with ischemic hepatitis.

651 **D.** (S&F, ch90)

Investigators at King College in London performed a multivariate analysis of clinical and biochemical variables and their relationship to mortality in 588 patients with acute liver failure. In this analysis, a major distinction was made between acetaminophen toxicity and other causes of acute liver failure. For liver failure due to acetaminophen toxicity, the King's College criteria for liver transplantation were as follows: (1) pH less than 7.3 or arterial lactate greater than 3.5 mmol/L at 4 hours or arterial lactate greater than 3.0 mmol/L at 12 hours or (2) INR greater than 6.5 (prothrombin time longer than 100 seconds), (3) serum creatinine greater than 3.4 mg/dL, and (4) stage 3 or 4 encephalopathy.

652 **A.** (S&F, ch76)

Although histologic evidence of liver injury will develop in approximately one half of the patients within the first year after liver transplantation, severe graft dysfunction rarely occurs in the short term. With longer follow-up (5 to 7 years) after transplantation, HCV-related graft cirrhosis will develop in a substantial proportion of patients, ranging from 8% to 30%. Once the patient has reached the stage of clinically compensated cirrhosis, the risk of decompensation is approximately 40% per year.

653 **E.** (S&F, ch77)

HEV is an RNA virus endemic to developing countries such as the Indian subcontinent, Southeast Asia, and Central Asia. Outbreaks of HEV infection have been reported from northern and western parts of Africa and the Middle East. Two small outbreaks were reported to have occurred in Mexico, one in 1986 and one in 1987. Overall attack rates range from 1% to 15% and are higher among adults. The outbreaks have been characterized by a particularly high attack rate and mortality among pregnant women. The most recognizable form of HEV infection is acute enteric hepatitis. The clinical manifestations are similar to those of acute HAV infection. The onset of HEV infection is usually insidious, has a prodromal phase lasting 1 to 4 days, and is characterized by a combination of flu-like symptoms, fever, chills, abdominal pain, anorexia, nausea, aversion to smoking, vomiting, clay-colored stools, dark urine, diarrhea, arthralgias, asthenia, and transient macular skin rash. Acute HAV infection is less likely in this patient given the presence of IgG antibody to HAV. The correct answer is HEV infection.

654 **A.** (S&F, ch79)

Clonorchiasis typically presents with fever, abdominal pain, and diarrhea. Chronic manifestations correlate with fluke burden and are dominated by hepatobiliary features: fever, right upper quadrant pain, tender hepatomegaly, and eosinophilia. If the worm burden in the bile ducts is heavy, chronic or intermittent biliary obstruction can ensue, with frequent cholelithiasis, cholecystitis, jaundice, and ultimately, recurrent pyogenic cholangitis. Longstanding infection leads to exuberant inflammation, resulting in periportal fibrosis, marked biliary epithelial hyperplasia and dysplasia, and ultimately, a substantially increased risk of cholangiocarcinoma. Cholangiocarcinoma should be suspected in infected persons with weight loss, jaundice, epigastric pain, or abdominal mass.

655 **D.** (S&F, ch80)

Portal vein obstruction results from thrombosis, constriction, or invasion of a portal vein. The resulting portal hypertension leads to splenomegaly and formation of portosystemic collaterals and esophageal, gastric, duodenal, and jejunal varices. In most cases of portal vein thrombosis there is an identifiable cause such as systemic hypercoagulability or local factors such as inflammation, trauma, or malignancy. The results of liver function tests are usually normal. Doppler ultrasonography is highly sensitive for portal vein thrombosis: It typically shows an echogenic thrombus in the portal vein, extensive collateral vessels in the porta hepatis, and an enlarged spleen, although occasionally the portal vein cannot be visualized by this technique.

656 **A.** (S&F, ch68)

The portal vein supplies 70% of the blood flow to the hepatic parenchyma. The common hepatic artery arises from the celiac artery. The cystic arteries usually arise from the right hepatic artery. Arterial ligation is usually well tolerated by persons with normal liver function.

657 **B.** (S&F, ch74)

Administration of serum immunoglobulin (IG) and the first dose of HAV vaccine, along with good handwashing and other infection control practices are the mainstays of preventing HAV infection. When IG is used for postexposure prophylaxis, it should be given within 2 weeks of exposure. In these cases, the recommended dose is 0.02 mL/kg by intramuscular injection.

Although considered safe, IG can cause fever, myalgias, and pain at the injection site. Postexposure prophylaxis with IG can be accompanied safely with initiation of active immunization with the vaccine, and this course is recommended rather than IG alone.

658 **C.** (S&F, ch82)

Of the listed choices, only pioglitazone has been shown in clinical trials to result in significant improvement in the histologic appearance of the liver in cases of nonalcoholic fatty liver disease (NAFLD). The findings in these clinical trials are preliminary, however, and will require confirmation. Insulin has not been shown to be useful in treating NAFLD. Leptin is not available for treatment of NAFLD. Ursodiol was found in a large prospective clinical trial not to alter the histologic appearance of the liver in cases of NAFLD. Vitamin E lowered ALT levels in some trials, but it did not have any effect on the histologic appearance of the liver.

659 **D.** (S&F, ch81)

Pentoxifylline can reduce inflammation by inhibiting the synthesis of tumor necrosis factor (TNF). The safety and efficacy of pentoxifylline for alcoholic hepatitis were studied in a randomized controlled trial conducted in the year 2000 that involved 101 patients. All patients had severe alcoholic hepatitis as judged by a discriminant function greater than 32; 49 were treated with pentoxifylline (400 mg orally three times a day) for 4 weeks, and 52 received placebo. Pentoxifylline did not cause a significant decrease in plasma TNF levels in treated patients. It did, however, afford a survival benefit and significant protection against the hepatorenal syndrome. The 4-week mortality rate in the placebo group was 46.1%, as would be predicted by the discriminant function. In the pentoxifylline group, the mortality rate over the same interval was 24.5%. In addition, pentoxifylline reduced the frequency of hepatorenal syndrome from 34.6% to 8.2%. The mechanism of action of pentoxifylline may be related to its beneficial effects on the microcirculation, particularly within the kidney. These promising results require confirmation.

660 **C.** (S&F, ch92)

This patient's alkaline phosphatase level indicates bile duct obstruction or injury. The ultrasound results do not suggest large bile duct obstruction; however, the histological findings strongly suggest obstruction, so lack of obstruction must be confirmed by endoscopic retrograde cholangiopancreatography (ERCP). Another reason to perform ERCP is that it would identify anastomotic strictures that may be present patient as a consequence of surgery.

661 **E.** (S&F, ch80)

Veno-occlusive disease (VOD) is characterized by occlusion of the terminal hepatic venules and hepatic sinusoids. VOD most commonly occurs after bone marrow transplantation. A variety of antineoplastic drugs have been implicated as causes for VOD, including gemtuzumab ozogamicin, actinomycin D, dacarbazine, cytosine arabinoside, mithramycin, and 6-thioguanine. Classically, VOD presents with mild hyperbilirubinemia (concentration more than 2 mg/dL), painful hepatomegaly, weight gain, and ascites. On liver biopsy, sinusoidal dilatation and severe hepatic congestion will be seen, the results of progressive occlusion of the sinusoids and venules. Inflammation is notably absent in VOD.

662 **A.** (S&F, ch73)

The pathognomonic lesion of cystic fibrosis, focal biliary cirrhosis (FCC), presumably results from defective function of the cystic fibrosis gene product, which is expressed in bile duct cells. Obstruction of small bile ducts leads to chronic inflammatory changes, bile duct proliferation, and portal fibrosis. At autopsy, FCC has been identified in 25% to 30% of individuals more than 1 year of age with cystic fibrosis. Progression to multilobular biliary cirrhosis occurs in approximately 10% of individuals with cystic fibrosis and leads to typical symptoms of portal hypertension such as splenomegaly and variceal bleeding. Hepatic steatosis also develops in roughly one half of patients, but this development does not appear to correlate with progressive liver disease.

663 **B.** (S&F, ch72)

This patient has Wilson disease and is presenting with fulminant hepatic failure with severe coagulopathy and encephalopathy. Acute intravascular hemolysis is usually present in this situation. Unlike fulminant viral hepatitis, Wilson disease is usually characterized by disproportionately low serum aminotransaminase levels, and the serum alkaline phosphatase level is in the normal or even low range. The serum bilirubin level is disproportionately elevated secondary to hemolysis. These patients do not respond well to chelation therapy and require urgent transplant evaluation.

664 **A.** (S&F, ch73)

Plasma ammonia levels are generally dramatically elevated in patients with urea cycle defects,

sometimes to more than 2000 μmol/L (3400 μg/dL), with normal being 50 μmol/L (85 μg/dL) or less. This patient's blood gas values reflect respiratory alkalosis, which is secondary to hyperventilation triggered by the effects of ammonia on the central nervous system. Serum levels of liver enzymes are usually normal or minimally elevated in such cases. Citrulline levels are barely detectable in patients with ornithine transcarbamylase (OTC) or carbamyl phosphate synthetase (CPS) deficiencies but are markedly elevated in those with argininosuccinate synthetase (AS) and argininosuccinate lyase (AL) deficiencies.

665 **C.** (S&F, ch79)

Human infections with *Trichinella spiralis* are usually due to consumption of raw or undercooked pork containing *T. spiralis* larvae, which are released in the small intestine, penetrate the mucosa, and disseminate through the circulation. The larvae may then enter the myocardium, cerebral spinal fluid, brain, and, less often, liver and gallbladder. From these locations, the larvae re-enter the circulation and reach striated muscle, where they become encapsulated. Clinical manifestations of infection develop when the worm burden is high and include diarrhea, fever, myalgias, periportal edema, and leukocytosis with marked eosinophilia. The diagnosis is suggested by a characteristic history in a patient with fever and eosinophilia. A muscle biopsy may help to confirm the diagnosis. Treatment consists of glucocorticoids to relieve allergic symptoms, followed by albendazole 400 mg per day for 3 days or mebendazole 200 mg per day for 5 days.

666 **B.** (S&F, ch81)

Liver biopsy is viewed by many authorities as the standard for diagnosing alcoholic liver injury. Indeed, in one study as many as 20% of cases of alcoholic liver disease were misdiagnosed by clinical criteria alone. Although the true error rate in diagnosis by clinical criteria alone is probably closer to 10%, liver biopsy is still quite useful for diagnosis and for prediction of prognosis. Among the most common histologic features of alcoholic liver disease are (1) steatosis, (2) ballooning degeneration of hepatocytes, (3) presence of Mallory's bodies, (4) neutrophilic inflammation, and (5) pericellular fibrosis.

667 **D.** (S&F, ch86)

Ursodeoxycholic acid (UDCA) occurs naturally in small quantities in human bile. It is the only medication approved by the U.S. Food and Drug Administration for the treatment of primary biliary cirrhosis (PBC). Several mechanisms for the protective actions of UDCA have been proposed, including inhibiting the absorption of toxic, hydrophobic, endogenous bile salts; stabilizing hepatocyte membranes against toxic bile salts; replacing endogenous bile acids, some of which may be hepatotoxic, with the nonhepatotoxic UDCA; and reduction in expression of major histocompatibility complex class I and class II antigens. Administration of UDCA to patients with PBC leads to a rapid improvement in the results of liver function tests. UDCA therapy also leads to improvement in several histologic features of PBC such as interface hepatitis, inflammation, cholestasis, bile duct paucity, and bile duct proliferation. UDCA significantly decreases the risk of developing gastroesophageal varices and delays progression to cirrhosis. One study predicted probabilities of 4%, 12%, and 59% for development of cirrhosis after 5 years of therapy with UDCA in patients with stage 1, 2, or 3 PBC.

668 **B.** (S&F, ch88)

Diuretics are the mainstay of treatment for ascites due to cirrhosis. Therapy with spironolactone alone requires several days to induce weight loss. Although spironolactone alone has been shown to be superior to furosemide alone in the treatment of cirrhotic ascites, the author's preference is to start daily administration of both spironolactone and furosemide on the first hospital day. Repeated doses of intravenous furosemide for the patient with cirrhosis can lead to crescendo azotemia and then to an erroneous diagnosis of hepatorenal syndrome.

669 **E.** (S&F, ch76)

Factors associated with spontaneous resolution of acute HCV include young age at infection, female gender, absence of parenteral transmission, and presence of symptoms and jaundice. At least three studies have indicated that delaying therapy until 2 to 4 months after the onset of acute hepatitis C virus infection does not alter the effectiveness of antiviral therapy in achieving sustained virologic response.

670 **C.** (S&F, ch78)

Like transfusion-transmitted virus (TT virus; TTV), SEN virus can be transmitted by both parenteral and fecal-oral routes. Neither virus causes chronic infection or end-stage liver disease. Most studies have shown no association between infection with either TTV or SEN virus and mortality or the response to treatment of chronic HCV infection.

671 **E.** (S&F, ch83)

Numerous environmental substances can cause induction or inhibition of microsomal enzymes and thereby alter concentrations of drugs and other substances metabolized by the cytochrome P450 (CYP) pathway. For example, chemicals in cigarettes and cannabis induce CYP1A2 activity and alcohol affects CYP2E1 and possibly CYP3A4. Several drugs are also potent inducers of CYP enzymes. Isoniazid induces CYP2E1, and phenobarbital and phenytoin increase the expression of multiple CYP enzymes. Rifampicin is a potent inducer of CYP3A4, and so too is hypericum, the active ingredient of St. John's wort, a commonly used herbal medication.

672 **E.** (S&F, ch87)

TIPS has been used for control of variceal bleeding, as well as the prevention of variceal rebleeding when pharmacologic and endoscopic therapy have failed, especially in patients with Child-Pugh class B or C disease in whom refractory bleeding is more commonly encountered. When bleeding from varices cannot be controlled in spite of two endoscopic sessions within a 24-hour period, TIPS placement is the usual treatment of choice. A surgical portosystemic shunt may be preferred to a TIPS in patients with excellent liver synthetic function, as indicated by Child-Pugh class A status, when the surgical expertise is available to place this type of shunt.

673 **D.** (S&F, ch76)

Factors associated with a better outcome include low serum levels of HCV RNA, viral genotype other than 1, absence of cirrhosis, female gender, and age younger than 40 years. African-American ethnicity has have been shown to be associated with a poor response to interferon monotherapy as well as to combination therapy.

674 **A.** (S&F, ch83)

Amiodarone is an iodinated benzofuran derivative used for therapy-resistant ventricular tachyarrhythmias. Adverse effects lead to discontinuation of therapy in 25% of patients and include pulmonary infiltrates, worsening cardiac failure, hypothyroidism, peripheral neuropathy, nephrotoxicity, and corneal deposits, but liver disease is one of the most serious. The spectrum of abnormalities includes abnormal liver tests in 15% to 80% of patients and clinically significant liver disease in 0.6%, including rare cases of acute liver failure. The most common finding on histologic evaluation of the liver is steatohepatitis; cirrhosis is present in 15% to 50% of persons with steatohepatitis.

675 **E.** (S&F, ch87)

Neither the optimal interval nor the most cost-effective method of surveillance for TIPS stenosis has been determined. Doppler ultrasound is generally used to identify TIPS stenosis, but this procedure has poor negative predictive value and barely acceptable positive predictive value. The best indicator of shunt stenosis is recurrence of the problem that necessitated TIPS placement. The only certain method of demonstrating shunt patency is by means of a TIPS venogram and measurement of the portocaval pressure gradient. An increase in the gradient to greater than 12 mmHg would warrant dilatation of the stent or placement of additional stents.

676 **D.** (S&F, ch89)

Hepatorenal syndrome should be suspected in any patient with acute or chronic liver disease and portal hypertension when there is a rise in serum creatinine to above 1.5 mg/dL. In general, hepatorenal syndrome occurs in patients with relatively advanced liver disease, and the risk is increased for patients with hyponatremia, high plasma renin activity, and small liver size. However, neither the etiology of the liver disease nor the patient's Child-Pugh class has significant predictive value.

677 **D.** (S&F, ch92)

The period immediately following liver transplantation is characterized by acid/base abnormalities, fluid shifts, and abnormalities in liver enzyme levels. The most important indicators of graft function are clinical and include the patient's mental status and, in those with a t-tube, the amount and character of bile production.

678 **D.** (S&F, ch68)

During the development of cirrhosis the sinusoids acquire some features of systemic capillaries; the space of Disse becomes widened with collagen, basement membrane material is deposited, and endothelial fenestrations become smaller and less numerous, all leading to decreased transport across sinusoidal walls.

679 **A.** (S&F, ch71)

Those in whom hereditary hemochromatosis is diagnosed most frequently have the genotype C282Y/C282Y or C282Y/H63D

680 **B.** (S&F, ch75)

The incubation period (time from acute exposure to clinical symptoms) of hepatitis B infection ranges between 60 and 180 days. The clinical presentation varies, from asymptomatic infection to cholestatic hepatitis with jaundice and, rarely, liver failure. In patients with acute infection, HBsAg and markers of active viral replication (HBeAg titer and burden of HBV DNA as determined by hybridization assays) become detectable approximately 6 weeks after inoculation, before the onset of clinical symptoms or biochemical abnormalities. These tests remain positive throughout the prodromal phase and during the early clinical phase of the illness. Biochemical abnormalities usually coincide with the prodromal phase of the acute illness and may persist for several months. With the onset of symptoms, IgM anti-HBc becomes detectable. Detectable levels of IgM anti-HBc may persist for many months, and detectable levels of IgG anti-HBc may persist for many years, if not a lifetime. Anti-HBs is the last serologic marker to become detectable and its appearance (as HBsAg titers fall) indicates that the infection is resolving. Much has been made of the serologic window when neither HBsAg nor anti-HBs is detectable and IgM anti-HBc is the only marker of acute infection. However, with the ability of currently available serologic assays to detect low levels of marker proteins, this window occurs rarely.

681 **B.** (S&F, ch79)

Bacillary angiomatosis is an infectious disorder that primarily affects persons with AIDS or other immunodeficiency states. The causative agents have been identified as the gram-negative bacillus *Bartonella henselae* and, in some cases, *B. quintana*. Infection is frequently associated with exposure to cats. Multiple red, papular skin lesions most often are present in cases of bacillary angiomatosis, but disseminated infection with or without skin involvement also has been described. The bacilli can infect liver, lymph nodes, pleura, bronchi, bones, brain, bone marrow, and spleen. Additional manifestations of infection include persistent fever, bacteremia, and sepsis. Hepatic infection should be suspected in patients with otherwise unexplained elevations in serum aminotransaminase levels.

682 **D.** (S&F, ch69)

Pores of the nuclear envelope are associated with a large number of proteins that are organized in an octagonal array. The nuclear pore complex (NPC) is a large macromolecule assembly that protrudes into both the cytoplasm and the nucleoplasm. Bidirectional nucleocytoplasmic transport occurs through the central aqueous channel in the NPC.

683 **B.** (S&F, ch82)

Magnetic resonance imaging (MRI), ultrasonography (US), and computed tomography (CT) are all sensitive for detection of hepatic fat, but noneis able to distinguish simple steatosis from steatohepatitis. Liver biopsy remains the only reliable tool to make this distinction.

684 (S&F, ch69) Answers: 1-**B**; 2-**D**; 3-**A**; 4-**C**

Bile duct epithelial cells, or cholangiocytes, line the bile ducts, which are not mere passive conduits for biliary drainage but play an active role in the secretion and absorption of biliary components and in regulating the composition of the extracellular matrix.

Hepatic sinusoidal cells, unlike capillary endothelial cells, do not form intracellular junctions but simply overlap each other. The specialized endothelial lining of hepatic sinusoids serves as a selective barrier between blood and the hepatocytes.

Kupffer cells are highly active in removing from portal blood (draining the intestines) any particulate matter and toxic or foreign substances.

Hepatic stellate cells are important sources of paracrine, autocrine, juxtacrine, and chemoattractant factors that maintain homeostasis in the microenvironment of the hepatic sinusoid. Following liver injury, the hepatic stellate cells become activated to myofibroblasts, a central event in hepatic fibrogenesis.

685 **D.** (S&F, ch78)

Herpes simplex virus (HSV) hepatitis is seen in neonates, pregnant women, and immunocompromised patients and can be aggressive and possibly life-threatening. Mucocutaneous lesions are present in only one half of the cases; therefore, a high index of clinical suspicion is important in making a timely diagnosis. Hepatitis is more common with acute infection than with reactivation. The individual with HSV hepatitis typically presents with fever, leukopenia, and markedly elevated aminotransaminase levels. Disseminated intravascular coagulation and jaundice may also be seen. Liver biopsy is essential for diagnosis, particularly during pregnancy. Focal or extensive hemorrhagic or coagulative necrosis is seen with few inflammatory infiltrates. Intranuclear inclusions (Cowdry type A inclusions) may be identified in hepatocytes at the margins of the necrosis. In addition, some multinucleated periportal hepatocytes show a ground-glass appearance suggestive of viral inclusions. Electron microscopy, immunohistochemical

staining, and polymerase chain reaction (PCR) amplification techniques can be used to confirm the diagnosis.

686 **D.** (S&F, ch87)

The hyperdynamic circulation of cirrhosis is characterized by peripheral and splanchnic vasodilation, reduced mean arterial pressure, and increased cardiac output. Vasodilation, particularly in the splanchnic bed, allows for greater inflow of systemic blood into the portal circulation. It is important to note that the generation of excess nitric oxide and ensuing vasodilation, hyperdynamic circulation, and hyperemia that occur in the splanchnic and systemic circulation are in contrast to the changes that occur in the hepatic circulation where nitric oxide deficiency contributes to increased intrahepatic resistance.

687 **A.** (S&F, ch91)

Fibrolamellar hepatocellular carcinoma typically arises in young patients, has an approximately equal sex distribution, does not secrete alpha fetoprotein (AFP), is not caused by chronic HBV or HCV infection, and almost always arises in a noncirrhotic liver.

688 **A.** (S&F, ch79)

In the past, most cases of pyogenic liver abscess occurred in young patients as a consequence of appendicitis complicated by pyelophlebitis (portal vein inflammation). This presentation is less common today as a result of earlier diagnosis and effective antibiotic therapy for portal vein inflammation. Most cases of pyogenic liver abscess today are cryptogenic or occur in older men with underlying biliary tract disease. Infections of the biliary tract (cholangitis/cholecystitis) are the most common identifiable sources of pathogens causing liver abscess. Infection of the liver may occur via the bile duct, along a penetrating vessel, or from an adjacent septic focus. Less commonly, liver abscess is a complication of bacteremia arising due to underlying abdominal disease, such as diverticulitis, perforated or penetrating peptic ulcer, gastrointestinal malignancy, inflammatory bowel disease, or peritonitis. Rarely abscess in the liver is a complication of bacterial endocarditis or the result of penetration of a foreign body through the wall of the colon.

689 **D.** (S&F, ch72)

Penicillamine, although effective in treating Wilson's disease, can have very serious adverse side effects. Adverse reactions include rash, pemphigus, and elastosis perforans serpiginosa.

Other effects include minor to severe proteinuria, leukopenia, or thrombocytopenia. Aplastic anemia occurs rarely and does not always reverse when penicillamine is stopped. Nephrotic syndrome, Goodpasture's syndrome, a myasthenia syndrome, and a systemic disease resembling lupus have been reported. These severe side effects require immediate discontinuation of the medicine and initiation of treatment with an alternative chelating agent.

690 **A.** (S&F, ch76)

In contrast to the high efficiency of perinatal transmission of HBV from mothers to infants, the efficiency of perinatal transmission of HCV is low, with a risk estimated to range from 0% to 10%. There is considerable controversy as to whether the rate of vertical transmission is higher when the mother is coinfected with HIV, as suggested in early studies. However, in a recent large study of 370 anti–HCV-positive women, 4% were coinfected with HIV but did not transmit HCV to their infants. Interestingly, all women were on antiretroviral therapy during pregnancy, and this therapy was believed to reduce HIV-related immunosuppression. Data regarding the risk associated with vaginal delivery as opposed to caesarean delivery are controversial. The risk posed to the infant from breast-feeding is believed to be negligible. Further studies are needed, however, to delineate the time of infection (in utero or at the time of delivery), the importance of breast-feeding in neonatal transmission, and the natural history of HCV infection in children.

691 **D.** (S&F, ch84)

There are various phases of acute hepatic injury from chemical toxins. Phosphorus poisoning is most likely to present with the syndrome described in the question.

692 **B.** (S&F, ch74)

HAV infection with prolonged cholestasis occurs rarely but can promptthe (inappropriate) performance of invasive diagnostic procedures because the diagnosis of acute hepatitis may not be readily considered in patients who have had jaundice for several months, even when they have detectable levels of anti-HAV immunoglobulin M (IgM). The cholestatic variant of HAV infection is not associated with increased mortality. The treatment is symptomatic.

693 **E.** (S&F, ch70)

ALT is a cytosolic enzyme, whereas AST is present as both cytosolic and mitochondrial isoenzymes.

Elevated levels of these enzymes in serum is believed to be the result of leakage from damaged cells and thus reflects hepatocyte injury. These enzymes are elevated in many forms of liver disease, especially those that are associated with significant hepatocyte necrosis, such as acute viral hepatitis and chemical or ischemic injury. Extreme aminotransaminase elevations (greater than 2000 U/L) occur only in a few conditions, namely drug hepatotoxicity, viral hepatitis, hepatic ischemia, and autoimmune hepatitis. In the case described, ischemia is the most likely of these differential diagnoses.

694 **B.** (S&F, ch83)

According to Hy's rule, the propensity of a drug to cause acute liver disease is related to the frequency of its association with hyperbilirubinemia or with an elevation of the serum ALT level to 8-fold or more above the upper limit of normal. The actual liver failure rate is about 10%. Thus, if, as in the scenario described, 2 cases of jaundice associated with drug-induced liver injury were reported among 2500 patients in phase II clinical trials, acute liver failure would be expected in every ~12,500 subjects who take the drug during the marketing phase.

695 **B.** (S&F, ch87)

Ligation initially should be at the bleeding site or immediately below the bleeding site. Other large varices should also be banded in the same session. If active bleeding is not noted, then ligation is carried out beginning at the gastroesophageal junction and proceeding proximally at a distance of every 2 cm in a spiral fashion. If bleeding obscures the varices, then multiple bands are placed at the gastroesophageal junction circumferentially until bleeding can be controlled, but the long-term risks of esophageal stricture increase in such patients. Bleeding can be controlled in up to 90% of patients by a combination of pharmacologic and endoscopic methods.

696 **E.** (S&F, ch88)

The diagnosis of secondary bacterial peritonitis requires the presence of at least two of the following three criteria: total protein more than 1 g/dL, glucose more than 50 mg/dL, and LDH more than the upper limit of normal for serum.

697 **E.** (S&F, ch79)

The treatment of choice for schistosomiasis is praziquantel, 60 mg/kg in three divided doses 4 hours apart on a single day or, for patients who cannot tolerate praziquantel, oxamniquine, 15 to 60 mg/kg per day for 1 or 2 days.

698 **D.** (S&F, ch82)

To date, no pharmacologic intervention has shown a conclusive benefit in the management of nonalcoholic fatty liver disease (NAFLD). Treatment of underlying disorders, such as diabetes mellitus, obesity, and hyperlipidemia, has been shown to promote normalization of liver function test results, and in some studies, to improve findings on liver histology evaluations. Bariatric surgery has not been shown to predictably improve the histologic appearance of the liver in cases of NAFLD.

699 **B.** (S&F, ch84)

Pyrrolizidine alkaloids are found in approximately 3% of all flowering plant species throughout the world, including comfrey and Jamaican bush teas, and their ingestion, often as medicinal teas or in other formulations, can produce acute and chronic liver disease, including veno-occlusive disease. The remainder of the choices cause acute hepatocellular injury.

700 **A.** (S&F, ch91)

Chronic ulcerative colitis is a risk factor for primary sclerosing cholangitis, which is, in turn, a risk for cholangiocarcinoma. In the Far East, the most common risk factors for cholangiocarcinoma are chronic biliary infections, especially infections with *Clonorchis sinensis*.

701 **A.** (S&F, ch73)

Congenital erythropoietic porphyria (CEP) is a rare form of porphyria that is inherited in autosomal recessive fashion. The gene mutation causes a deficiency of uroporphyrinogen III cosynthase, which mainly affects the erythropoietic tissue. Affected patients typically present in the first year of life with blisters and disfiguring skin lesions in exposed areas. Infants may present with pink urine and photosensitivity. As patients age, erythrodontia, a pathognomonic red or brownish discoloration of the teeth, is frequently seen. CEP can be distinguished clinically from hepatoerythropoietic porphyria (HEP) by the variable presence of a Coombs-negative hemolytic anemia, which can be quite severe. Splenomegaly is common.

702 **D.** (S&F, ch72)

For pregnant patients with Wilson disease, treatment must be continued throughout pregnancy. There is a risk of postpartum hepatic decompensation if treatment is stopped altogether during pregnancy. Although there have been reports of women who continued penicillamine during pregnancy being delivered of healthy babies, treating the mother with zinc alone during pregnancy may be associated with a lower risk for adverse drug effects on the development of collagen in the fetus. Severe collagen defects have occasionally been reported in the offspring of women who continued penicillamine during pregnancy; in these cases, the effects in the offspring could be due in part to copper deficiency from prolonged aggressive treatment of the mother as well as from teratogenic effects of penicillamine.

703 **B.** (S&F, ch70)

Levels of alkaline phosphatase (AP) up to three times normal are relatively nonspecific and occur in various liver diseases. Striking elevations of AP are seen predominantly with infiltrative hepatic disorders (for example, primary or metastatic tumor) or biliary obstruction, either within the liver (e.g., primary biliary cirrhosis, PBC) or in the extrahepatic biliary tree. The level of AP cannot be used to distinguish reliably between intra- and extrahepatic duct obstruction or hepatic infiltration. Hepatic gamma glutamyl transpeptidase (GGTP) is derived from hepatocytes and biliary epithelia but, like AP, GGTP is found in many extrahepatic tissues, including the kidney, spleen, pancreas, heart, lung, and brain. However, it is not found in appreciable quantities in bone, and it is thus helpful in confirming the hepatic origin of an elevated AP level.

704 **E.** (S&F, ch76)

HCV infection is strongly implicated in the pathogenesis of essential mixed cryoglobulinemia and membranoproliferative glomerulonephritis, presumably by immune complex deposition. Anti-HCV antibodies are found in serum in 50% to 90% of patients with essential mixed cryoglobulinemia. Furthermore, cryoglobulins are found in approximately one half of patients infected with HCV. Many studies have found HCV RNA concentrated in cryoprecipitate. Clinical symptoms develop in only 25% to 30% of HCV-infected patients with cryoglobulinemia, with symptoms ranging from fatigue, arthralgias, or arthritis to purpura, Raynaud's phenomenon, vasculitis, peripheral neuropathies, and glomerulonephritis.

705 **C.** (S&F, ch79)

In the United States, amebiasis is a disease of young, often Hispanic, adults. Amebic liver abscess is the most common extraintestinal manifestation of amebiasis. Typical symptoms include abdominal pain, fever, malaise, myalgias, and arthralgias. During its life cycle, *Entamoeba histolytica* exists in trophozoite or cyst form. After infection, amebic cysts pass through the gastrointestinal tract and become trophozoites in the colon, where they invade the mucosa and produce typical "flask-shaped" ulcers. The organism is carried by the portal circulation to the liver, where an abscess may develop. Aspiration of this abscess may yield a reddish brown, pasty ("anchovy paste") aspirate in which trophozoites are rarely identified.

706 A. (S&F, ch77)

Acute HEV infection is usually self-limiting. A few patients have a prolonged course with marked cholestasis, including persistent jaundice lasting 2 to 6 months, prominent itching, and marked elevation of alkaline phosphatase, which resolves spontaneously. Chronic hepatitis or cirrhosis does not occur.

707 B. (S&F, ch87)

Recommended clinical treatment in this case would be to use somatostatin or octreotide in combination with endoscopic management of variceal bleeding. Nonselective beta-blocker drugs such as propranolol and nadolol are recommended as prophylaxis against a first variceal bleed in selected patients with portal hypertension. Nitrates are no longer recommended, either alone or in combination with beta blockers for primary prophylaxis. For secondary prophylaxis, isosorbide mononitrate may be added to beta-blocker therapy if the beta-blocker drugs have not resulted in an appropriate decrease in HVPG. Terlipressin, although not currently available in the United States, would be preferred to vasopressin due to its better safety profile and studies showing longer survival of patients with variceal bleeding treated with terlipressin. Losartan has not been shown in randomized controlled trials to promote a clinically significant reduction in portal pressure.

708 B. (S&F, ch77)

HEV transmission is predominantly via the fecal-oral route. Most reported outbreaks have been related to consumption of fecally contaminated drinking water. Recurrent epidemics are probably related to continuous fecal contamination of water. Person-to-person transmission is distinctly uncommon during epidemics and secondary attack rates among household contacts are only 0.7% to 2.2%. Although transmission by ingestion of undercooked meat or by receiving

a blood transfusion has been reported, the frequency of infection by these mechanisms is low.

709 C. (S&F, ch83)

Isoniazid-induced liver injury was first described in the 1970s, but deaths from this condition still occur. Hepatitis develops in approximately 21 of every 1000 persons exposed to isoniazid; 5% to 10% of cases are fatal. The risk and severity of isoniazid-induced hepatitis increase with age; the risk is 0.3% in the third decade of life and increases to 2% or higher after age 50 years. The overall frequency is the same in men and women, but 70% of fatal cases occur in women; African-American and Hispanic women may be at particular risk. There is no relationship to dose or blood level.

710 A. (S&F, ch81)

Women are more susceptible to serious alcoholic liver injury than men. Not only are women at increased risk of alcoholic liver injury, but they also exhibit a tendency toward disease progression even with abstinence. This gender-specific difference in the risk of alcoholic liver disease is unexplained. Accelerated alcoholic liver injury in women may be related to gender-specific differences in fatty acid metabolism. If the fatty acids that accumulate in liver cells as a result of impaired beta oxidation are not converted to triglyceride, they can induce liver injury. This problem may be circumvented by diversion of the fatty acids to alternative routes of metabolism, such as cytochrome P-4504A1–mediated omega hydroxylation. This compensatory pathway is efficiently up-regulated in male rats fed alcohol, but not in female rats fed alcohol. Fatty acid binding capacity is also reduced in female rats after long-term ethanol feeding. This reduced binding capacity may contribute to fatty acid toxicity.

711 A. (S&F, ch82)

Patient-related risk factors for nonalcoholic fatty liver disease (NAFLD) include obesity, insulin resistance, and dyslipidemia.

712 A. (S&F, ch87)

In patients receiving drug therapy to decrease the risk of variceal rebleeding who do have a rebleed, variceal ligation should be carried out. Similarly, in patients who have undergone variceal ligation and have recurrent bleeding, beta-blocker therapy should be added. Patients who have a variceal rebleed despite undergoing both pharmacologic and endoscopic treatment require placement of a portosystemic shunt. The surgical shunt offered is typically a distal splenorenal shunt in patients with Child-Pugh class A disease. In other patients, a TIPS is recommended.

713 **C.** (S&F, ch70)

Unconjugated hyperbilirubinemia (i.e., indirect bilirubin fraction more than 85% of the total serum bilirubin) results from either increased bilirubin production or inherited or acquired defects in hepatic uptake or conjugation. Of note, chronic hemolysis cannot account for a sustained elevation of serum bilirubin to concentrations greater than 5 mg/dL in the presence of normal hepatic function. The remaining choices are causes of conjugated bilirubin elevations.

714 **D.** (S&F, ch73)

Variegate coproporphyria is the only example given of an acute porphyria; the other conditions listed are cutaneous porphyrias. The signs and symptoms of the acute neurovisceral attacks that occur in the four acute porphyrias vary considerably. Abdominal pain is present in more than 90% of patients, followed by tachycardia and dark urine in about 80% of patients. The other acute porphyrias are alanine dehydratase deficiency, acute intermittent porphyria, and hereditary coproporphyria.

715 **E.** (S&F, ch79)

A history of exposure to the pathogen in a patient with hepatomegaly and an abdominal mass is highly suggestive of hepatic echinococcosis, although the suspicion must be confirmed, most importantly by radiology and serology tests. In cases of infection, ring-like calcifications can be seen in up to one fourth of hepatic cysts delineated by plain abdominal radiographs. On both ultrasound and CT, intracystic septations and daughter cyst formation may be seen in about one half of the cysts. CT may show avascular cysts with ring enhancement.

716 **A.** (S&F, ch75)

HBV is considered the most infectious of the listed viruses.

717 **D.** (S&F, ch75)

In Asia, the most common route of HBV transmission is vertical. In the United States, spread of infection is predominantly by horizontal routes, and adults and adolescents are at greatest risk of acquiring HBV infection. However, children of certain ethnic groups are at

substantial risk for infection, probably from both vertical transmission and horizontal spread in early childhood from mothers and other family members. Because the vast majority of these infections are subclinical, the true epidemiology of HBV infection in the United States is not known.

718 **D.** (S&F, ch69)

The liver plays a central role in the synthesis of fatty acids for storage in distal sites and in the transport of lipids within the body. To transport lipids in the circulation, the liver synthesizes and extracts a large number of apolipoproteins. Apolipoproteins, in combination with triglycerides, phospholipids, cholesterol and its esters, and lecithins, constitutes circulating lipoproteins. In addition to these protein and lipid synthesizing functions, the liver expresses cell surface receptors for circulating lipoproteins and modulates intravascular levels of these important macromolecules.

Lipoprotein lipase (LPL) is synthesized in fat and muscle cells; after synthesis, it traverses endothelial cells and binds to the luminal surface of the capillary bed. Found in adipose, lung, and muscle tissues, LPL promotes lipolysis of triglycerides present in very-low-density lipoproteins (VLDLs), chylomicrons, or high-density lipoprotein (HDL). Regulation of LPL involves multiple stimuli, including fasting and levels of various fatty acids, hormones, and catecholamines.

719 **D.** (S&F, ch69)

Tight junction complexes between neighboring hepatocytes separate the sinusoidal space from the bile canaliculi. Disruption of tight junctions can permit regurgitation of biliary solutes into the bloodstream. The liver's unique sinusoidal structure is well suited for the bidirectional transfer of a variety of solutes, including macromolecules, across the sinusoidal membrane. The low pressure allows blood to percolate slowly through the sinusoids and hepatic acinus. Fenestrae within the sinusoidal endothelium and the absence of a basement membrane permit direct contact of the portal blood with the hepatic sinusoidal surface in the subsinusoidal vascular space, referred to as the space of Disse. Microvilli on the hepatic sinusoidal plasma membrane further facilitate interchange of nutrients between sinusoidal blood and hepatocytes.

720 **D.** (S&F, ch73)

The initial treatment for porphyria cutanea tarda (PCT) should be to remove any offending agent.

Historically, the treatment has been phlebotomy to decrease iron overload and siderosis. This may give relief of cutaneous symptoms in 4 to 6 months. Chloroquine complexes with uroporphyrin and aids its excretion, but caution must be utilized during chloroquine therapy because this drug is potentially hepatotoxic. Intravenous administration of hematin, a congener of heme, has been shown to decrease the drive for heme synthesis and its abnormal byproducts. It also can have a dramatic effect on the neurological symptoms, especially if given early in an attack. Because of the wavelengths absorbed by the porphyrias, these patients are at risk of injury from exposure not only to sunlight, but also to incandescent and fluorescent lights. Special sunscreen lotions must be used that block light with wavelengths between 400 and 410 nm.

721 **E.** (S&F, ch75)

HBV is most prevalent in people born in or descending from residents of regions where HBV is highly endemic. High levels of virus in serum (as indicated by serum tests positive for HBV DNA and HBeAg) have been associated with an increased risk of transmission by needle-stick exposure and by vertical routes. Infants born to HBeAg-positive mothers who have high levels of viral replication (HBV DNA level more than 80 pg/mL) have a 70% to 90% risk of perinatal infection unless precautions are taken. In contrast, the risk of mother-to-infant transmission from HBeAg-negative mothers is substantially lower (10% to 40%). Infection occurs through occult inoculation of the infant at the time of birth or shortly thereafter. IgM anti-HBc is not detectable in cord blood, so infection is unlikely to have occurred in utero. Even with active and passive immunization, 5% to 10% of babies may acquire HBV infection at birth.

722 **B.** (S&F, ch81)

Roughly 18% to 25% of alcoholics are infected with the hepatitis C virus (HCV). In alcoholics with liver disease, the frequency of HCV infection is even higher: some studies report seropositivity rates of 40% or more. The combination of alcohol use and HCV infection significantly accelerates the progression of liver disease over that seen with either insult alone. One study indicates that HCV infection in alcoholics increases the probability of development of cirrhosis 8- to 10-fold. This association may be related to the effects of alcohol on HCV replication or on the host immune response to the virus.

723 **A.** (S&F, ch75)

The risk of chronicity after acute HBV infection is low in immunocompetent adults. The risk of chronic infection is greatly increased in patients whose immune systems have a reduced ability to recognize and clear viral infection (e.g., those on chronic hemodialysis or who are receiving immunosuppressant medications to prevent rejection of a transplanted organ or who are undergoing cancer chemotherapy). Patients with concomitant HIV infection are also at significant risk of developing chronic infection (20% to 30% of these patients continue to test HBsAg-positive after acute infection). The risk of chronicity in those who acquire the infection neonatally is extremely high (up to 90%), presumably because neonates have an immature immune system. One possible mechanism is that the fetus is sensitized in utero to HBV by exposure to viral proteins that cross the placenta. Those who acquire HBV infection in early childhood, before the age of 6 years, have a lower yet nevertheless significant risk of chronic infection (approximately 30%).

724 **E.** (S&F, ch73)

Even though liver disease is often (but not always) mild during infancy and childhood, patients with α_1-antitrypsin (α_1-AT) deficiency have an 8-fold increased risk of developing cirrhosis during adulthood, with 37% of all patients who test positive for PiZZ having histological evidence of cirrhosis at autopsy. Histopathologic features of α_1-AT deficiency change as the patient ages. In infancy, the liver biopsy may show bile duct paucity, intracellular cholestasis with or without giant-cell transformation, mild inflammatory changes, or steatosis, with few of the characteristic PAS-positive, diastase-resistant globules. These inclusions are most prominent in periportal hepatocytes, but may also be seen in Kupffer cells.

725 **B.** (S&F, ch75)

HBV infection is most prevalent among people born in regions where HBV is highly endemic and among the descendants of such individuals. High levels of virus in serum (as indicated by positive results on serologic tests for HBV DNA and HBeAg) have been associated with an increased risk of transmission by needle-stick exposure and by vertical routes. Infants born to HBeAg-positive mothers who have high levels of viral replication (HBV DNA level greater than 80 pg/mL) have a 70% to 90% risk of perinatal acquisition of HBV infection in the absence of interventions. In contrast, the risk of mother-to-infant transmission of HBV infection when the mother is HBeAg-negative is substantially lower (10% to 40%). Infection occurs through occult inoculation of the infant at the time of birth or shortly thereafter. IgM anti-HBc is not detectable in the cord blood of these infants, so intrauterine infection is unlikely to have occurred. Even with active and passive immunization, 5% to 10% of babies may acquire HBV infection at birth.

726 **B.** (S&F, ch81)

Men who drink more than 80 grams of ethanol (eight 12-ounce beers, 1 L of wine, or 1/2 pint of distilled spirits) per day are at substantial risk for development of clinical liver disease. Liver disease is two to four times more likely to develop in women who drink excessively than in men who drink excessively. In 1997, investigators examined the relationship between ethanol intake and alcoholic liver disease in entire populations rather than individuals. The results indicate that the risk of liver disease begins at relatively low levels of alcohol consumption (30 g/day). This finding has led to a general recommendation that the maximal safe level of ethanol consumption is 20 g/day of ethanol, or two "drinks" per day.

727 **D.** (S&F, ch75)

Patients with chronic liver disease, particularly those with established cirrhosis, are at increased risk of developing hepatocellular carcinoma (HCC). The risk of developing HCC is increased 10- to 390-fold in patients with chronic HBV infection compared with those who test HBsAg-negative, and it is greater in those who acquired HBV infection perinatally than in those who acquired the infection as adults. In regions where HBV is endemic, HCC is the leading cause of cancer-related deaths.

728 **B.** (S&F, ch68)

The caudate lobe of the liver is posterior to the transverse fissure. At the porta hepatis, the portal vein travels behind the hepatic artery and the bile duct. The falciform ligament contains the round ligament, which contains the obliterated umbilical vein. The fibrous capsule on the posterior aspect of the liver reflects on the diaphragm and posterior abdominal wall and leaves a bare area where the liver is in continuity with the retroperitoneum.

729 **D.** (S&F, ch83)

Hepatic stellate cells (formerly referred to as fat-storing or Ito cells) are the principal liver cell type involved in matrix deposition and hepatic fibrosis. Stellate cells are activated in methotrexate-induced hepatic fibrosis, and the possibility that vitamin A, drugs, or drug metabolites can transform stellate cells into collagen-synthesizing myofibroblasts is of considerable interest.

730 **E.** (S&F, ch86)

Primary biliary cirrhosis (PBC) is an autoimmune liver disease that generally affects middle-aged women from a variety of racial groups. It is the most frequently diagnosed cholestatic chronic liver disease in adults in the United States. It is characterized by ongoing inflammatory destruction of the intralobular bile ducts that leads to chronic cholestasis and biliary cirrhosis. The patient with PBC typically presents with symptoms of fatigue or pruritus. Other symptoms include right upper quadrant abdominal pain, anorexia and jaundice. Widespread use of screening laboratory tests has lead to the diagnosis of PBC at an asymptomatic stage in up to 60% of patients with this condition. Such patients are identified by incidental findings of elevated serum alkaline phosphatase and anti-mitochondrial antibody (AMA) levels in a serum specimen obtained during a routine health evaluation. In the case presented here, the results of the patient's blood tests for markers of viral hepatitis are consistent with a past history of vaccination against hepatitis B virus.

731 **B.** (S&F, ch83)

Death from isoniazid-induced hepatitis has been associated with a longer duration of therapy or continued ingestion of isoniazid after the onset of symptoms. Thus, most deaths from isoniazid-induced hepatitis could be prevented if patients report symptoms early and isoniazid is discontinued. Recovery is rapid if isoniazid is discontinued before severe liver injury is established. Management of liver failure is supportive; transplantation is indicated in the most severe cases.

Prevention is the best approach to managing isoniazid-induced liver failure, and it is critical to determine whether the risks of isoniazid prophylaxis outweigh those of reactivation of latent tuberculosis. The optimal approach to monitoring for isoniazid toxicity is uncertain; the onset of severe hepatotoxicity may be rapid, so monitoring for adverse effects of isoniazid by measuring serum ALT levels every other week or monthly will not always be effective. The most effective means of prevention is educating the patient to be vigilant for and to quickly report symptoms, no matter how nonspecific, that could indicate drug toxicity.

732 **A.** (S&F, ch87)

Endoscopic variceal ligation is associated with fewer complications than sclerotherapy, and requires fewer sessions for variceal obliteration. Specifically, esophageal variceal ligation during an acute bleed is not associated with the sustained elevation in HVPG seen with sclerotherapy.

Compared to sclerotherapy, endoscopic band ligation of varices is less often associated with local complications such as esophageal ulcers, strictures, and dysmotility. However, ulcers that occur as a complication of banding can be large and potentially serious when gastric fundal varices have been banded. Now that over-tubes are not used, the mechanical complications of mucosal tear, or even esophageal perforation, are uncommon.

733 **E.** (S&F, ch88)

A urine sodium/potassium ratio less than 1 in a randomly obtained urine specimen suggests compliance with a low-salt diet and inadequate natriuresis despite diuretic therapy. The doses of both diuretics must be increased. Very-low-sodium diets are unrealistic for outpatients.

734 **A.** (S&F, ch92)

The risk of recurrent cirrhosis in persons who have undergone liver transplantation because of liver failure caused by HCV is estimated to be 20% to 30% over 5 years. A small percentage of patients will suffer so-called cholestatic fibrosing hepatitis, leading to rapid graft loss and death.

735 **D.** (S&F, ch89)

Ammonia levels should be measured whenever hepatic encephalopathy is suspected, both for diagnostic purposes and as a general guide to treatment. However, normal values do not exclude the diagnosis of encephalopathy and should not delay initiation of ammonia-lowering therapy. Approximately one fourth of patients will have non-nitrogenous causes of encephalopathy, such as adverse reactions to a sedative medication or a fluid or electrolyte imbalance. In light of the potential involvement of the GABA receptor complex in encephalopathy, it is not surprising that patient responses to treatment are similar whether encephalopathy is due to elevated ammonia levels or another cause. Other diagnostic tests, including measurement of glutamine levels in the spinal fluid and electroencephalography (EEG), can help to confirm, but alone are not sensitive or specific enough to establish, the diagnosis of encephalopathy.

736 **C.** (S&F, ch87)

Currently available data do not support endoscopic variceal ligation as the preferred method for primary prophylaxis against variceal bleeding. Beta-blocker therapy is less expensive and less invasive, and it may reduce risks of bleeding from gastric varices and portal hypertensive gastropathy. However, band ligation is the only option for patients with high-risk varices who have contraindications to beta-adrenergic blocker therapy or are intolerant of this therapy or whose condition has not responded to beta-blocker therapy.

737 **A.** (S&F, ch76)

Since 1995, the incidences of infection by HCV genotypes 1a and 3a, which are common in injection drug users, have increased in frequency compared to the incidence of infection by HCV genotype 1b, which is usually transmitted in a blood transfusion.

738 **B.** (S&F, ch85)

Type I autoimmune hepatitis (AIH) can occur at any age and in either sex, although 78% of patients are women and the female:male ratio is 3.6:1. The clinical manifestations of AIH reflect chronic liver inflammation. Cholestatic features may be present, but they do not dominate the clinical picture. Similarly, manifestations of liver decompensation, such as ascites, hepatic encephalopathy, and variceal bleeding, are uncommon findings at the initial medical evaluation. At initial presentation, fatigability is the most frequently reported symptom (86%). Hyperbilirubinemia is present in 83% of patients and an elevated alkaline phosphatase level is found in 81%. Anti-smooth muscle antibodies, present in this patient, are characteristic of type I AIH. Liver/kidney microsome type 1 antibody is a classic finding in patients with type II AIH.

739 **B.** (S&F, ch88)

Among the choices listed, only cardiac ascites is associated with a serum-ascites albumin gradient (SAAG) of more than 1.1.

740 **B.** (S&F, ch91)

This incidentally discovered mass is likely to be a cavernous hemangioma, the most common benign tumor of the liver. Although the ultrasonographic appearance of this tumor is variable, the lesion is usually echogenic. Contrast-enhanced CT or MRI is diagnostic. Biopsy is unnecessary, and in fact, some reports on series of patients with this tumor have suggested that biopsy in these cases is associated with an increased risk of bleeding. Hemangioma rarely requires resection, which is usually only performed when a patient has severe symptoms or hemorrhage.

741 **B.** (S&F, ch81)

In a meta-analysis performed by Imperiale and McCullough, only when patients who had gastrointestinal hemorrhage were excluded from consideration did treatment improve the chances for survival. Glucocorticoids did not increase the risk of gastrointestinal hemorrhage, but bleeding was independently associated with such a high mortality risk that it overrode the beneficial effect of glucocorticoids. Poor renal function at the time of randomization to glucocorticoid therapy can also limit the benefit of this treatment. Patients with alcoholic hepatitis who had serum creatinine levels greater than 2.5 mg/dL were at high risk of progression to renal failure, and the short-term mortality in this group was 75%, with or without glucocorticoid therapy. When evaluating patients for glucocorticoid therapy, certain confounding illnesses should be considered contraindications to therapy; these illnesses include active infection, pancreatitis, and possibly insulin-dependent diabetes mellitus.

742 **A.** (S&F, ch74)

The highest rate of reported disease due to hepatitis A virus infection is among children between 5 and 14 years old, and 25% of reported cases are among persons aged 20 years or younger; however, HAV infection can occur at any age. The epidemiologic risk factors for HAV infection in the U.S. population in 2002 were reported to be as follows: unknown, 57%; sexual or household contact with a patient who has hepatitis A, 12%; international travel, 9%; male homosexual activity, 8%; injection drug use, 5%; child or employee in a day-care center, 1%; food or waterborne outbreak, 1%; contact with a day-care child or employee, 3%; and other contact with a patient who has hepatitis, 4%.

743 **C.** (S&F, ch89)

Clinical trials showed that desmopressin has beneficial effects on the coagulation cascade in patients with cirrhosis-related coagulopathy.

744 **A.** (S&F, ch87)

Variceal hemorrhage, hepatic encephalopathy, and ascites are the major complications of cirrhosis of the liver; all result from portal hypertension. Up to 25% of patients with newly diagnosed varices will have bleeding in the first 2 years. A good indicator of bleeding risk appears to be variceal size, with the risk of bleeding in the first 2 years being 7% in patients with varices less than 5 mm in diameter compared to 30% in patients with varices more than 5 mm in diameter. The most important predictor of bleeding, however, is the hepatic venous pressure gradient (HVPG), with risk of bleeding being virtually absent when this value is below 12 mmHg.

QUESTIONS

745 A 75-year-old white man with a history of congestive heart failure comes to the emergency department because of abrupt onset of left lower quadrant pain and bloody diarrhea. Medications include digoxin and furosemide. Physical examination reveals a temperature of 100.5°F. The heart rate is 110 beats/minute and the rhythm is irregular. The blood pressure is 136/85 mmHg. On abdominal palpation, moderate left lower quadrant tenderness is noted but no masses are felt. Rectal examination discloses bloody stool.

Hemoglobin is 13.0 g/dL. The leukocyte count is 14,000/mm³. Gentle flexible sigmoidoscopy reveals a normal rectum and a localized area of mucosal erythema, friability, edema, and submucosal hemorrhage in the mid sigmoid. A stool specimen tests positive for leukocytes but no infectious or parasitic agents are identified. Which of the following is the best plan of management at this time?

A. Laparotomy
B. Mesenteric angiography
C. Computed tomography (CT) of the abdomen and pelvis
D. Mesalamine and prednisone therapy
E. Supportive care and observation

746 A 65-year-old woman is found to have a malignancy in the sigmoid colon. CT shows no evidence of metastasis and after evaluation of biopsy specimens obtained during left hemicolectomy, the cancer is determined to be Duke's stage B1. One year later, CT shows liver metastases. Resection of liver metastases would not be considered if:

A. Bilobar metastases are present
B. Two metastases are present
C. More than four metastases are present
D. No extrahepatic disease is present

747 Which of the following is the most accurate statement regarding chylomicrons?

A. Chylomicrons are the major triglyceride-rich lipoprotein exported from enterocytes during the fasting state.
B. The surface coat comprises triglycerides and the core consists of cholesterol esters and phospholipids.
C. The absence of apolipoprotein B (apo B) prevents synthesis and secretion of chylomicrons.
D. Chylomicrons are released across the enterocyte basolateral membrane.

748 The Rome II criteria for IBS are as follows: at least 12 weeks or more (nonconsecutive) in the last 12 months of abdominal pain or discomfort that has two of the three following features:

A. Looser stool at pain onset, more frequent stools at pain onset, abdominal distention
B. Passage of mucus, incomplete evacuation, abdominal distention
C. Pain relieved with defecation, onset associated with a change in stool frequency, onset associated with a change in stool form
D. Bloating, anal fissures, hemorrhoids from straining
E. Female gender, age younger than 30, pain relieved with defecation

749 Diversion colitis appears to be caused by:

A. Recurrence of inflammatory bowel disease (IBD)
B. Colonic epithelium changes due to luminal nutrient deficiency
C. Radiation
D. *Clostridium difficile* infection

750 Which of the following is the most common human protozoan enteropathogen worldwide that causes chronic diarrhea and intestinal malabsorption and contributes to retardation of growth and development in infants and young children?

A. *Isospora belli*
B. *Giardia lamblia*
C. *Cyclospora cayetanensis*
D. *Cryptosporidium parvum*

751 A 31-year-old man with no significant medical history is being evaluated for perianal pruritus. The patient reports that over the prior 6 months he has had worsening itching that occurs both after and unrelated to defecation. He has begun to vigorously clean his perianal area with a washcloth and soap several times daily, especially after bowel movements, without significant relief. The patient has no history of diarrhea, rectal bleeding, discharge, incontinence, or proctalgia. He denies participation in anal intercourse. The patient consumes approximately six alcohol-containing beverages weekly and three to five cups of coffee daily.

An examination of the man's perianal area demonstrates no external hemorrhoids, anal fissure, skin tags, fistula tracts, or anal warts. No masses are appreciated upon digital rectal examination. A stool sample is brown and tests negative for occult blood. A flexible sigmoidoscopy demonstrates normal rectosigmoid mucosa without evidence of internal hemorrhoids. What is the most likely etiology for the patient's symptoms?

A. Human papilloma virus (HPV) infection
B. Perianal Crohn's disease
C. Anal fissure
D. Idiopathic pruritus ani
E. Anal cancer

752 A 64-year-old white woman with hypertension and non–insulin-dependent diabetes mellitus diagnosed 11 years previously is now referred for evaluation of abdominal discomfort and loose bowel movements. The patient reports postprandial bloating followed by loose bowel movements that she describes as "oily." She reports subjective weight loss over the past year. She denies a history of excessive alcohol consumption. Laboratory tests show macrocytic anemia with a hemoglobin of 9.7 g/dL and mean corpuscular volume (MCV) of 106/mL. There is also evidence of mild hypocalcemia. Sudan stain of a stool specimen is positive for the presence of fecal fat.

Small intestinal bacterial overgrowth (SIBO) is suspected. A glucose breath test is ordered. Which of the following statements regarding the glucose breath test is most accurate?

A. In the presence of bacterial overgrowth, glucose absorption in the upper small intestine is greatly increased.
B. Within 2 hours of the ingestion of the glucose substrate, a rise of 20 parts per million of hydrogen in exhaled breath is regarded as diagnostic of SIBO.
C. Patient preparation is not important for this test.
D. In general, breath testing in cases of suspected SIBO is prohibitively expensive and therefore the glucose breath test is not widely used.

753 Infectious diseases caused by the following organisms are definitely linked to the etiology of Crohn's disease:

A. *Chlamydia*
B. *Listeria*
C. *Pseudomonas*
D. Paramyxovirus (measles virus)
E. None of the above

754 The most common symptom(s) early in the course of acute mesenteric ischemia (AMI) is (are):

A. Abdominal distention
B. Fever
C. Abdominal pain
D. Nausea and vomiting
E. Bloody diarrhea

755 The treatment of familial adenomatous polyposis (FAP) with the nonsteroidal anti-inflammatory drug sulindac has shown some benefit. Which of the following statements is *true* regarding sulindac?

A. Sulindac may decrease the number but not the size of polyps.
B. Sulindac may decrease the size but not the number of polyps.
C. Maintenance therapy with sulindac does not protect against the development of rectal cancer.
D. When the drug is discontinued, the positive effects are irreversible.
E. Sulindac has beneficial effects on upper gastrointestinal (GI) neoplasia, similar to the effects on FAP.

756 A 2-month-old child is referred by his pediatrician for evaluation of episodic vomiting, abdominal distention, and constipation. According to his parents, he has had "trouble with constipation" since coming home from the hospital and produces a small, hard bowel movement every "few days." Prior to bowel movements, he is "very fussy" with a visibly distended abdomen. In addition, he occasionally vomits bilious material. On digital rectal examination, there is forceful expulsion of gas and scant stool is found. Regarding the pathogenesis of the most likely diagnosis:

A. It results from the failure of splanchnic cells to migrate during organogenesis, resulting in an absence of ganglion cells in the submucosal plexus.
B. There is an absence of ganglion cells in the distal colon, resulting in a failure of the involved segment to relax, resulting in a functional colonic obstruction.
C. A genetic basis for this disease has not yet been identified.
D. The abnormality is easily diagnosed by superficial rectal biopsy.

757 The accuracy of fecal occult blood testing for colorectal cancer is not affected by:

A. Rehydration
B. Ascorbic acid
C. Tocopherol
D. Ingestion of red meat
E. Nonsteroidal anti-inflammatory drugs

758 Mucosal folds of the small intestine are called:

A. Appendices epiploicae
B. Columns of Morgagni
C. Haustral folds
D. Plicae circularis
E. Rugae

759 Which of the following drugs stimulates small intestinal motility when given after a meal?

A. Clonidine
B. Octreotide
C. Calcium channel antagonists
D. Antiparkinsonian drugs
E. Opiate analgesics

760 Which of the following carbohydrates cannot be absorbed intact and requires hydrolysis by brush border enzymes in the duodenum and jejunum?

A. Fructose
B. Galactose
C. Glucose
D. Lactose

761 Appendicitis is epidemiologically best linked to:

A. African countries
B. People between the ages of 15 and 19 years old
C. Women
D. The third most common reason for presenting with acute abdominal symptoms to an emergency department in a developed country
E. None of the above

762 A 40-year-old man has a history of familial adenomatous polyposis treated by total proctocolectomy with ileoanal anastomosis 15 years previously. At a follow-up examination, he denies any history of problems and none are found on the physical exam. Upper GI endoscopy with a side-viewing scope to view the ampulla and a capsule endoscopy are recommended. Which of the following statements is *true* regarding extracolonic tumors in patients with familial adenomatous polyposis?

A. Gastric polyps frequently occur and are usually adenomas.
B. Gastric cancer occasionally occurs.
C. Gastric carcinoids cause significant morbidity.
D. Duodenal adenomas may occur in 60% to 90% of patients and duodenal cancer in 4% to 12%.
E. Ileal and jejunal adenomas occur in up to 75% of patients.

763 The most common anatomic position of the appendix relative to the cecum is:

A. Anterior
B. Lateral
C. Medial
D. Retrocecal
E. Retrocolic

764 The risk factor most strongly associated with IBS is:

A. Depression
B. Food intolerance
C. Bacterial gastroenteritis
D. Hypochondria
E. Oral glucocorticoid use

765 Which of the following statements about melanosis coli is *false?*

A. It is secondary to chronic use of anthraquinone laxatives.
B. Lipofuscin pigment is the etiologic agent.
C. Melanin pigment causes the discoloration.
D. It usually disappears within 1 year of stopping laxatives.

766 Which of the following is the most common cause of vitamin B_{12} malabsorption?

- **A.** Pancreatic insufficiency
- **B.** Bacterial overgrowth syndrome
- **C.** Crohn's disease involving the terminal ileum
- **D.** Pernicious anemia
- **E.** Ileal resection

767 Which of the following is a true statement regarding risk factors for small bowel adenocarcinomas?

- **A.** Only patients with FAP develop adenocarcinomas of the duodenum.
- **B.** A diet high in animal fat and protein is not associated with small bowel adenocarcinomas.
- **C.** DNA adducts (chemical bonds between a carcinogen and DNA) are as common in small-bowel as they are in large-bowel adenocarcinomas.
- **D.** Min mice are a model for studying various carcinogens and their effects on crypt cells.
- **E.** The relative resistance of the small bowel to the development of adenocarcinomas is believed to be due in part to fewer bacteria and rapid transit of contents.

768 Extraintestinal manifestations of celiac sprue include all of the following except:

- **A.** Iron deficiency anemia
- **B.** Ataxia
- **C.** Osteopenia
- **D.** Dermatitis herpetiformis
- **E.** Uveitis

769 Tropical sprue is predominantly a disease of southern and Southeast Asia, Central and South America, and:

- **A.** Africa
- **B.** Australia
- **C.** Caribbean Islands
- **D.** Hawaii

770 A well-established therapy for enteropathy-type intestinal T-cell lymphoma (ETL) includes (see figure):

- **A.** Glucocorticoid drugs
- **B.** Azathioprine
- **C.** Cyclosporine
- **D.** None of the above

771 The enteric nervous system includes all of the following except:

- **A.** Myenteric plexus
- **B.** Interneurons

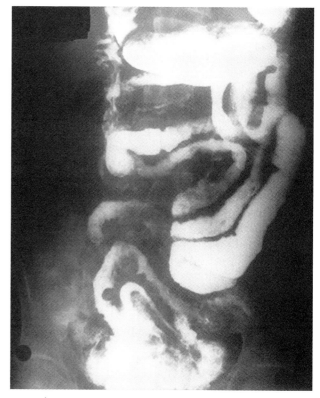

Figure for question **770**

- **C.** Submucosal plexus
- **D.** Vagus nerve

772 Regarding reperfusion injury, which of the following statements is *true?*

- **A.** It is the major cause for injury after a prolonged episode of ischemia.
- **B.** It results in the production of superoxide, hydrogen peroxide, and hydroxyl radicals.
- **C.** Thiopurine methyltransferase is the rate-limiting enzyme involved in the production of these oxygen radicals.
- **D.** Leukotriene B1 is a major cytokine involved in this type of injury.

773 With regard to the enteric motor nervous system, the excitatory neurotransmitter is:

- **A.** Adenosine triphosphate (ATP)
- **B.** Acetylcholine (Ach)
- **C.** Epinephrine
- **D.** Nitric oxide (NO)
- **E.** Vasoactive intestinal peptide (VIP)

774 Regarding familial visceral myopathy, which of the following statements is *true?*

- **A.** It is a disease characterized by degeneration of gastrointestinal neurons.

B. It is a primary disorder of the interstitial cells of Cajal.
C. Hirschsprung's disease is a form of this disorder.
D. Patients may exhibit mitochondrial DNA abnormalities and histologically it is characterized by degeneration and fibrosis of gastrointestinal smooth muscle.
E. It is the most common cause for chronic intestinal pseudo-obstruction.

775 The outer longitudinal muscular bands that characterize the colon and distinguish it from the small intestines are the:

A. Appendices epiploicae
B. Columns of Morgagni
C. Haustra
D. Plicae circularis
E. Taenia coli

776 The following test has *not* been widely advocated for colorectal cancer screening:

A. Yearly fecal occult blood test (FOBT)
B. Flexible sigmoidoscopy every 5 years
C. Optical colonoscopy every 10 years
D. Double-contrast barium enema every 5 to 10 years
E. Virtual colonoscopy every 5 to 10 years

777 The internal anal sphincter (IAS) and external anal sphincter (EAS) both have critical roles in regulating defecation. The IAS is composed of smooth muscle with a high resting tone that is modulated by sympathetic and parasympathetic innervations. The EAS:

A. Is composed of striated muscle under voluntary control and is innervated by the lumbar plexus, similar to the more proximal colon.
B. Is composed of striated muscle under voluntary control and is innervated by the pudendal nerve (S3 and S4) similar to the other pelvic floor muscles.
C. Is composed of smooth muscle with a high resting tone that is modulated by sympathetic and parasympathetic innervations.
D. Is composed of smooth muscle with a high resting tone that is modulated by the pudendal nerve (S3 and S4) similar to other pelvic floor muscles.

778 Patients with ulcerative proctitis typically complain of:

A. Severe abdominal pain
B. Bloody diarrhea
C. Nausea and vomiting
D. Tenesmus

779 A patient with diffuse ulcerations of the small intestine, celiac disease refractory to gluten withdrawal, and intestinal villous atrophy most likely has:

A. Enteropathy-type intestinal T-cell lymphoma (ETL)
B. Crohn's disease
C. Ulceration induced by use of nonsteroidal anti-inflammatory drugs (NSAIDs)
D. Whipple's disease

780 Which of the following statements is *not* true about fistulae in patients with diverticulitis?

A. Fistulae occur in fewer than 5% of patients with diverticulitis.
B. Colovesicular fistulae are the most common.
C. There is a 2:1 female:male predominance.
D. Colovaginal fistulas represent 25% of all cases.
E. None of the above

781 Which of the following statements is *true* about small bowel obstruction (SBO) secondary to hernias?

A. Internal hernias are a more common cause for obstruction than external hernias.
B. Hernias have a high risk of strangulation.
C. Inguinal hernias are more common in young adults.
D. Hernias are the most common cause for small bowel obstruction.
E. Internal hernias are always congenital.

782 A 50-year-old woman presents for colorectal cancer screening. Her father had colon cancer diagnosed at age 45 and her sister at age 55. Her colonoscopy reveals a cecal adenocarcinoma. Which of the following statements is *not* true regarding this patient's syndrome?

A. It is inherited in an autosomal dominant fashion.
B. It causes fewer than 1% of all colorectal cancers.
C. There is increased frequency of cancer of the female genital tract.
D. About 80% of the colon cancers are caused by germline mutations in the *hMSH2* or *hMLH1* genes.
E. There is a predominance of proximal tumors.

783 The prevalence of celiac sprue in first-degree relatives of those with this disease is roughly:

A. 1:200
B. 1:100
C. 1:50
D. 1:20

784 Which of the following statements describing the effects of cholera is *true?*

A. Cholera produces a cytoxin that impairs absorption and damages mucosa.
B. Cholera produces an enterotoxin that increases cyclic adenosine monophosphate and thus increases secretion.
C. Sodium-nutrient pathways (i.e., the sodium-glucose pathway) are never damaged by toxin.
D. Cholera toxin blocks electroneutral sodium chloride absorption.

785 Which of the following would stimulate absorption from gastrointestinal mucosa?

A. Increase in cyclic adenosine monophosphate (cAMP)
B. Decrease in cyclic adenosine monophosphate (cAMP)
C. Increase in cyclic guanosine monophosphate (cGMP)
D. Increase in Ca^{++} and/or activation of protein kinase C

786 The gold standard for the diagnosis of Whipple's disease is:

A. Sputum analysis
B. Stool analysis
C. Serologic tests for antibodies
D. Biopsy of the duodenum with subsequent polymerase chain reaction (PCR) amplification

787 Which of the following is an accurate statement regarding the relationship between small intestinal bacterial overgrowth (SIBO) and chronic liver disease?

A. SIBO is more common in patients with advanced liver disease.
B. SIBO does not occur in cirrhotic patients in the absence of portal hypertension.
C. The etiology of SIBO in patients with chronic liver disease is likely related to motility disturbances.
D. Liver transplantation improves small bowel dysmotility in cirrhotic patients.
E. All of the above

788 The risk of colorectal cancer in patients with ulcerative colitis (UC) is:

A. 20% at 20 years
B. 50% after 35 years
C. 7% to 10% at 20 years
D. 2% to 3% per year after 8 or 10 years

789 A 64-year-old with a history of multiple medical problems was admitted for pyelonephritis 5 days ago and now has diarrhea. The bowel movements are loose, greenish, mucus-like, and heme-positive. What is the most likely pathogen in this case?

A. *Clostridium difficile*
B. *Salmonella*
C. Rotavirus
D. Amebiasis

790 In a patient suspected of having colon ischemia who undergoes colonoscopy within 48 hours of the onset of symptoms, typical findings would include:

A. A single line of erythema with ulceration oriented along the long axis of the colon (colon single-stripe sign, CSSS)
B. "Thumbprinting"
C. Extensive rectal involvement with a single, deep ulceration
D. Stricture formation in the sigmoid colon

791 Inhibitory neural reflexes play a role in postoperative ileus by:

A. Norepinephrine release by efferent sympathetic splanchnic nerves inhibiting acetylcholine release from excitatory neurons in the myenteric plexus
B. Serotonin release from neurons, causing a direct inhibition of peristalsis
C. Somatostatin-induced inhibition of acetylcholine release
D. Nitrous oxide production within the myenteric plexus
E. Reduction of endogenous opioids within myenteric plexus neurons

792 The proposed mechanisms for acute intestinal pseudo-obstruction include which of the following?

A. Excess sympathetic motor input to the gut
B. Excess nitrous oxide release from inhibitory motoneurons
C. Decreased stimulation of peripheral opioid receptors by endogenous or exogenous opioids
D. Reflex motor excitation through splanchnic afferents in response to noxious stimuli
E. Reduced inflammatory response with reduced release of inflammatory mediators

793 Which of the following statements about small intestinal bacterial overgrowth is most accurate?

A. Small intestinal bacterial overgrowth is the most common cause of malabsorption in developed countries.
B. Many patients may have nonspecific symptoms, similar to those of IBS.

C. The gold standard for diagnosis is the ^{14}C-xylose breath test.

D. Treatment with antibiotics such as metronidazole, amoxicillin/clavulanate, or ciprofloxacin is usually ineffective.

794 Sensory innervation of the colon is via:

A. Spinal efferent neurons with nerve cell bodies in the lumbar dorsal root ganglion (DRG).

B. Spinal efferent neurons with nerve cell bodies in the celiac and superior mesenteric ganglia and paravertebral chain ganglia.

C. Spinal afferent neurons with nerve cell bodies in the lumbar dorsal root ganglion (DRG).

D. Spinal afferent neurons with nerve cell bodies in the celiac and superior mesenteric ganglia and paravertebral chain ganglia.

795 Which of the following is the most common cause of small intestinal bacterial overgrowth?

A. Disorders affecting small intestinal peristalsis, such as diabetes mellitus and scleroderma

B. Proton-pump inhibitor use

C. Anatomic abnormalities resulting from abdominal surgery, such as a blind loop

D. Atrophic gastritis

796 A 40-year-old man with a history of asthma visits a physician in the southeastern United States complaining of a serpiginous urticaria rash. He just finished a course of glucocorticoid medication for his asthma and is complaining of abdominal pain, nausea, and worsening shortness of breath. He is admitted to the hospital and administered broad-spectrum antibiotics. Which study is *not* sensitive for the diagnosis of the intestinal worm causing this patient's symptoms?

A. Enzyme-linked immunoassay (ELISA) for immunoglobulin G (IgG)

B. Examination of a stool smear cultured on an agar plate

C. Intestinal biopsy

D. Examination of a stool smear for rhabditiform larvae

797 Randomized controlled trials of fiber supplementation therapy and diet manipulation for IBS have shown that:

A. Wheat bran is better than placebo

B. Fiber supplementation benefits constipation and diarrhea-predominant IBS equally

C. The key to fiber supplementation is to start at high doses and then taper to the lowest effective dose

D. In most patients a lactose-free diet does not improve typical IBS symptoms

E. Exclusion of foods to which the patient has a positive IgG antibody response may provide benefit in both diarrhea- and constipation-predominant IBS

798 A 56-year-old white woman with gastric adenocarcinoma localized to the proximal stomach is scheduled to undergo a total gastrectomy. Which of the following is least likely to be a complication of this operation?

A. Carbohydrate malabsorption

B. Protein malabsorption

C. Fat malabsorption

D. Vitamin B_{12} malabsorption

E. Iron malabsorption

799 Multichannel intraluminal impedance (MII) is a technique:

A. That measures intraluminal pressures to determine the bolus progression along the intestines.

B. That measures differential conductivities of luminal contents to monitor the bolus progression along the intestines.

C. That measures differential conductivities of luminal contents to monitor intraluminal pressures.

D. That measures differential resistances of luminal contents to monitor the bolus progression along the intestines.

800 Which of the following environmental factors has/have been associated with Crohn's disease?

A. Occupations that do not involve outdoor physical labor

B. Oral contraceptives

C. Nonsteroidal anti-inflammatory drugs (NSAIDs)

D. Bottle-feeding babies

E. All of the above

F. None of the above

801 Several symptoms are thought *not* to be associated with IBS and in the presence of these so-called alarm features, the physician considering a diagnosis of IBS should investigate for an organic disease. Which of the following "alarm features" does *not* discriminate between IBS and organic disease?

A. Unexplained weight loss

B. History of rectal bleeding

C. Nighttime or nocturnal symptoms

D. New onset of symptoms in an older-age patient

E. Dysphagia

802 A 40-year-old man developed diarrhea 6 hours after eating fried rice in a Chinese restaurant. Examination of a stool specimen shows no leukocytes. What is the most likely diagnosis?

A. *Bacillus cereus* infection
B. *Shigella flexneri* infection
C. *Salmonella typhi* infection
D. *Yersinia enterocolitica* infection
E. *Clostridium difficile* infection

803 A 25-year-old woman complains that she has passed worms in her stool. She recently returned from a trip to Alaska where she frequently consumed salmon. *Diphyllobothrium latum* infection is diagnosed. Which of the following statements is *true* regarding this infection?

A. The pathogen is one of the smallest parasites that infects humans.
B. The infection is acquired by eating undercooked or raw saltwater fish.
C. The treatment is ivermectin.
D. Patients are usually symptomatic.
E. Vitamin B_{12} deficiency may occur.

804 Regarding the prevalence of acquired primary lactase deficiency (adult-type hypolactasia), among which of the following groups does lactase persistence predominate?

A. Adults of Chinese heritage
B. Adults of Western European heritage
C. Adults of Native American heritage
D. Adults of Jewish heritage
E. Adults of Southern Italian heritage

805 A 25-year-old woman with a 10-year history of Crohn's disease without perianal involvement whose disease is mildly active is contemplating starting a family. It would be accurate to tell the patient:

A. She has a significantly lower chance of becoming pregnant
B. If she becomes pregnant, a cesarean section is recommended
C. Her risk of having a child with a birth defect is higher than average
D. She has a 33% chance that Crohn's disease will remain stable, a 33% change that it will get better, and a 33% chance that it will worsen during the pregnancy.

806 In the fed state, peristalsis, a coordinated contractile pattern, moves chyme along the small intestine to facilitate digestion and nutrient absorption. In the fasting state:

A. The small intestine has very little motor activity because luminal contents are required to stimulate motor function.

B. Peristalsis continues unchanged, regardless of luminal contents.
C. "Fast" peristalsis is replaced by "slow" peristalsis.
D. Interdigestive motor cycles (IDMCs) are complex patterns of contractions that periodically sweep along the small intestine.

807 Gastrointestinal stromal tumors (GISTs) are associated with a poorer prognosis if they:

A. Express the c-kit mutation
B. Are located in the stomach
C. Are greater than 2.5 cm in size
D. Have a low mitotic count
E. Have a low proliferative index

808 Risk factors for the development of colonic adenomas include all of the following *except:*

A. Diet high in fat
B. Obesity
C. Cigarette smoking
D. Excess alcohol intake
E. High vitamin C intake

809 An 18-year-old man presents with abdominal pain, bloody diarrhea, nausea, and fever. He remembers eating a hamburger a few days ago. The results of laboratory testing of a serum sample show hemoglobin (Hgb) of 9 mg/dL, white blood cell (WBC) count of 12,000/µL, platelet count of 100,000/µL, blood urea nitrogen (BUN) level of 20 mg/dL, and creatinine level of 3 mg/dL. What is the most likely etiologic pathogen?

A. *Salmonella*
B. *Campylobacter*
C. *E. coli* O157:H7
D. *Yersinia*

810 Carcinoid tumors of the small intestine:

A. Are the least common malignancy in the small intestine
B. Are almost always located in the proximal small intestine
C. Are generally greater than 5 cm at time of diagnosis
D. Are multifocal in 30% of patients
E. Are most common in adults younger than 50 years old

811 The prevalence of celiac sprue in the general population is roughly:

A. 1:3000
B. 1:1000
C. 1:100
D. 1:10

812 Which of the following statements about fluid load of the gastrointestinal tract is *false?*

A. The salivary glands produce 1500cc of fluid daily.
B. The stomach produces 2500cc of fluid daily.
C. Bile amounts to 1000cc daily.
D. Pancreatic secretions amount to 1500cc daily.

813 The following therapy should reduce the duration of postoperative ileus:

A. Nonsteroidal anti-inflammatory drug therapy
B. Thoracic epidural injections with bupivacaine
C. Intravenous administration of erythromycin
D. Intravenous administration of metoclopramide
E. Placement of a nasogastric tube for decompression

814 A 51-year-old man presents to the emergency department with abdominal pain, fever, and mild rectal bleeding 1 day after undergoing a screening colonoscopy, the results of which were normal. A radiographic "obstruction series" showed no obstruction of the gastrointestinal tract. CT showed mild thickening of the sigmoid colon. Which is the most likely diagnosis?

A. Perforation of the colon
B. *C. difficile* colitis
C. Ischemic colitis
D. Glutaraldehyde colitis

815 *C. difficile* diarrhea and colitis are caused by toxins, not by bacterial invasion of the colonic mucosa. All of the following statements about *C. difficile* colitis are true *except:*

A. *C. difficile* produces two structurally similar protein exotoxins, toxins A and B, which are the major known factors of this bacterium.
B. Toxin A is an inflammatory enterotoxin.
C. Toxin B is an extremely potent cytotoxin but has minimal enterotoxin activity in animals.
D. Toxin A is 10 times more potent than toxin B in causing injury and electrophysiologic changes in human colonic explants in vitro.
E. Toxin B is considered to be a major factor in the pathogenesis of *C. difficile*–associated diarrhea and colitis in patients.

816 Colonic smooth muscle possesses intrinsic, oscillatory activity (even when external neural activity is blocked) that includes large-amplitude, slow membrane potential oscillations called slow waves and small-amplitude, rapid membrane potential oscillations called:

A. Accelerated or fast waves
B. Giant motor complexes (GMCs)
C. Myenteric potential oscillations (MPOs)
D. Migrating motor complexes (MMCs)

817 Which of the following statements is *not* true about listeriosis?

A. The vehicles of infection are raw and pasteurized milk and soft cheeses.
B. Listeriosis usually is a systemic disease.
C. It rarely causes death.
D. Neurologic sequelae may occur.

818 *Isospora belli* and *Cyclospora cayetanensis* share the following characteristics:

A. Do not test positive with acid-fast stains
B. Are readily killed by trimethoprim-sulfamethoxazole in immunocompetent patients
C. Cause protracted illness in immunocompetent and immunocompromised hosts
D. Cause peripheral eosinophilia with Charcot-Leyden crystals in the stool

819 A 50-year-old man who has had ulcerative colitis (UC) for 30 years was hospitalized 10 days ago for the third time in 18 months. His condition has not improved since admission. His past medical history is notable for previous treatment for tuberculosis (TB). Laboratory results show a hemoglobin level of 9.0mg/dL, white blood cell count of 15,000/uL, albumin level of 3.0, and a cholesterol level of 110. The next best step in this patient's management should be:

A. Administer cyclosporine 4mg/kg intravenously by continuous infusion
B. Check a chest x-ray and if there are no signs of TB, start infliximab (Remicade)
C. Perform total proctocolectomy with ileal pouch anal anastomosis (IPAA)
D. Administer intravenous heparin
E. None of the above

820 Which of the following statements is *false* regarding traveler's diarrhea?

A. Antibiotic treatment will decrease the duration of diarrhea.
B. Prophylactic treatment with antibiotics can effectively prevent more than 80% of cases of traveler's diarrhea.
C. Prophylactic antibiotic therapy is recommended for anyone traveling to third-world countries.
D. Rifaximin is an effective antibiotic for treatment.

821 Which of the following statements is *true* regarding other treatments for IBS?

A. Tricyclic antidepressants should not be used because the doses required exceed standard antidepressant drug dosing recommendations.
B. Selective serotonin reuptake inhibitors (SSRIs) may be more beneficial in patients with constipation-predominant IBS because they accelerate small bowel transit.
C. Colchicine has been used to treat diarrhea-predominant IBS.
D. Octreotide increases intestinal transit, secretion, and sensation in patients with IBS.
E. Clonidine may be useful in treating constipation-predominant IBS.

822 Motor activity in the small intestine is dependent upon all of the following *except:*

A. Colonic distention
B. Intraluminal osmolality
C. Intraluminal pH
D. Nifedipine use
E. Underlying medical disease, such as systemic sclerosis

823 Which of the following statements is *true* regarding Gardner's syndrome?

A. Hamartomatous polyps are present and have malignant potential.
B. Osteomas of the mandible and skull and dental abnormalities may be present.
C. Congenital hypertrophy of the retinal pigmented epithelium may be present and causes significant change in vision.
D. Desmoid tumors may occur; however, they are virtually always benign.
E. The inheritance pattern is autosomal recessive.

824 The single best test to make the diagnosis of Crohn's disease is:

A. Upper GI small-bowel follow-through
B. Small-bowel wireless capsule endoscopy (CAM)
C. Colonoscopy
D. CT
E. None of the above

825 The most common presentation for benign small-bowel neoplasms is:

A. Small bowel obstruction
B. Overt GI bleeding
C. Occult iron-deficiency anemia
D. Perforation
E. Unexplained weight loss

826 Celiac sprue is associated with all of the following autoimmune disorders *except:*

A. Sclerosing cholangitis
B. Ulcerative proctitis
C. Insulin-dependent diabetes mellitus
D. Hypothyroidism
E. Wegener's granulomatosis

827 What is the single most important independent determinant of adenoma prevalence?

A. Patient age greater than 60 years
B. Family history of colon cancer
C. Family history of adenomas
D. Race
E. Gender

828 A 46-year-old man with a history of cirrhosis of the liver secondary to hepatitis C virus infection who is on a liver transplant list is advised by his physician to avoid eating raw seafood because it may contain which of the following pathogens that can cause lethal infection in those with liver disease?

A. Rotavirus
B. Calicivirus
C. *C. difficile*
D. *Vibrio vulnificus*
E. Enterotoxigenic *E. coli*

829 The human leukocyte antigens (HLAs) HLA DQ2 and HLA-DQ8 are associated with which one of the following disorders?

A. Tropical sprue
B. Ulcerative colitis
C. Crohn's disease
D. Celiac sprue

830 Which of the following statements is *false* regarding hyperplastic polyps?

A. There is a distal predominance of hyperplastic polyps.
B. There is little, if any, intrinsic malignant potential.
C. Serrated adenomas should be treated as adenomatous polyps and not as hyperplastic polyps.
D. The majority of diminutive polyps in the rectosigmoid are hyperplastic.
E. Hyperplastic polyps do not usually coexist with adenomatous polyps in those with a strong family history of colon cancer or hereditary nonpolyposis colorectal cancer (HNPCC).

831 A 32-year-old African-American woman is evaluated for complaints of crampy abdominal pain, bloating, watery diarrhea, and excessive flatulence. These symptoms have occurred over several years and typically develop 30 minutes to

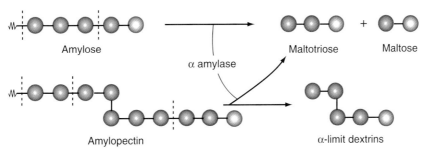

Figure for question **834**. (From Gray GM: Carbohydrate absorption and malabsorption. In Johnson LR [ed]: Physiology of the Gastrointestinal Tract. New York, Raven Press, 1981, p 1064.)

1 hour after consumption of foods such as milk, cheese, and ice cream. She denies weight loss, melena, or hematochezia. There is no family history of inflammatory bowel disease or gastrointestinal malignancy. A diagnosis of lactose malabsorption is suspected. Which of the following test results would support this diagnosis?

A. An increase in breath hydrogen concentration of more than 20 parts per million over baseline 15 minutes after ingestion of 50 g of lactose

B. An increase in breath hydrogen concentration of more than 20 parts per million over baseline 90 minutes after ingestion of 50 g of lactose

C. An increase in serum glucose concentration of more than 20 mg/dL over baseline 30 minutes after ingestion of 50 g of lactose

D. A fecal pH greater than 5.5

832 Each of the following statements is true about *Bacillus anthracis except:*

A. The endospore-contaminated meat from infected animals is the primary mode of transmission of gastrointestinal anthrax.

B. The clinical manifestations include bloody diarrhea and diffuse abdominal pain.

C. More than 50% of episodes are fatal.

D. Ampicillin is the drug of choice.

E. Ascites may be present.

833 Observations about drug therapy for IBS have shown that:

A. Anticholinergics are most useful for those with postprandial pain when taken prior to eating.

B. Sublingual anticholinergics are more effective than oral ones.

C. Loperamide is effective for abdominal pain and bloating as well as for diarrhea.

D. Stimulant laxatives are not safe and should not be used by patients with constipation-predominant IBS.

E. Codeine phosphate has low risks for side effects and for dependency.

834 Which of the following statements is the *most* accurate regarding the roles of salivary and pancreatic amylase in starch digestion (see figure)?

A. Salivary amylase is the major enzyme of starch digestion.

B. Rapid swallowing of poorly chewed foods may result in suboptimal salivary amylase activity.

C. Pancreatic and salivary amylase produce glucose monomers from starch.

D. Most of the activity of pancreatic amylase occurs at the brush border membrane of enterocytes into the portal venous system.

835 Paraneoplastic visceral neuropathy is associated with:

A. Gastric carcinoma

B. Breast cancer

C. Small-cell carcinoma of the lung

D. Prostate carcinoma

E. Metastatic ovarian cancer

836 A patient with Crohn's disease who has just undergone ileal resection is complaining of diarrhea. He is prescribed a bile acid binding resin, but his diarrhea worsens. The most likely explanation is:

A. Bile acid binding resins cause diarrhea.

B. Patients with ileal resection frequently develop bacterial overgrowth.

C. The bile acid binder has further depleted the bile acid pool.

D. Bile acid binders may cause vitamin deficiencies.

E. The patient increased his consumption of poorly digested carbohydrates.

837 Which of the following statements is *true* regarding the Manning criteria for IBS?

A. It is only useful in women.

B. It includes five major and five minor criteria.

C. Three or more criteria correctly made the diagnosis of IBS in more than 90% of patients.

D. All criteria have been shown to be statistically significant discriminators.
E. It is named for Peyton Manning who suffers from IBS and is a major supporter of IBS research.

838 A 65-year-old man presents to the emergency department with hematochezia. Recently, he had started taking ibuprofen for treatment of arthritis. Initially, he is hemodynamically unstable and receives volume rescusitation with saline and blood. Nasogastric lavage reveals bilious material. After stabilization, a colonoscopy reveals pandiverticulosis. There was no evidence of bleeding in the cecum, but fresh blood and clots were seen in the right, transverse, descending, and rectosigmoid colon without an obvious focal source. Due to continued profuse bleeding, an angiogram was ordered. It is *most* likely that bleeding will be found to originate from which artery?

A. Left gastric artery arising from the celiac artery
B. Left colic artery arising from the inferior mesenteric artery
C. Middle colic artery arising from the superior mesenteric artery
D. Superior rectal artery arising from the inferior mesenteric artery
E. Inferior pancreaticoduodenal artery arising from the superior mesenteric artery

839 Neoplasms of the small intestine can arise from any of the cells comprising this organ. Gastrointestinal stromal tumors (GISTs) are believed to arise from which cells?

A. Fibroblasts
B. Smooth muscle cells
C. Mucosal glands
D. Mesenchymal cells
E. Argentaffin cells

840 Therapy for tropical sprue would include nutritional support as well as a trial of:

A. Tetracycline
B. Amoxicillin
C. Metronidazole
D. A gluten-free diet

841 Which of the following statements about anal cancer is *most* accurate?

A. Anal cancers are among the most frequently encountered gastrointestinal malignancies.
B. In the United States, the annual incidence of anal cancer is increasing.
C. The majority of anal cancers are adenocarcinomas.
D. Most patients with anal cancer are asymptomatic.

842 A patient with steatorrhea, anorexia, abdominal cramps, and bloating who was recently in Southeast Asia undergoes small bowel imaging. The results (see figure) are most consistent with:

A. Crohn's disease
B. Ulcerative colitis
C. Irritable bowel syndrome
D. Tropical sprue

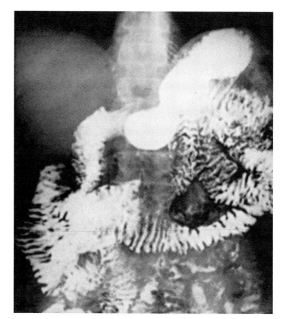

Figure for question **842**

843 Which of the following gastrointestinal signaling agents has been shown to increase appetite?

A. Apolipoprotein A IV (apo A IV)
B. Cholecystokinin (CCK)
C. Ghrelin
D. Leptin
E. Peptide tyrosine-tyrosine (PYY)

844 Colon cancer is the result of multiple genetic alterations during the progress of the adenoma/carcinoma sequence. Which of the following statements regarding these alterations is *true?*

A. Point mutations of the tumor suppressor gene K-ras occur.
B. The tumor suppressor gene *APC* is located on chromosome 18.
C. The tumor suppressor gene *DCC* (deleted in colon cancer) is located on chromosome 18.
D. Loss of the oncogene p53 probably occurs as a late step in the adenoma/carcinoma sequence.
E. The DNA mismatch repair gene is altered in patients with sporadic colorectal cancer.

845 The autonomic nervous system (ANS) consists of both sympathetic and parasympathetic pathways. Sympathetic stimulation:

A. Decreases smooth muscle activity and increases sphincter tone.
B. Increases smooth muscle activity and decreases sphincter tone.
C. Decreases both smooth muscle activity and sphincter tone.
D. Increases both smooth muscle activity and sphincter tone.

846 The gastrointestinal tract is primarily derived from the embryonic:

A. Allantoic duct
B. Ectoderm
C. Endoderm
D. Mesoderm
E. Vitelline duct

847 The classic findings on x-ray for a sigmoid volvulus are as follows:

A. A distended, ahaustral colonic loop with a bent inner-tube appearance with the apex directed toward the patient's right shoulder
B. A distended colonic loop with a bent inner-tube appearance with the apex directed toward the patient's left lower quadrant
C. A diffusely dilated colon with air throughout with a coffee-bean appearance of a distended cecum
D. A colon cut-off sign at the splenic flexure
E. Nonspecific bowel gas pattern

848 A 40-year-old man traveled on a cruise ship from Florida to the Caribbean. After a few days he developed vomiting and diarrhea. The diarrhea is watery and nonbloody. Many other passengers had similar symptoms. Which of the following organisms is probably responsible for the infection?

A. *Shigella*
B. *C. difficile*
C. Norwalk virus
D. *Salmonella*

849 The most common cause for small bowel obstruction secondary to neoplasms is:

A. Carcinoid tumor
B. Advanced colorectal carcinoma
C. Metastatic breast cancer
D. Endometrial carcinoma
E. Melanoma

850 Which of the following is *not* a prognostic factor in colorectal cancer?

A. Lymphatic invasion
B. Size of the primary tumor
C. Perineural invasion
D. Venous invasion
E. Histologic grade

851 Where in the gastrointestinal tract does protein digestion begin?

A. Oropharynx
B. Stomach
C. Duodenum
D. Proximal third of the jejunum

852 The best predictor for a complete small bowel obstruction (SBO) versus a low-grade partial SBO is the:

A. Presence of feculent emesis
B. Presence of borborygmi
C. Lack of stool evacuation
D. Crampy abdominal pain occurring every 4 to 5 minutes
E. Differential air-fluid levels in the same small bowel loop with a mean air-fluid level diameter of 2.5 cm or greater

853 A 35-year-old man with longstanding Crohn's disease and a history of multiple small bowel resections was brought to the emergency department by his family because the patient has been acting bizarre and is confused. On physical examination, he has nystagmus, ophthalmoplegia, and an ataxic gait. The most likely diagnosis is:

A. Medication toxicity
B. Alcohol ingestion
C. Transient ischemic attack (TIA)
D. D-lactic acidosis
E. Vitamin B_{12} deficiency

854 The primary neurotransmitter of the parasympathetic nervous system is:

A. Acetylcholine
B. Epinephrine
C. Nitric oxide
D. Norepinephrine
E. Substance P

855 A 5-year-old child is presented because of fever, abdominal cramps, and diarrhea for 3 weeks. Microscopic examination of the stool shows leukocytes and erythrocytes. CT of the abdomen shows inflammation of the terminal ileum. What is the most likely diagnosis?

A. *E. coli* infection
B. *Yersinia enterocolitica* infection
C. *Salmonella* infection
D. *Shigella* infection
E. Rotavirus infection

856 Which of the following is more common in neuropathic as opposed to myopathic forms of chronic intestinal pseudo-obstruction (CIP)?

A. Colonic dilatation
B. Bacterial overgrowth
C. Air-fluid levels on obstruction series
D. Postprandial abdominal pain
E. Hyperactive bowel sounds

857 Which of the following statements about host defense factors is *false?*

A. Most bacterial pathogens are highly susceptible to low gastric pH.
B. Gastric mucus along with low pH acts as a first line of defense.
C. Resident microflora in the gut produce lactic acid and short-chain fatty acids, which are toxic to many bacterial pathogens.
D. Secretory immunoglobulin A (IgA) appears later than serum IgG in the time course of the body's defense against enteropathogens.
E. Breast-fed infants are less susceptible to bacterial diarrhea than are formula-fed infants.

858 Which of the following polyposis syndromes does not confer an increased risk of gastrointestinal cancers?

A. Turcot's syndrome
B. Peutz-Jegher's syndrome
C. Juvenile polyposis syndrome
D. Cowden's syndrome
E. Cronkhite-Canada syndrome

859 A 45-year-old man presents with a 2-week history of bloody diarrhea, abdominal pain, and a 10-pound weight loss 3 weeks after returning from Guatemala. CT shows a thickened cecum and right colon. Stool cultures are tested for ova and parasites but only white blood cells (WBCs) are found. Colonoscopy reveals right-sided colitis and analysis of a biopsy specimen from an ulcer edge shows trophozoites. Which of the following statements is *true* regarding the organism present in this case?

A. Acute necrotizing colitis/toxic megacolon occurs in 0.5% of cases.
B. In 30% of cases, a serum sample will test positive for the pathogen.
C. Examining a stool sample for ova and parasites is reliable for diagnosis.
D. In 90% of carriers, invasive disease will develop and should be treated.
E. About 10% of infected individuals will remain asymptomatic.

860 Which of the following statements regarding the composition of human enteric bacterial flora is most accurate?

A. Enteric flora are essentially identical in different individuals.
B. The composition of an individual's enteric flora is usually unstable throughout adulthood.
C. Environmental factors, including diet and sanitation, likely have a profound effect on early intestinal colonization with bacteria.
D. In adulthood, dietary fluctuations induce changes in the relative populations of the flora.
E. Most human enteric bacteria can be cultured.

861 The type of primary tumor that most often metastasizes to the small intestine is:

A. Lung cancer
B. Breast cancer
C. Melanoma
D. Colon cancer
E. Stomach cancer

862 A 47-year-old white man with a longstanding history of poorly controlled insulin-dependent diabetes mellitus complicated by chronic renal insufficiency, retinopathy, peripheral neuropathy, and peripheral vascular disease with prior right foot amputation is now being evaluated for diarrhea. He reports four to eight loose bowel movements daily with occasional episodes of fecal incontinence over the last year. What is a likely mechanism of this patient's chronic diarrhea?

A. Reduced pancreatic exocrine function
B. Rapid gastric emptying secondary to autonomic neuropathy
C. Rapid intestinal transit secondary to autonomic neuropathy
D. Small intestinal bacterial overgrowth
E. All of the above

863 Which of the following statements is *true* regarding the incidence of colorectal cancer?

A. Colorectal cancer mortality has decreased and the colorectal cancer incidence has increased among U.S. adults since 1985.
B. Colorectal cancer mortality and incidence among U.S. adults have decreased since 1985.
C. Colorectal cancer incidence is higher in whites.
D. Colorectal cancer mortality is higher in whites.
E. Colorectal cancer risk doesn't change significantly in populations that migrate from areas of low risk to areas of high risk.

864 Dermatitis herpetiformis is closely linked to which disease?

A. Celiac sprue
B. Tropical sprue
C. Crohn's disease
D. Ulcerative colitis

865 Which of the following statements is *false* regarding enteritis necroticans?

A. It is caused by strains of *C. perfringens* type A.
B. It is associated with consumption of poorly cooked pork.
C. Life-threatening complications like intestinal perforation, sepsis, and hemorrhage can result.
D. It is rarely encountered in the United States.

866 Each of the following statements about intestinal adaptation after partial intestinal resection is true *except:*

A. The remaining small bowel frequently grows in length and diameter.
B. Initiating postoperative oral feeding enhances the crypt cell production rate.
C. Adaptive changes are more prominent in the jejunum than in the ileum.
D. Mean stool volume generally decreases over time.
E. Adaptive changes are thought to be mediated by growth factors.

867 The treatment of patients with complete SBO is as follows:

A. Urgent early laparotomy
B. Conservative management and laparotomy if the patient develops signs of strangulation
C. Urgent surgery only in patients with inguinal hernias
D. Capsule endoscopy followed by surgery if the capsule gets stuck
E. Therapeutic gastrografin enteroclysis

868 A 35-year-old man with acquired immune deficiency syndrome (AIDS) presents with abdominal pain, diarrhea, hematochezia, and fever. Physical examination shows a palpable rectal mass. Colonoscopy shows a yellowish, sessile, ulcerated plaque. Histology reveals macrophages with voluminous cytoplasm containing von Hansemann bodies (intracellular organisms) and Michaelis-Gutmann bodies (intracytoplasmic concentric laminated inclusion bodies). What is the most likely diagnosis?

A. Crohn's disease
B. Whipple's disease

C. Malakoplakia
D. Reticulum cell sarcoma

869 Risk factors for the development of pseudomembranous enterocolitis in the absence of *C. difficile* infection include which of the following?

A. Intestinal surgery
B. Intestinal ischemia
C. Neonatal necrotizing enterocolitis
D. Intestinal obstruction
E. All of the above

870 Which of the following well-studied screening tools for colon cancer is likely to have the *best* sensitivity and specificity for polyps smaller than than 1 cm?

A. CT colonography
B. Barium enema
C. Sigmoidoscopy
D. Fecal occult blood testing
E. Colonoscopy

871 Which of the following statements regarding management of mild to moderately severe *C. difficile* diarrhea and colitis reflects sound clinical judgment?

A. Antimotility agents such as loperamide or narcotics are best avoided.
B. Vancomycin at doses of 125 mg four times a day may be as effective as doses of 500 mg four times per day.
C. Avoid metronidazole and warfarin due to prolongation of the prothrombin time.
D. Vancomycin should not be administered intravenously for *C. difficile* colitis.
E. All of the above.

872 Which of the following conditions is associated with adenomatous colon polyps?

A. Prostate cancer
B. Parathyroid adenomas
C. Ureterosigmoidostomy
D. Squamous carcinoma of the skin
E. *Staphylococcus* bacteremia

873 A 50-year-old man with a history of total gastrectomy for malignancy presents to the emergency department with nausea and vomiting, followed by abdominal cramps and diarrhea. When questioned about his recent food intake, he reports having eaten two half-boiled eggs 7 hours prior to his visit. Stool studies reveal multiple polymorphonuclear (PMN) leukocytes and red blood cells (RBCs). Which of the following statements is *false* regarding *Salmonella?*

A. The major route of spread of *Salmonella* is flies, food, fingers, feces, and fomites.
B. The two most common serotypes in the United States are *S. enteritidis* and *S. typhimurium*.
C. The most common syndrome caused by *Salmonella* is typhoid.
D. Patients with sickle cell disease are more prone to salmonella osteomyelitis.

874 A 12-year-old child is brought to his pediatrician with symptoms of profound fatigue. His physical examination shows resting tachycardia. The results of routine laboratory studies show a normal coagulation profile, thyroid profile, and a normal WBC count and differential, but his hemoglobin level is 8.6 grams (MCV 83). On further questioning, the child reports "seeing red" in his stool "about once a week for the past month." A rectal exam is performed and reveals strongly heme-positive brown stool. Among other diagnoses, Meckel's diverticulum is considered. Which of the following statements is *true* concerning this diagnosis?

A. It is found equally in male and female patients.
B. It is rarely diagnosed before the third decade of life.
C. It presents commonly with painless maroon stools.
D. Massive bleeding is common.

875 In this patient, the most appropriate initial diagnostic test is:

A. Esophagogastroduodenoscopy (EGD)
B. Colonoscopy
C. Laparotomy or laparoscopy
D. Tc-99 Meckel's scan with cimetidine administration
E. Visceral angiography

876 Intestinal pseudo-obstruction is a syndrome:

A. Of impaired intestinal propulsion resembling intestinal obstruction without a mechanical cause
B. Involving the large colon only
C. That is chronic only
D. With a unique and specific pathophysiology
E. That occurs primarily secondary to a myopathy

877 Regarding 5-aminosalicylic acid (5-ASA) compounds:

A. They are all approved by the U.S. Food and Drug Administration (FDA) for Crohn's disease
B. As a family, all 5-ASAs appear to have similar efficacy

C. They are effective for severe disease.
D. There does not appear to be any benefit with doses larger than 2 grams

878 A 50-year-old man who emigrated recently from India presents with weight loss, abdominal pain, and a mass in the right lower quadrant. The mass in the right lower quadrant is *not* typical on presentation with which of the following?

A. Intestinal tuberculosis
B. Cecal carcinoma
C. Crohn's disease
D. Amebiasis
E. Syphilis

879 What is the diagnostic study of choice in patients with colonic Dieulafoy-type lesion?

A. Colonoscopy
B. Selective mesenteric angiography
C. Barium enema
D. Exploratory laparotomy

880 Which of the following chronic conditions has been associated with small intestinal bacterial overgrowth?

A. Celiac sprue
B. Chronic pancreatitis
C. Radiation enteritis
D. Chronic renal failure
E. All of the above

881 The following statements regarding *Entamoeba histolytica* are true *except*:

A. Ten percent of infected patients develop invasive disease
B. It has a two-stage life cycle: infectious cyst and motile trophozoite
C. The cecum and ascending colon are the most commonly affected sites
D. Ninety percent of infected individuals remain asymptomatic
E. Persons with AIDS are at increased risk for invasive amebiasis

882 All of the following statements are true about the typical presentation of acute diverticulitis in Westerners *except*:

A. Left lower quadrant (LLQ) abdominal pain is common.
B. The rectal exam may disclose tenderness or a mass.
C. Acute appendicitis is the misdiagnosis most frequently made in patients with diverticulitis.
D. Right lower quadrant (RLQ) abdominal pain is a more common presentation in Asians.
E. The WBC count is infrequently elevated.

883 Celiac sprue is an allergy to which of the following?

A. Barley, oats, and rye
B. Wheat, rye, and barley
C. Oats, wheat, and rye
D. Wheat, oats, and hops

884 Regarding scleroderma:

A. The small bowel is the primary gastrointestinal organ involved
B. Longitudinal muscles are more involved than circular muscles
C. Pneumatosis cystoides intestinalis is a common association
D. Bacterial overgrowth is an uncommon consequence
E. There is absence of the interdigestive migratory motor complex (MMC)

885 Which of the following statements regarding anal fissures is most accurate?

A. Most anal fissures are located in the anterior position of the anus.
B. The etiology of anal fissures is likely related to trauma during defecation and reduced blood flow to the posterior anoderm.
C. Patients with anal fissures commonly report the painless passage of bright red blood during defecation.
D. Digital rectal examination must be performed during the initial evaluation of a patient with a suspected anal fissure.

886 The most accurate characterization of p-ANCA as it relates to ulcerative colitis (UC) is:

A. It is present in nearly 100% of patients
B. The level of p-ANCA correlates with disease activity
C. Patients who test positive for p-ANCA have a lower instance of pouchitis following ileal pouch anal anastomosis (IPAA)
D. p-ANCA has no pathological role but likely serves as a marker of susceptibility of genetically distinct subsets of UC

887 A 39-year-old woman has rectal pain. She describes a sensation of aching and tenderness high in the rectum that often occurs while she is seated at her desk at work. The symptoms are often exacerbated by defecation. When the pain begins she attempts to achieve relief by walking around the office. The episodes typically last from 30 minutes to an hour. They have been occurring several times monthly over the past 2 years. She does not report diarrhea, constipation, or blood per rectum.

A digital rectal examination is performed. Anal sphincter tone is normal. A tight, slightly tender band is noted in the posterior and lateral rectum. A stool sample was brown and tested negative for occult blood. On flexible sigmoidoscopy the rectosigmoid mucosa appears normal. What is the most likely diagnosis?

A. Proctalgia fugax
B. Coccygodynia
C. Levator ani syndrome
D. Pruritus ani

888 The enteric nervous system is modulated by sympathetic and parasympathetic inputs. Which of the following statements is most accurate?

A. Sympathetic activation inhibits colonic motor activity, reduces colonic blood flow, and inhibits secretion to minimize fluid loss.
B. Sympathetic activation stimulates colonic motor activity, enhances colonic blood flow, and stimulates secretion to maximize fluid loss.
C. Parasympathetic activation inhibits colonic motor activity, reduces colonic blood flow, and inhibits secretion to minimize fluid loss.
D. Parasympathetic activation stimulates colonic motor activity, enhances colonic blood flow, and stimulates secretion to maximize fluid loss.

889 Which of the following are risk factors for *C. difficile* infection?

A. Presence of inflammatory bowel disease
B. Older patient age
C. Currently receiving antineoplastic therapy
D. Infection with human immunodeficiency virus (HIV)
E. All of the above

890 Which of the following statements about lipid digestion and absorption is *most* accurate?

A. Most lipid digestion occurs in the stomach and most dietary lipid is absorbed in the duodenum.
B. Most lipid digestion occurs in the duodenum and most dietary lipid is absorbed in the jejunum.
C. Most lipid digestion occurs in the jejunum and most dietary lipid is absorbed in the ileum.
D. Most lipid digestion occurs in the ileum and most dietary lipid is absorbed in the colon.

891 The most effective treatment for solitary rectal ulcer syndrome is:

A. Cortisone enemas
B. Mesalamine suppositories
C. Mesalamine enemas
D. Biofeedback

892 Which of the following statements is *most* accurate regarding complicated appendicitis?

A. The perforation rate is 10% to 30%.
B. Perforation rates vary widely with age but this condition is most common at extremes of age.
C. The risk of perforation increases particularly after 24 hours of illness.
D. Perforation is often a consequence of delay in diagnosis.
E. All of the above.

893 Which haplotypes are commonly seen in patients diagnosed with celiac disease?

A. HLA-DQ2 and HLA-DQ6
B. HLA-DQ6 and HLA-DQ8
C. HLA-DQ8 and HLA-DQ2
D. HLA-DQ3 and HLA-DQ6

894 A 27-year-old man on a visit to India developed diarrhea 10 days into the trip. Regarding the pathogenesis of traveler's diarrhea, which one of the following statements is *false?*

A. The most common cause is *Campylobacter*.
B. The infectious agent is identified in most of the cases.
C. The major determinant of risk is the destination of the traveler.
D. Younger travelers have the highest risk.
E. The patient's country of origin can be a factor in the diarrhea.

895 A 75-year-old woman presents with chronic intermittent abdominal pain, distention associated with nausea, and vomiting. Imaging reveals a smooth stricture in the proximal ileum measuring 5 to 6cm in length. The most likely diagnosis is:

A. Crohn's disease
B. Idiopathic joint ileitis
C. Lymphoma
D. Small bowel adenocarcinoma
E. Focal segmental ischemia (FSI)

896 Which of the following statements about the appendix is *not* well documented in the literature?

A. Appendectomy may protect against the development of ulcerative colitis.
B. The vast majority of appendiceal tumors are carcinoid tumors.
C. At birth, an individual's lifetime risk of appendicitis is about 1 in 12.
D. The greatest risk of appendicitis is in the first decade of life.
E. Persons between the ages of 10 and 30 have the lowest rates of perforation (10% to 20%).

897 The optimal treatment for familial adenomatous polyposis is:

A. Total abdominal colectomy with creation of a Hartman's pouch
B. Total proctocolectomy with creation of an ileostomy or ileoanal pouch
C. Subtotal colectomy with ileorectal anastomosis
D. Partial colectomy of polypoid tumor-containing colon
E. Left hemicolectomy

898 A 39-year-old homosexual man is evaluated for the complaint of anal bleeding. He reports that for several months he has noticed the passage of blood-streaked stool and blood on the toilet paper. Furthermore, he describes a lump-like sensation in his anal region exacerbated by defecation. He has no history of hemorrhoids.

A digital rectal examination and anoscopy are performed, which demonstrate a firm 2-cm mass at the level of the dentate line. A biopsy confirms a diagnosis of squamous cell carcinoma. CT of the abdomen and pelvis does not demonstrate abdominopelvic lymphadenopathy or evidence of metastatic disease. What is the most appropriate initial treatment for this lesion?

A. Wide local excision
B. Abdominal-perineal resection
C. Combined radiation and chemotherapy with 5-fluorouracil and mitomycin
D. Wide local excision followed by adjuvant radiation and chemotherapy

899 As feces enter the rectum, the rectoanal inhibitory reflex:

A. Causes both the internal anal sphincter (IAS) and external anal sphincter (EAS) to relax, leading to defecation.
B. Causes both the internal anal sphincter (IAS) and external anal sphincter (EAS) to contract, maintaining continence.
C. Causes the internal anal sphincter (IAS) to relax, allowing feces into the proximal anal canal, while continence is maintained by contraction of the external anal sphincter (EAS).
D. Causes the external anal sphincter (EAS) to relax, allowing feces into the proximal anal canal, while continence is maintained by contraction of the internal anal sphincter (IAS).

900 About 15% to 30% of patients with *C. difficile* infection have a relapse after successful treatment with metronidazole or vancomycin. The best approach for treating a relapse is:

A. Extend treatment for 30 days
B. Increase the dose of the antibiotic
C. Add cholestyramine to bind the toxin
D. Treat with a second course of the same antibiotic used in the initial attack but extend the treatment to 14 days.

901 Which of the following statements about the mechanisms by which various organisms cause diarrhea is *false?*

A. *E. coli* heat-stable enterotoxin increases intracellular levels of cGMP.
B. *Vibrio cholerae* toxin increases levels of cyclic guanidine monophosphate (cGMP).
C. NSP4 enterotoxin released by rotavirus leads to an increase in intracellular calcium.
D. *Salmonella typhimurium* activates NF-kappaB and interleukin-8 (IL-8) secretion.
E. *Clostridium difficile* toxins A and B disrupt cytoskeletal architecture.

902 Short bowel syndrome (intestinal failure) generally occurs when there is at most:

A. 500 cm of intestine
B. 400 cm of intestine
C. 300 cm of intestine
D. 200 cm of intestine
E. 100 cm of intestine

903 Each of the following statements regarding severe pseudomembranous colitis is true *except:*

A. It occurs in only 3% to 5% of cases.
B. Mortality is as high as 65%.
C. Diarrhea may be minimal or absent.
D. Vancomycin is often used as first-line therapy.
E. Vancomycin should be administered intravenously (IV) to patients with ileus.

904 Regarding laboratory findings in patients with ischemic bowel:

A. A normal white blood cell count excludes the diagnosis
B. D-lactate levels rise early in the course of the condition
C. Elevations in amylase are secondary to ischemic pancreatitis
D. The sensitivity and specificity of serum markers have not been established

905 A 60-year-old white woman with known sigmoid diverticulosis presents with left lower quadrant (LLQ) pain and fever. Acute diverticulitis is suspected. The best test to confirm the diagnosis is:

A. Barium enema
B. Computed tomography with contrast

C. Ultrasound
D. Colonoscopy
E. Magnetic resonance imaging (MRI)

906 What minimal cecal diameter warrants consideration for decompression in patients with acute intestinal pseudo-obstruction during the first 72 hours after treatment of potential causes?

A. More than 6 cm
B. More than 9 cm
C. More than 12 cm
D. More than 15 cm
E. More than 18 cm

907 Adenomas with advanced pathology are considered to have a higher risk of harboring invasive carcinoma. Which of the following is *not* an adenoma with advanced pathology?

A. A tubular adenoma with mild dysplasia
B. A 1-cm villous adenoma
C. A 1-cm flat adenoma with high-grade dysplasia
D. A 2-cm tubulovillous adenoma with high-grade dysplasia
E. A 2-cm serrated adenoma with high-grade dysplasia

908 Overall, the best initial test to assess for suspected intestinal ischemia is:

A. Duplex ultrasound
B. Plain films
C. Tagged red blood cell scan
D. CT

909 A 30-year-old man presents with a 7-day history of watery diarrhea, nausea, and abdominal discomfort after returning from a summer camping trip in the Midwest. A modified acid fast stain of his stool is positive for a small intracellular protozoon. The treatment that is most consistently effective for this infection is:

A. Iodoquinol
B. Ciprofloxacin
C. Metronidazole
D. Nitazoxanide

910 A 25-year-old man with no previous history of illness presents with a 4-week history of abdominal pain, rectal burning, and diarrhea. Microscopic examination of a stool specimen reveals multiple polymorphonuclear leukocytes and red blood cells. Which of the following pathogens is likely to have caused his symptoms and signs, which are similar to those of ulcerative colitis?

A. Rotavirus
B. *Shigella*
C. *Salmonella*
D. *Yersinia*
E. *E. coli*

911 Which region of the bowel is most often affected by celiac sprue?

A. Stomach
B. Duodenum
C. Jejunum
D. Ileum

912 Symptoms of rectal ulceration, erythema or a mass associated with straining at defecation, rectal prolapse, and a feeling of incomplete evacuation are most consistent with:

A. Solitary rectal ulcer syndrome
B. Ulcerative proctitis
C. Crohn's disease
D. Hemorrhoids

913 A primarily myopathic cause for chronic intestinal pseudo-obstruction is:

A. Diabetes mellitus
B. Parkinson's disease
C. Scleroderma
D. Multiple sclerosis
E. Osgood-Schlatter disease

914 A 35-year-old man has ileocolonic Crohn's disease that is not improving with 5-aminosalicylic acid (5-ASA) therapy and two attempts at tapering glucocorticoid drug therapy. The decision is made to try infliximab. The recommended schedule for infliximab infusion is:

A. A single 5-mg/kg infusion, repeated every 8 weeks
B. A single 10-mg/kg infusion, repeated every 8 weeks
C. A single 5-mg/kg infusion, repeated as needed
D. Three infusions of 5 mg/kg each administered at 6-week intervals, and then a 5-mg/kg infusion approximately every 8 weeks.

915 Regarding familial visceral neuropathies:

A. They are genetic diseases characterized by degeneration of the interstitial cells of Cajal
B. They are genetic diseases characterized by degeneration of the myenteric plexus
C. They are disorders for which there is effective therapy and a good prognosis
D. They are inherited with incomplete penetrance, and most affected persons are asymptomatic
E. They only involve the small intestine

916 A 60-year-old Guatemalan man moved to the United States a few months ago and now presents with dysphagia and shortness of breath. A chest x-ray shows evidence of congestive heart failure and an enlarged esophagus. Which of the following statements regarding the protozoon infection that caused this illness is *false?*

A. Megacolon can occur, leading to constipation.
B. A bite from the reduviid bug is responsible for transmission.
C. Manometric findings may be indistinguishable from achalasia.
D. Trimethoprim-sulfamethoxazole for 4 weeks readily treats infection with this organism.
E. The diagnosis can be made by examining blood smears for the organism.

917 Levels of which of the following vitamins tend to be high in patients with small intestinal bacterial overgrowth?

A. Vitamin B_{12}
B. Folate
C. Thiamine
D. Nicotinamide
E. Vitamin D

918 A barium-contrast radiograph (see figure) in a patient with diarrhea and dermatitis herpetiformis is consistent with which of the following?

A. Crohn's disease
B. Ulcerative colitis
C. Ulcerative enteritis
D. NSAID-induced ulcerations of the small bowel

919 Whereas in children intussusception is rarely caused by an anatomical abnormality, in adults the most common cause is:

A. Small bowel neoplasm
B. Meckel's diverticulum
C. Crohn's disease
D. Idiopathic small bowel ulcers
E. Vascular ectasias

920 Familial adenomatous polyposis is the most common adenomatous polyposis syndrome. Which of the following statements is *true* regarding this syndrome?

A. Polyps usually are present at birth.
B. One mutated *APC* gene is inherited as a germline mutation and adenomas develop when a second allele is mutated or lost.
C. It is inherited in an autosomal recessive pattern.

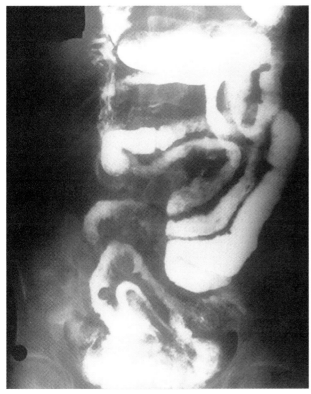

Figure for question **918**. (Courtesy of Christophe Cellier, MD, PhD, Paris).

D. There is approximately 40% to 50% penetrance.

E. The polyps are virtually all villous in nature.

921 A 60-year-old man with emphysema who is being treated with glucocorticoid medications presents with diarrhea mixed with blood. A plain x-ray of the abdomen shows radiolucent clusters or streaks along the bowel. Colonoscopy shows multiple cysts. What is the most likely diagnosis?

A. Colonic tumor

B. Pneumatosis cystoides intestinalis

C. Ischemic colitis

D. *C. difficile* colitis

922 A 53-year-old Chinese immigrant develops abdominal pain, fever, and malaise. He has been in the United States for 10 years. Liver enzymes are elevated and an ultrasound shows a dilated bile duct. Which of the following statements about his condition is *true?*

A. *Opisthorchis viverrini* is a closely related parasite that also markedly increases the risk of cholangiocarcinoma.

B. Eosinophilia is not present.

C. The diagnosis cannot be made by stool examination.

D. Albendazole is the drug of choice.

923 The neurotransmitter that is believed to play a major role in the manifestations of IBS is:

A. Norepinephrine

B. Nitrous oxide

C. 5-Hydroxytryptamine

D. Acetylcholine

E. γ-Aminobutyric acid (GABA)

924 Which of the following statements about clinical features of *Campylobacter* gastroenteritis is *false?*

A. Diarrhea, fever, abdominal pain, and bloody stools are common.

B. Constitutional symptoms such as headache and myalgias are frequent.

C. Fecal leukocytes are absent.

D. There may be associated pancreatitis and cholecystitis.

925 A 52-year-old man comes to the emergency department complaining of four episodes, the first 3 hours earlier, in which the sensation of urgency to defecate was followed by the painless passage of large amounts of bright red blood and clots. He denies associated abdominal pain, hematemesis, or fever. There is no history of peptic ulcer disease or significant lower gastrointestinal tract hemorrhage. The prior evening he passed a soft brown nonbloody bowel movement.

The patient reports a history of prolapsed hemorrhoids that were treated by a colorectal surgeon with rubber band ligation one week earlier. After the procedure, he experienced mild rectal discomfort that resolved with the use of ibuprofen. Three days ago, he resumed daily ingestion of an enteric-coated aspirin tablet. What is the most likely etiology of this patient's gastrointestinal bleeding?

A. Peptic ulcer disease

B. Ischemic colitis

C. Sloughing of necrotic hemorrhoidal tissue

D. Diverticular bleeding

926 All of the following may point to a diagnosis of *Ascaris* infection *except:*

A. Results of endoscopy

B. Results of barium studies

C. Peripheral eosinophilia

D. Results of endoscopic retrograde cholangiopancreatography (ERCP)

E. Findings on direct examination of smears of the stool

927 Nutritional deficiencies that result in anemia, stomatitis, glossitis, pigmentation of the skin, and edema caused by hypoproteinemia are consistent with which of the following infections?

A. Enterotoxigenic *Escherichia coli* infection
B. *Campylobacter* infection
C. *Shigella* infection
D. Tropical sprue

928 Oculomasticatory myorhythmia and oculofacial skeletal myorhythmia are characteristic CNS signs of what disease?

A. Celiac sprue
B. Crohn's disease
C. Ulcerative colitis
D. Whipple's disease

929 The most common cause of small bowel obstruction is:

A. Gallstone ileus
B. Inguinal hernia
C. Intra-abdominal adhesions
D. Neoplasms
E. Crohn's disease

930 A 35-year-old homosexual man complains of 3 weeks of diarrhea, bloating, and fatigue. He recently returned from a camping trip in the Rocky Mountains. Which of the following is true regarding his infection with *Giardia lamblia?*

A. Paromomycin may be used to treat infections due to this organism, except in women who are pregnant.
B. The organisms are eradicated in 80% to 95% of cases by a 5-day course of metronidazole.
C. This parasite is rarely encountered in the United States except in the Midwest.
D. Prolonged lactose intolerance does not occur after infection with this organism.

931 The most common cause of ileus is:

A. Abdominal surgery
B. Metabolic abnormalities
C. Drug reactions
D. Gastroenteritis
E. Inactivity

932 Which of the following medications is *not* used to treat chronic diabetic diarrhea?

A. Loperamide
B. Metronidazole (Flagyl)
C. Clonidine
D. Octreotide

933 The main treatment for celiac sprue is:

A. Avoidance of gluten
B. Glucocorticoid drugs

C. Cyclosporine
D. Tetracycline

934 A patient develops a small bowel obstruction soon after laparoscopic cholecystectomy. The most likely cause for this postoperative obstruction is:

A. Richter's hernia
B. Inguinal hernia
C. Intra-abdominal adhesions
D. Small bowel volvulus
E. Metastatic gallbladder cancer

935 Complications of celiac sprue include which of the following?

A. T-cell lymphoma, ulcerative jejunoileitis, and collagenous sprue
B. Collagenous sprue, B-cell lymphoma, and ulcerative jejunoileitis
C. Colon cancer, ulcerative jejunoileitis, and B-cell lymphoma
D. T-cell lymphoma, colon cancer, and collagenous sprue

936 Which of the following is a metabolic property of enteric flora?

A. Biotransformation of bile acids
B. Breakdown of plant polysaccharides
C. Production of short-chain fatty acids from carbohydrates
D. Conversion of prodrugs into active metabolites
E. All of the above

937 Which of the following statements about Hartnup disorder is true?

A. It results from a congenital defect of intestinal transport of free neutral amino acids.
B. It is demonstrates an autosomal dominant pattern of inheritance.
C. Most patients suffer from severe protein malnutrition.
D. A low-protein diet has been shown to improve symptoms.

938 A patient's symptoms are suspected to be due to acute appendicitis. The *most* accurate statement regarding laparoscopic versus open appendectomy is:

A. Laparoscopic procedures are safer than open procedures for perforated appendicitis
B. He will return to normal activity 1 month sooner than with an open appendectomy
C. Laparoscopic appendectomy takes less time to perform and is associated with lower costs

D. The wound infection risk is 50% lower with a laparoscopic procedure but there maybe an increased risk of intra-abdominal abscess

939 The risk for small bowel obstruction due to adhesions is higher in patients who have undergone:

A. Appendectomy
B. Subtotal colectomy
C. Cholecystectomy
D. Tubal ligation
E. Laparoscopic Heller myotomy

940 A 50-year-old man with ulcerative colitis that had been asymptomatic for the past 12 months complains of crampy lower abdominal pain, low-grade fever, headache, and multiple episodes of bloody diarrhea that have lasted 10 days. Tests for bowel infection are negative. The most recent colonoscopy, performed a year ago, revealed pancolitis. Which of the following is most likely to control this patient's acute symptoms?

A. Mesalamine suppositories
B. Mesalamine enemas
C. Azathioprine
D. Balsalazide
E. Oral glucocorticoid medications

941 Polyarthralgias involving the knees, ankles, elbows, or fingers; uveitis; weight loss; diarrhea; abdominal pain; and skin hyperpigmentation are all associated with which one of the following diseases?

A. Whipple's disease
B. Hemochromatosis
C. Irritable bowel syndrome
D. Alpha-1 antitrypsin deficiency

942 Which of the following is more characteristic of mechanical obstruction of the GI tract than chronic intestinal pseudo-obstruction (CIP)?

A. Dysphagia
B. Constipation
C. Urinary retention
D. Symptom-free periods between attacks
E. Cachexia

943 A 30-year-old white woman presents to the emergency department complaining of acute colicky right lower quadrant pain, nausea, low-grade fever, loose nonbloody diarrhea, and abdominal distention. An "obstruction" radiography series reveals a partial small bowel obstruction. The most likely diagnosis in this case is:

A. Acute appendicitis
B. Ulcerative colitis

C. Crohn's disease
D. Infection with *E. coli* 0157-H7

944 A 20-year-old man presents with fever, headache, and abdominal pain 1 week after a visit to India, where he did not take any precautions to avoid ingesting contaminated food or water. His temperature is 101°F, his heart rate is 80 beats/minute, he has erythematous spots on his cheeks, and mild splenomegaly is noted. What is the most likely diagnosis?

A. Typhoid
B. Cholera
C. Amebiasis
D. Traveler's diarrhea

945 The imaging study most often used to diagnose small bowel neoplasms is:

A. CT of the abdomen
B. Upper GI small bowel series
C. Angiography
D. MRI of the abdomen
E. Barium enema

946 A possible pathophysiologic mechanism for Crohn's disease is "immune tolerance." This refers to:

A. Mediating gut inflammation via CD41 helper T-cells
B. Modification of intestinal barrier function
C. Programmed over-responsiveness to a persistent stimulus
D. Expression of adhesion molecules

947 A 50-year-old Brazilian man presents with symptoms of an upper GI bleed. Upper GI endoscopy reveals esophageal varices, which are treated. He has been living in the United States for 10 years, denies ethanol abuse, and tests negative for infection with hepatitis A, B, or C virus. Splenomegaly is present. His alkaline phosphatase and gamma-glutamyl transferase levels are mildly elevated but levels of other liver enzymes and albumin, and his prothrombin time are normal. Thrombocytopenia and eosinophilia are present. Which of the following statements about this patient's disease is *true?*

A. The organism is transmitted by a reduviid bug.
B. Albendazole is the treatment.
C. Katayama fever is the classic presentation of acute infection.
D. Liver biopsy is diagnostic.
E. Cirrhosis develops in most patients.

948 A 25-year-old man complains of diarrhea for the last 2 months, since he returned from a trip to

Mexico. Which of the following is least likely to be the cause of this patient's diarrhea?

A. *Bacillus cereus*
B. *Salmonella*
C. *Shigella*
D. *Giardia*
E. Post-dysenteric irritable bowel syndrome

949 Periodic acid–Schiff staining of a patient's specimen (see figure) reveals:

A. *Giardia* infection
B. *Cryptosporidium* infection
C. Whipple's disease
D. *Yersinia* infection

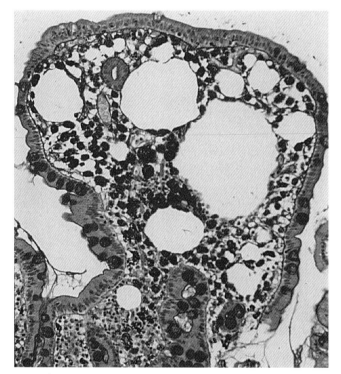

Figure for question **949**

950 Complications of short bowel syndrome include which of the following?

A. Gallstones
B. Cirrhosis
C. Calcium oxalate kidney stones
D. All of the above
E. None of the above

951 An 80-year-old woman with coronary artery disease complains to her primary care doctor that she has had abdominal pain for the past 4 to 6 months. Typically, it occurs 30 minutes postprandially and usually resolves in 1 to 3 hours. The severity of the pain has increased and she is losing weight. Physical examination reveals a cachectic woman, but no abnormality is found

on abdominal examination. The additional symptom that would be *most* suggestive of a diagnosis of chronic mesenteric ischemia is:

A. Intermittent nausea and vomiting
B. Bloating
C. Fear of eating resulting in weight loss
D. Diarrhea

952 Solitary rectal ulcers are most often located:

A. On the posterior wall, 2 to 3 cm from the anal verge
B. On the posterior wall, 7 to 10 cm from the anal verge
C. On the anterior wall, 2 to 3 cm from the anal verge
D. On the anterior wall, 7 to 10 cm from the anal verge

953 *Ascaris lumbricoides* is harbored by up to 25% of the world's population. Of the following statements, the one that is *false* regarding the clinical presentation of infection caused by this organism is:

A. Most infected persons have no symptoms
B. Biliary obstruction and jaundice may occur
C. Intestinal obstruction may occur
D. Pneumonia may occur
E. Disease usually develops even in those with light worm burdens

954 Tropical enteropathy has been detected in most tropical regions of Asia, the Middle East, the Caribbean, Central and South America, and:

A. Africa
B. Australia
C. New Zealand
D. Hawaii

955 Patients with IBS are at increased risk for:

A. Ischemic colitis
B. Colon cancer
C. Ulcerative colitis
D. Antibiotic-associated colitis
E. Pancreatic cancer

956 The following therapies have been shown in large, randomized controlled trials to be effective for UC:

A. Antibiotics
B. Probiotics
C. Methotrexate
D. Nicotine transdermal
E. None of the above

957 A 60-year-old man complains of abdominal pain, nausea, vomiting, and diarrhea 2 days after he attended a barbeque. Several others who attended the barbeque also became sick, and all of those who are sick ate sausage. The patient's subsequent symptoms include high fever, myalgias, and periorbital edema. Of the following statements, the one that is *not* true regarding this patient's infection is:

A. Development of myositis is typical
B. Eosinophilia and elevated levels of creatinine phosphokinase (CPK) may occur
C. Diagnosis may be made by examining stool samples
D. Larvae may be seen on muscle biopsy
E. Treatment with albendazole for 10 to 15 days is effective

958 Which of the following statements about the epidemiology of *Shigella* is *false?*

A. *S. dysenteriae,* also known as the Shiga bacillus, produces the most severe form of dysentery.
B. *S. flexneri* is the most common serotype in the United States.
C. *S. flexneri* is the most common serotype in tropical countries.
D. *S. sonnei* produces the mildest disease.

959 In patients with presumed IBS without alarm features the only test that has proven cost-effective for screening and that is recommended is:

A. SeCAT test for bile salt malabsorption
B. Test to detect p-ANCA and ASCA characteristic for patients with IBD
C. Test for anti-endomysial or tissue transglutaminase antibody for celiac disease
D. Serum test for trypsinogen level indicative of chronic pancreatitis
E. Lactose breath test

960 The IBD-1 locus in people with IBD has been linked to Crohn's disease. The IBD-1 locus has been identified as the *NOD-2* gene also known as the *CARD-15* gene. Characteristics of the *NOD-2/CARD-15* gene include:

A. Persons with disease-associated allelic variants have a 40-fold increased relative risk of Crohn's disease
B. Heterozygous individuals have a 30-fold increased risk
C. Colonic location of disease is more common
D. The gene product is a mitochondrial protein

961 A 20-year old woman is admitted with a 7-day history of 10 to 15 episodes of bloody diarrhea daily, fever, and abdominal pain. Stool samples obtained at multiple times test negative for infectious organisms. The next best step to

confirm the diagnosis of ulcerative colitis should be:

A. Full colonoscopy
B. CT
C. Serum test for p-ANCA/ASCA
D. Flexible sigmoidoscopy without preparation

962 The gold standard for diagnosis of celiac sprue is:

A. Characteristic findings on small bowel biopsy
B. Presence of anti-endomysial antibodies
C. Presence of anti-tissue transglutaminase antibodies
D. Resolution of symptoms on a gluten-free diet

963 Which of the following is *most* important in differentiating early postoperative SBO from postoperative ileus?

A. Abdominal distension and pain
B. Nausea and vomiting
C. Occurrence of obstructive symptoms after initial return of bowel function and resumption of oral intake
D. Type of surgery performed
E. Cumulative dose of narcotics used postoperatively

964 Which of the following is most useful in differentiating Crohn's disease from ulcerative colitis?

A. Predominantly left-sided disease
B. Rectal involvement
C. Perianal complications
D. Shape of the colon ulcers

965 The mechanism of action of 5-ASA compounds include(s):

A. Inhibition of T-cell proliferation
B. Presentation of antigen to T-cells and antibody production by B-cells
C. Inhibition of macrophages and neutrophil adhesion
D. Decreased production of interleukin-1 (IL-1) and tumor necrosis factor (TNF)
E. All of the above

966 Regarding the occurrence of psychologic/psychiatric disorders in those with IBS, data have shown that:

A. Patients with IBS are less likely to report greater lifetime and daily stressful events than are those with organic disease
B. Patients with IBS report a history of sexual, physical, or emotional abuse more often than those without IBS
C. When reported, adult stressful events are more important than childhood stressful events

D. In animal studies, stress has no effect on colonic motility

E. A history of abuse is associated with rectal hypersensitivity

967 Which of the following statements is true concerning the epidemiology of *Tropheryma whippelii* infection?

A. It is more common in women in the sixth decade of life.

B. It is more common in men in their sixth decade of life.

C. It is more common in women in the third decade of life.

D. It is more common in men in the third decade of life.

968 Nonoperative management of partial SBO is warranted because:

A. Surgery increases the risk of recurrent SBO

B. In most patients the condition will improve with nonsurgical management

C. Gangrenous complications do not occur in patients presenting with partial SBO

D. Partial SBO can always be distinguished from complete SBO by radiologic studies

E. Oral Gastrografin is the treatment of choice, obviating the need for surgery

969 A 55-year-old man with hypertension undergoes colonoscopy. A 2-cm pedunculated sigmoid polyp is removed completely and histopathologic evaluation shows it to be a well-differentiated carcinoma extending to within 2.5 mm of the margin of a villous polyp that extends into the submucosa. No evidence is found of lymphatic and or blood vessel involvement. What is recommended next?

A. Resection of the sigmoid colon

B. Short-term follow-up colonoscopy

C. Left hemicolectomy

D. Colonoscopy in 3 years

E. Chemotherapy

970 Current recommendations for treatment of Whipple's disease are as follows:

A. Penicillin G plus streptomycin, followed by trimethoprim-sulfamethoxazole

B. Ciprofloxacin

C. Albendazole

D. Augmentin

971 The primary manometric abnormality seen in myopathic forms of CIP is:

A. Decreased amplitude of contractions in the affected small bowel segment

B. Increased amplitudes of gastric antral contractions

C. Disorganization and incoordination of motor activity with normal amplitudes of contractions

D. Absent or abnormal migrating motor complex (MMC) activity

E. Cluster contraction pattern in the diseased segment

972 Screening recommendations for members of families with hereditary nonpolypoid colon cancer (HNPCC) do *not* include:

A. Colonoscopy every 2 years

B. Genetic testing

C. Colonoscopy beginning at age 25

D. Yearly sigmoidoscopy starting at puberty and then colonoscopy every 2 years starting at age 40

973 Which of the following statements regarding anorectal abscesses is *most* accurate?

A. Most anorectal abscesses result from infection of the anal glands.

B. The most common type of anorectal abscess is the supralevator abscess.

C. The absence of abnormal findings on physical examination of the anorectum sufficiently rules out an anorectal abscess.

D. Small anorectal abscesses can often be treated with antibiotics alone.

974 A 56-year-old white man with a longstanding history of alcohol abuse and several prior episodes of acute pancreatitis complains that he has had loose, pale, greasy, foul-smelling stools every day for several months. A low serum level of which of the following may be suggestive of pancreatic exocrine insufficiency and steatorrhea?

A. Folate

B. Iron

C. β-carotene

D. Albumin

975 A patient with UC undergoes biopsy. The histologic features of the biopsy specimen (see figure) are characteristic of:

A. Dysplasia, low-grade

B. Dysplasia, high-grade

C. Acute colitis

D. Superimposed cytomegalovirus (CMV) infection

E. Chronic quiescent UC

976 The most accurate statement regarding pouchitis is:

A. The underlying disease has no role in the future development of pouchitis

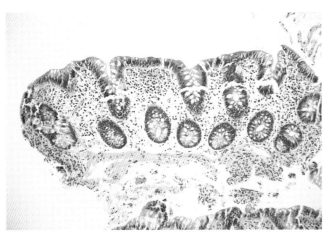

Figure for question **975**

B. Loperamide is the treatment of choice
C. The villous architecture is distorted and colonic metaplasia is present in biopsy specimens from most pouches, even in the absence of severe acute inflammation
D. It will occur in 90% of patients
E. Metronidazole is the only effective antibiotic

977 Which of the following genetic findings has been associated with IBD?

A. *NOD 2/CARD 15* gene
B. IBD-2 locus on chromosome 12
C. *C3435T*
D. HLA DR1, 2, 3
E. All of the above

978 The "target lesion sign" is an attenuated area on CT consistent with an intraluminal soft-tissue mass with an eccentrically placed fatty area. This sign represents:

A. A Meckel's diverticulum
B. An intussusception
C. A carcinoid tumor
D. Acute appendicitis
E. SBO secondary to internal hernia

979 A 25-year-old man with a history of anxiety disorder is concerned about his family history of colon polyps. His father developed colonic adenomas in his 70s. His paternal uncle developed polyps in his 60s, and his sister had colon polyps in her mid-40s. He is very anxious to learn how he might decrease his risk of colon adenomas. Which of the following has *not* been shown to decrease the risk of colon adenomas?

A. High-fiber diet
B. Low-carbohydrate diet
C. Calcium supplementation
D. Physical activity
E. Aspirin therapy

980 A 40-year-old man with refractory ulcerative colitis was admitted to the hospital for intravenous administration of glucocorticoid drugs. After 7 days, he is still having bloody diarrhea and abdominal pain. The decision is made to initiate cyclosporine therapy. This treatment:

A. Takes at least 4 weeks to begin having an effect
B. Can be utilized, at low doses, for maintenance therapy
C. Should not be utilized if the patient's serum cholesterol level is below 120 mg/dL
D. Does not require monitoring of the drug level

981 IBS is:

A. The functional gastrointestinal disorder most frequently seen in gastrointestinal practices
B. Associated with abdominal pain that is continuous and not relieved with defecation
C. Not associated with noncolonic symptoms such as headache, backache, or impaired sleep
D. Not seen in patients with inflammatory bowel disease
E. Most prevalent among middle-aged people

982 Which of the following laboratory test results are most supportive of a diagnosis of cobalamin deficiency?

A. Normal serum methylmalonic acid level, normal serum homocysteine level
B. Elevated serum methylmalonic acid level, normal serum homocysteine level
C. Normal serum methylmalonic acid level, elevated serum homocysteine level
D. Elevated serum methylmalonic acid level, elevated serum homocysteine level

983 A 40-year-old white man is hospitalized for his first attack of ulcerative colitis. What are the chances he will require a colectomy during this admission?

A. 80%
B. 60%
C. 40%
D. 10% or less

984 A 16-year-old boy presents with RLQ pain and fever. Acute appendicitis is suspected. The best test to confirm the diagnosis is:

A. Plain radiography
B. Ultrasound
C. Complete blood count (CBC)
D. Measurement of C-reactive protein (CRP) level
E. CT

985 There is no genetic test to identify increased risk for colorectal cancer in:

A. Patients at increased risk of sporadic colorectal cancer
B. Families with FAP
C. Families suspected of HNPCC
D. Family members of a colorectal cancer patient whose tumor exhibits microsatellite instability

986 The smooth-muscle cells within each muscle layer of the small intestine form a syncytium. Their activity is locally coordinated by the:

A. Enteric nervous system
B. Extrinsic neurons
C. Intrinsic neurons
D. Interstitial cells of Cajal
E. Myenteric plexus

987 The concept that ulcerative colitis is an autoimmune disease is supported by its association with other autoimmune diseases. These disorders include:

A. Thyroid disease
B. Diabetes mellitus
C. Pernicious anemia
D. All of the above
E. None of the above

988 Epidemiologic studies in patients with IBS have found that:

A. There is 2:1 male predominance
B. Women have slower colonic transit and smaller stool output than men
C. The prevalence is greater among African-American individuals than among white persons
D. IBS is not seen in China or Japan
E. The prevalence is higher in Hispanic compared to non-Hispanic populations

989 The most predominant feature of tropical sprue in patients in Asia and the Caribbean is:

A. Bloody diarrhea
B. Fat malabsorption
C. Hyperpigmentation
D. Alopecia

990 A 2-day-old child has recurrent bilious vomiting and is refusing feedings. Among other diagnoses, intestinal atresia is considered. This congenital abnormality:

A. Most often occurs in the duodenal bulb.
B. Most often occurs in the distal duodenum and in most such cases is contiguous with or distal to the ampulla of Vater.
C. Most often occurs in the ileum and usually involves the ileocecal valve.
D. Most often occurs in the colon and usually involves the "watershed" territory, the region

between that supplied by the superior and that supplied by the inferior mesenteric artery.

991 Which of the following statements is *true* regarding a diverticular abscess?

A. *E. coli, Streptococcus* spp., and *Bacteroides fragilis* most often grow on cultures of abscess fluid.
B. Small pericolic abscesses can be treated with broad-spectrum antibiotic drugs and bowel rest.
C. CT-guided percutaneous drainage may eliminate the need for a multiple-stage procedure with colostomy.
D. An urgent surgical procedure is required in 20% to 25% of cases.
E. All of the above.

992 Which of the following statements is *true* about small bowel neoplasms?

A. Small bowel neoplasms are diagnosed more often in female patients.
B. Small bowel neoplasms are the second most common GI malignancy.
C. Most small bowel neoplasms are malignant.
D. Small bowel neoplasms are more frequently diagnosed in young adults.
E. The most common small bowel malignancies are sarcomas.

993 Thiopurine methyltransferase (TMPT) is the enzyme that:

A. Converts 6-mercaptopurine (6-MP) to its inactive metabolites
B. May be helpful to evaluate prior to initiating immunomodulatory therapy
C. Is associated with genetic polymorphism
D. May interact with mesalamine to increase levels of thioguanine (6-TG)
E. All of the above

994 Which of the following statements regarding the Schilling test for vitamin B_{12} malabsorption is *most* accurate?

A. The Schilling test results are abnormal in patients with dietary vitamin B_{12} deficiency.
B. In patients with pernicious anemia, the results of the Schilling test normalize after oral administration of intrinsic factor.
C. In patients with ileal disease, the results of the Schilling test normalize after oral administration of intrinsic factor.
D. Pancreatic exocrine insufficiency does not cause Schilling test results to be abnormal.

995 The hallmark serologic abnormality in patients with paraneoplastic visceral neuropathy is:

A. Presence of antinuclear antibody to ribonucleoprotein

B. Presence of antineuronal nuclear (anti-Hu) antibody

C. Elevated creatine phosphokinase (CPK) level

D. Abnormal creatine kinase level

E. Presence of antiactin antibodies

996 A young patient with Crohn's disease presents with morning stiffness improved by exercise and gradually increasing low back pain. The patient undergoes imaging of the lumbosacral spine (see figure). Which of the following statements is *most* accurate regarding this patient's condition?

A. It is more common than peripheral arthropathy.

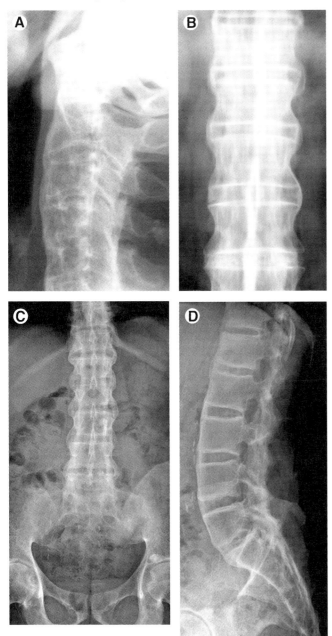

Figure for question **996**. (From Mansour M, Cheema G, Naguwa S, et al: Ankylosing spondylitis: A contemporary perspective on diagnosis and treatment. Semin Arthritis Rheum 36(4):210-223, 2007.)

B. Up to 75% of those with Crohn's disease may test positive for HLA-B27.

C. Uveitis is often associated with this condition.

D. Most patients with this entity are symptomatic.

997 Yellow plaque-like lesions (lymphangiectasias) of the distal duodenum and jejunum (see figure) with associated diarrhea are common in what disorder?

A. Whipple's disease

B. Crohn's disease

C. Ulcerative colitis

D. Celiac sprue

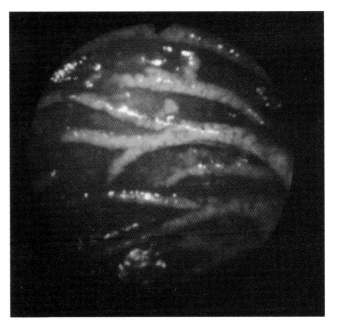

Figure for question **997**

998 A 38-year-old man reports that several times weekly he sees a small amount of blood in the toilet bowl and on the toilet paper after passage of hard, formed stool. This has been occurring for approximately 2 years. He denies rectal pain but reports frequent straining with defecation. He does not use stool softeners or laxatives. He has no family history of colorectal cancer.

On rectal examination, there are no external hemorrhoids, fissures, or masses. His stool is brown and tests negative for occult blood. A flexible sigmoidoscopy is performed and reveals small- to medium-sized internal hemorrhoids. What is the appropriate first step in treatment of the hemorrhoids?

A. Introduction of a high-fiber diet and routine intake of 6 to 8 glasses of fluid daily

B. Sclerotherapy with injection of sterilized arachis oils containing 5% phenol

C. Rubber band ligation

D. Cryotherapy

E. Surgical hemorrhoidectomy

999 Which statement is true regarding microsporidiosis?

A. *Enterocytozoon bieneusi* infection accounts for 90% of the cases and responds well to albendazole.
B. It occurs primarily in patients with impaired cell-mediated immunity.
C. Microsporida are identified in fewer than 10% of patients with AIDS who have chronic diarrhea.
D. Unlike cryptosporidiosis, microsporidiosis is not associated with sclerosing cholangitis.
E. Highly active antiretroviral therapy (HAART) to improve immune system function is not helpful in the control of microsporidiosis in patients with AIDS.

1000 A 50-year-old woman with severe diarrhea-predominant IBS is prescribed Alesetron for management of the diarrhea. Significant constipation develops within the first few days of Alesetron use. Regarding IBS and colon ischemia:

A. There does not appear to be an increased risk of colon ischemia with the use of this 5-hydroxytryptamine-3 (5-HT-3) receptor antagonist
B. Dosage reduction is all that is required
C. There is a three to four times increased risk of colon ischemia in patients with diarrhea-predominant IBS who are prescribed alesetron
D. Colon ischemia generally occurs in male patients with IBS rather than in female patients

1001 Which of the following statements regarding vitamin B_{12} deficiency caused by small intestinal bacterial overgrowth is *most* accurate?

A. Vitamin B_{12} deficiency is caused by bacterial consumption of the vitamin within the intestinal lumen.
B. SIBO causes mucosal damage and greatly reduces the number of ileal binding sites for vitamin B_{12}.
C. Aerobic organisms are responsible for the vitamin B_{12} deficiency.
D. During the Schilling test, vitamin B_{12} deficiency is reversible by the addition of intrinsic factor.

1002 A 51-year-old man who has had UC for 30 years undergoes his yearly surveillance colonoscopy. Based on the histopathologic appearance of biopsy specimens (see figure), the following is recommended:

A. Repeat colonoscopy in 1 year
B. Repeat colonoscopy now to confirm findings and location
C. Obtain a second pathologist's opinion regarding the biopsy results and if the first

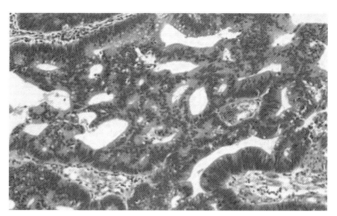

Figure for question **1002**

pathologist's findings are confirmed, recommend colectomy
D. Remove the colon segment where the biopsy was performed

1003 Which one of the following factors causes a relative increase in the rate of gastric emptying (see figure)?

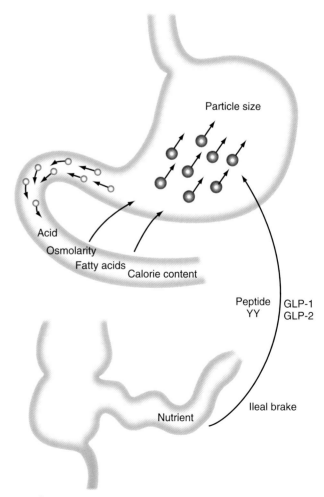

Figure for question **1003**

A. An acidic pH of the duodenal luminal contents

B. Ingestion of a high-calorie meal

C. Ingestion of a meal with a high viscosity

D. The presence of nutrients in the ileum and colon

1004 Diarrhea due to cryptosporidiosis may be most severe in which group?

A. HIV-positive men with CD4 counts greater than 700

B. Patients with immunoglobulin deficiency

C. Women of child-bearing age

D. Teenagers

1005 Small bowel x-rays (see figure) from an upper GI small bowel follow-through study in a patient with Crohn's disease indicate:

A. There is a loss of haustra

B. Transmural edema is responsible for separated bowel loops

C. Aphthous ulcers are present

D. There is cobblestoning, an early finding

1006 Vasoconstriction that is the result of occlusion of a major vessel occurs:

A. Immediately, elevating the pressure in the vascular bed and thus reducing collateral flow

B. After several hours, elevating the pressure in the vascular bed and reducing collateral flow

C. After 24 hours and is readily reversible but has little to do with progressive bowel ischemia, even if cardiac function is fully restored

D. Has little to do with progressive bowel ischemia even if cardiac function is fully restored

1007 A 40-year-old white man who has had ulcerative colitis for 15 years complains of pruritus and jaundice for the past several days. He denies any abdominal pain or fever. He has been taking mesalamine, 4 grams daily, for 3 years without problems. He has two semi-formed stools daily, without blood and with only occasional mucus. A colonoscopy performed a year ago showed quiescent UC and there was no evidence of dysplasia on multiple biopsies. The patient is found to have an elevated alkaline phosphatase level (500 U/L). Based on the results of ERCP (see figure), he is started on ursodeoxycholic acid, 1200 mg a day. The serum direct bilirubin was 6.0.

The prothrombin time was 13.0 seconds. An ultrasound reveals mildly dilated intrahepatic ducts. The most appropriate way to manage this patient's jaundice and pruritus is:

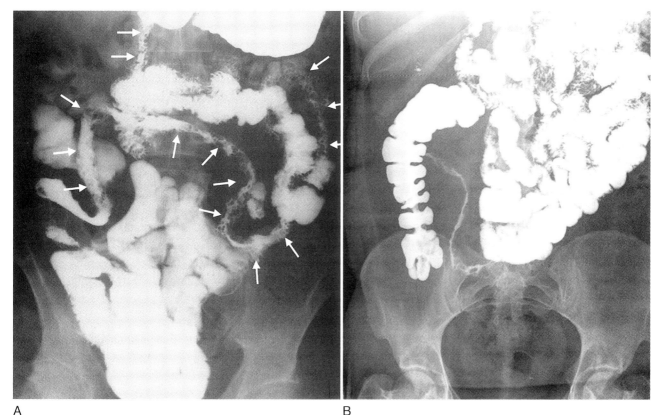

A   B

Figure for question **1005**. (*A* and *B*, Courtesy of Jack Wittenberg, MD, Boston, MA.)

A. A trial of high-dose glucocorticoid drug therapy
B. Total colectomy
C. Cholestyramine, 4 grams twice daily
D. Repeat ERCP with dilation of the dominant stricture
E. Referral for evaluation for liver transplantation

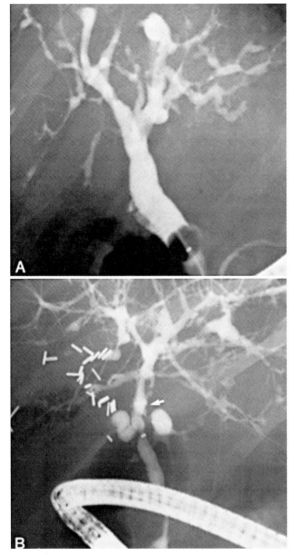

Figure for question **1007**

A. Recurrence of viral gastroenteritis
B. Superimposed bacterial infection
C. Ulcerative proctitis
D. Colon ischemia

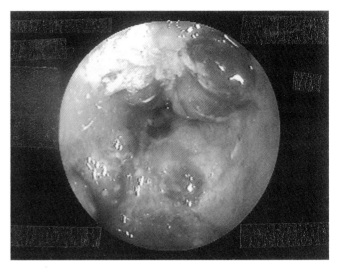

Figure for question **1008**

1008 A 71-year-old woman comes to the emergency department because of severe nausea, vomiting, and diarrhea determined to be secondary to viral gastroenteritis. Her blood pressure is 70/50 mmHg and she is administered intravenous fluid. One day later, she returns to the emergency department complaining of sudden onset of crampy left lower quadrant pain and passage of bloody diarrhea. Sigmoidoscopy findings (see figure) indicate that her new symptoms are likely due to:

1009 A 25-year-old pregnant woman presents with abdominal pain and diarrhea. Which of the following statements is *false?*

A. Malaria, amebiasis, and *Giardia* can cause diarrhea and abdominal pain.
B. *Campylobacter* infections may cause spontaneous abortion, prematurity, neonatal sepsis, neonatal enterocolitis, and death.
C. Septicemia due to shigellosis occurs more often in neonates than in adults.
D. Trimethoprim-sulfamethoxazole (TMP-SMX) is the drug of choice for treating diarrhea in pregnant women.

1010 Which of the following statements is accurate regarding asymptomatic diverticulosis presenting as an incidental finding?

A. There is no clear indication for any therapy or follow-up.
B. It is widely accepted that a high-fiber diet is effective in decreasing the risk of new symptomatic diverticulosis.
C. Diets high in fat and red meat are associated with an increased risk of diverticular disease.
D. A positive fecal occult blood test should not be attributed to diverticulosis.
E. All of the above

1011 Which of the following statements regarding colorectal cancer is *true?*

A. Colorectal cancer is second only to lung cancer as a cause of cancer death in the United States.

B. Annually, 0.6% of the United States population will develop colorectal cancer.
C. The incidence of colorectal cancer is higher in men.
D. Colorectal cancer incidence and mortality have risen since 1985 in the United States.

1012 A 50-year-old man presents to the emergency department with nausea, vomiting, abdominal cramps, diarrhea, and diplopia. On examination his heart rate is 45 beats/minute and his blood pressure is 90/60 mmHg. He reports having eaten red snapper in a local restaurant 6 hours before. Which of the following is the most likely cause of his symptoms?

A. Ciguatera poisoning
B. Scombroid poisoning
C. *Vibrio vulnificus* infection
D. *Salmonella* infection

1013 Paneth cells:

A. Are the primary cells of the acid-producing oxyntic gland.
B. Are associated with lymphoid follicles of the small intestine and colon and process and present antigens to lymphocytes, macrophages, and other immune cells.
C. Are primarily located in the proximal small intestine where they produce alkaline-rich secretions to neutralize acidic gastric effluent.
D. Possess abundant eosinophilic granules containing the bactericidal enzyme, lysozyme.
E. Secrete pepsinogen, the inactive precursor of pepsin.

1014 In acute mesenteric venous thrombosis:

A. Thrombolytic agents are commonly utilized
B. Intravenous heparin for 7 to 10 days has been shown to improve survival
C. One month of warfarin is usually adequate
D. Even if peritonitis is present, laparotomy is not necessary

1015 Treatment of small bowel ulcerations caused by NSAIDs includes:

A. NSAID avoidance, metronidazole, sulfasalazine
B. NSAID avoidance, metronidazole, imuran
C. NSAID avoidance, sulfasalazine, imuran
D. No specific therapy

1016 A 25-year-old male medical student who has had ileocecal Crohn's disease for 6 years comes to the office complaining of 1 to 2 weeks of progressive pain in the right flank along with additional discomfort in the right hip and thigh. He has taken mesalamine 2 grams daily since his original diagnosis and has intermittently been taking glucocorticoid drugs. He recently started taking 20 mg of prednisone daily due to increasing abdominal pain. On physical examination, the patient has a limping gait and is bending forward slightly at the waist. He has a low-grade fever (temperature 101°F). The abdominal examination reveals a slight fullness in the right lower quadrant with a mild to moderate amount of tenderness. There is no voluntary guarding or rebound. There is no evidence of edema of the right thigh or knee. His hemoglobin level is 12 mg/dL and his white blood cell count is 18,000/mm^3 with a left shift. Which of the following imaging studies is most likely to reveal the cause of this patient's complaints?

A. Plain x-rays of the lumbosacral spine
B. Computed tomography of the abdomen and pelvis
C. Colonoscopy
D. Joint aspiration
E. Intravenous pyelogram (IVP)

1017 Which of the following extraintestinal manifestations of ulcerative colitis does not correlate with the activity of the colitis?

A. Ankylosing spondylitis
B. Erythema nodosum
C. Episcleritis
D. Aphthous ulceration of the mouth
E. Peripheral arthropathy

1018 Local colonic motor activity is coordinated by the:

A. Enteric nervous system
B. Interstitial cells of Cajal
C. Parasympathetic nervous system
D. Sympathetic nervous system

1019 Adjuvant therapy with 5-fluorouracil (5-FU) and leucovorin is considered standard treatment for advanced colorectal cancer. It is *not* true that this regimen:

A. Prolongs disease-free survival
B. Is superior in convenience and efficacy compared to 5-FU and levamisole
C. Prolongs overall survival
D. Is standard treatment for stage 3 disease
E. Is standard treatment for stage 2, node-negative disease

1020 The first test that should be performed for the diagnosis of giardiasis is:

A. Stool enzyme-linked immunosorbent assay (ELISA) for giardiasis
B. Stool examination for ova and parasites
C. Duodenal aspirate or biopsy
D. Stool acid-fast staining

1021 A certain feature seen on endoscopy of a patient's proximal small bowel (see figure), is evidence of all of the following diseases *except*

A. Celiac sprue
B. Tropical sprue
C. Crohn's disease
D. *Giardia* infection

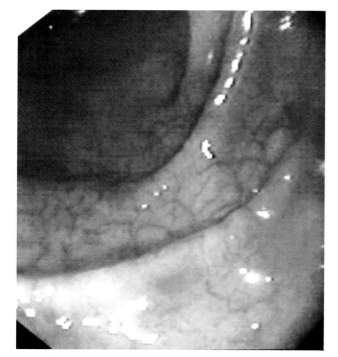

Figure for question **1021**

1022 A 15-year-old has periumbilical pain that migrates into the RLQ over the period of about a day. All of the following are likely presentations of appendicitis *except:*

A. "Downward" urge to defecate
B. Low-grade fever or chills
C. Pain elicited by internal or external rotation of the flexed right hip
D. Pain increased by passively flexing and extending the right hip in left lateral position
E. All of the above

1023 A 50-year-old man visiting Bangladesh has vomiting and diarrhea consisting of large volumes of "rice-water" stools. Stool analysis shows a sodium (Na) level of 124 mEq/L and potassium (K) of 16 mEq/L. Which of the following statements about the organism/infection causing this patient's symptoms is *false?*

A. Fecal outputs of 15 to 20 L/day are common.
B. The organism is not invasive.
C. Bloody diarrhea is common.
D. Bacteremia is rare.
E. Patients often present with profound dehydration and hypovolemic shock.

1024 Regarding serotonin (5-HT) receptor drugs for IBS:

A. Both 5-HT-4–receptor agonists and 5-HT-3–receptor antagonists have been associated with the development of ischemic colitis
B. Tegaserod (a 5-HT-3–receptor agonist) can be used in patients with alternating diarrhea and constipation
C. Alosetron (a 5-HT-3–receptor antagonist) is indicated in constipation-predominant IBS
D. Alosetron is no longer available in the United States
E. Tegaserod has been approved by the U.S. Food and Drug Administration (FDA) for both men and women

1025 The best treatment choice for patients with *Strongyloides* infection is:

A. Metronidazole
B. Albendazole
C. Ivermectin
D. Praziquantel
E. Mebendazole

1026 Visceral distention or discomfort of the small intestines is mediated by:

A. Sensory efferent neurons with cell bodies within the cerebellum
B. Spinal afferent fibers with cell bodies within the thoracic dorsal root ganglia and projections to the prevertebral ganglia and splanchnic nerves
C. The vagus nerve with cell bodies within the nodosa and jugular ganglia and projections to the intestinal wall
D. The vagus nerve with cell bodies within the dorsal root ganglia and projections to the intestinal wall

1027 A 25-year-old woman with Crohn's disease is complaining of a "rash" on her lower extremity. She has also had some increasing joint pain. The rash (see figure) is most consistent with:

A. Erythema nodosum
B. Metastatic Crohn's disease
C. Psoriasis
D. Pyoderma gangrenosum
E. Leukocytoclastic vasculitis

1028 The pathophysiologic defect in diabetes-induced CIP is:

A. Degeneration of the myenteric and submucosal plexuses
B. Demyelination of the proximal vagus and sympathetic nerves supplying the bowel
C. Primarily a degeneration of the circular and longitudinal muscles

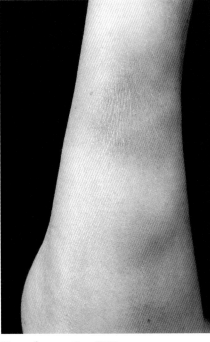

Figure for question **1027**

D. Proliferation of the interstitial cells of Cajal
E. Bile salt malabsorption

1029 Henoch-Schönlein purpura, which presents with a rash (see figure):

A. Typically affects adolescents 12 to 16 years of age
B. Is characterized by immunoglobulin G (IgG) immune complexes
C. Can be associated with intussusception
D. Manifests as palpable purpura, typically involving the upper extremities

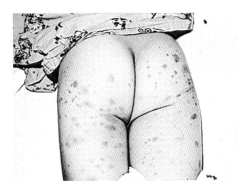

Figure for question **1029**

1030 A 56-year-old woman with rheumatoid arthritis presents with a 6-month history of diarrhea, abdominal cramping, and weight loss. The results of colonoscopy are unremarkable. On biopsy specimens a subepithelial collagen band of 12 μm is seen. All of the following drugs are commonly utilized to treat this patient's condition *except:*

A. Budesonide
B. 5-ASA
C. Remicade
D. Loperamide

1031 In addition to nutrient protein hydrolysis, a function of pancreatic proteases is:

A. Activating other pancreatic proteases from proenzymes
B. Splitting vitamin B_{12} from the R protein
C. Increasing the turnover of brush border membrane hydrolytic enzymes
D. Initiating the final steps in the processing of the sucrase-isomaltase complex
E. All of the above

1032 The risk of colorectal cancer is increased in patients with UC and:

A. Primary sclerosing cholangitis (PSC)
B. Short duration of disease
C. Left-sided disease
D. Older age at diagnosis
E. None of the above

1033 One of the postulated mechanisms for diarrhea-predominant IBS is:

A. An enhanced gastrocolonic response after a meal
B. Decreased high-amplitude propagated contractions (HPACs)
C. Reduced rectal sensitivity resulting in fecal urgency
D. Increased segmental nonpropulsive contractions
E. Hypertensive internal rectal sphincter

1034 All of the following congenital gastrointestinal anomalies result from abnormalities during the physiologic umbilical herniation *except:*

A. Gastroschisis
B. Inguinal hernia
C. Retrocecal appendix
D. Omphalocele

1035 A 25-year-old woman has rectal bleeding that she believes is due to a prolapsing external hemorrhoid. A colonoscopy is performed and reveals a single 1.5-cm juvenile polyp in the distal rectum. Which of the following is true?

A. Juvenile polyps are usually not single.
B. Juvenile polyps are classified as inflammatory polyps.
C. Juvenile polyps need not be removed.
D. Juvenile polyps have low to medium potential for becoming malignant.
E. Juvenile polyps, when multiple, have an increased risk of becoming cancerous.

1036 The histopathologic findings in a patient's biopsy specimen (see figure) are:

A. Typically seen in quiescent ulcerative colitis
B. Unique to Crohn's disease
C. Never found outside of the gastrointestinal tract
D. Sarcoid-like and consist of epithelioid histiocytes
E. Associated with leukotriene B4

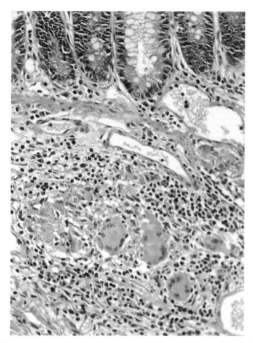

Figure for question **1036**. (Courtesy of Gregory Lauwers, MD, Boston, MA.)

1037 The intestine can tolerate what percent reduction in blood flow for as long as 12 hours without any change in histologic appearance being noted on light microscopy?

A. 10%
B. 25%
C. 50%
D. 75%
E. 90%

1038 Which of the following metabolites of ingested starch can be absorbed by colonic mucosa?

A. Polysaccharides
B. Disaccharides
C. Monosaccharides
D. Short-chain fatty acids

1039 The most common location of a nonspecific small bowel ulceration is:

A. Duodenal bulb
B. Treitz's ligament

C. Jejunum
D. Ileum

1040 Of all the following side effects associated with azathioprine and 6-MP, the one that is dose-dependent is:

A. Pancreatitis
B. Leukopenia
C. Fevers
D. Rash
E. Hepatitis

1041 The treatment of choice for acute mesenteric ischemia (AMI) without signs of peritonitis is:

A. Immediate laparotomy
B. Intravenous heparin
C. Hyperbaric oxygen
D. Selected mesenteric angiography with papaverine infusion

1042 The most common cause for large colon obstruction is:

A. Colon carcinoma
B. Volvulus
C. Stricture form diverticulitis
D. Crohn's disease
E. Fecal impaction

1043 The most common presenting symptom for a nonspecific small bowel ulceration is:

A. Abdominal pain
B. Perforation
C. Chronic gastrointestinal blood loss
D. Intermittent small bowel obstruction

1044 Which of the following statements is *not* true regarding dysplasia in adenomatous polyps?

A. Higher grades of dysplasia are more common in larger adenomas.
B. Adenomas with severe dysplasia are more likely to contain foci of invasive carcinoma.
C. Dysplasia is seen more commonly in villous adenomas than tubular adenomas.
D. Adenomas with villous content more commonly have higher grades of dysplasia.
E. Intramucosal carcinoma has a low risk of metastasis.

1045 A 60-year-old man with congestive heart failure and intermittent atrial fibrillation presents to the emergency department complaining of vague diffuse abdominal pain for the past month. He has lost 20 pounds in the last 3 months. He has a low-grade fever and mild-to-moderate diffuse abdominal pain without guarding or rebound. His stool is brown and tests heme-positive. The most likely diagnosis is:

A. Superior mesenteric artery embolus (SMAE)
B. Nonocclusive mesenteric ischemia (NOME)
C. Focal segmental ischemia (FSI)
D. Mesenteric venous thrombus (subacute)

1046 Regarding serologic markers in inflammatory bowel disease:

A. They are necessary to confirm a diagnosis
B. Negative markers rule out IBD
C. ASCA-positive patients have higher rates of surgery
D. Markers are more than 85% sensitive for IBD

1047 Which of the following have an increased occupational risk of Whipple's disease?

A. Dentists
B. Teachers
C. Farmers and carpenters
D. Sailors

1048 Which of the following has been shown to decrease mortality from colorectal cancer?

A. Yearly fecal occult blood testing
B. Double-contrast barium enema
C. Virtual colonoscopy
D. Yearly digital rectal examination

1049 Which of the following statements about diverticula is *false?*

A. Right-sided diverticula are more common than left-sided diverticula in Asian populations.
B. Diverticula are hernias of the mucosa and submucosa through a muscularis defect and are therefore pseudodiverticula.
C. Dietary factors are believed to play a major role in the pathogenesis of diverticula.
D. Rats fed low-fiber diets develop diverticula 45% of the time.
E. None of the above.

1050 The most accurate statement regarding the epidemiology of ulcerative colitis is:

A. There is a distinct South-North gradient
B. The overall incidence of ulcerative colitis is decreasing
C. Incidence rates among Jews in the United States are equal to those among non-Jewish white persons
D. Incidence rates are comparable between whites and people of color in the United States

1051 The intestinal pacemaker cells activating neuromuscular function are the:

A. Myenteric nerve cells
B. M cells

C. Interstitial cells of Cajal
D. Intraepithelial lymphocytes
E. Vagal crest cells

1052 A 30-year-old HIV-positive man presents with watery diarrhea, weight loss, and abdominal pain of 4 weeks' duration. His CD4 count is 50. Which treatment will have the greatest impact on the course of his *Cryptosporidium* infection?

A. HAART
B. Nitazoxanide
C. Paromomycin
D. Azithromycin

1053 A patient with ulcerative colitis has been on and off glucocorticoid drugs for the last 12 months. Nonglucocorticoid immunosuppressant drugs were added to the patient's regimen when it was impossible to taper glucocorticoid drugs, but symptoms have not remitted. On sigmoidoscopy, discrete deep ulcerations are seen. The next best step in this patient's care should be:

A. Increase the dose of glucocorticoid drug
B. Increase the dose of immunosuppressant drug
C. Add cyclosporine
D. Perform endoscopic biopsies of the mucosa and ulcer bed
E. Perform colectomy immediately

1054 Causes for focal segmental ischemia (FSI) of the small intestine include:

A. Atheromatous emboli
B. Strangulated hernia
C. Vasculitis
D. Radiation therapy
E. All of the above

1055 Amebiasis is not sensitive to:

A. Iodoquinol
B. Metronidazole
C. Paromomycin
D. Ciprofloxacin
E. Tinidazole

1056 The most common cause of short bowel syndrome in adults is:

A. Trauma
B. Crohn's disease
C. Radiation enteritis
D. Mesenteric infarction
E. Severe necrotizing enteric infection

1057 Infestations with the beef and pork tapeworms *Taenia saginata* and *Taenia solium* occur when people eat raw or undercooked meat. Which of the following statements is *true?*

A. Most people who are infested are symptomatic
B. Cysticercosis is a mild complication of *T. solium*
C. Neurocysticercosis is a rare cause of epilepsy in endemic areas
D. These tapeworms can be diagnosed by examination of stool samples
E. Praziquantel in a single oral dose is ineffective

1058 The bacterial pathogen that most often causes acute infectious diarrhea in travelers is:

A. *Shigella*
B. *Campylobacter*
C. Enterotoxigenic *Escherichia coli*
D. *Giardia*

1059 Features commonly associated with NSAID-induced small bowel ulceration include all of the following *except:*

A. Diaphragm-like strictures
B. Hypoalbuminemia
C. Anemia
D. Entero-entero fistulas

1060 Infections with which of the following have symptoms that can mimic those of UC?

A. *E. coli* 0157:H7
B. *C. difficile*
C. *Aeromonas hydrophila*
D. *Listeria monocytogenes*
E. All of the above

1061 The most accurate statement regarding the diagnostic test for *C. difficile* infection is:

A. Tissue culture cytotoxicity assay is the gold standard
B. Enzyme-linked immunoassay is highly sensitive for toxins but less specific than the cytotoxicity test

C. Stool culture for *C. difficile* has low sensitivity
D. Sigmoidoscopy evidence of a pseudomembrane is only seen in *C. difficile* colitis
E. Colonic mucosal biopsies may be confused with IBD

1062 The most common finding on plain x-rays of the abdomen early in the course of bowel ischemia is:

A. Free air under the diaphragm
B. No abnormality
C. Ileus
D. "Thumbprinting" of the right colon
E. Air in the portal vein

1063 Which group is at greatest risk for giardiasis in the United States?

A. Teenage children
B. Sexually active heterosexual men
C. Children in daycare
D. Those whose source of drinking water is a treated deep well

1064 The procedure of choice for most patients with chronic ulcerative colitis (CUC) or FAP is:

A. Ileal pouch anal anastomosis (IPAA)
B. Ileorectal anastomosis
C. Brooke ileostomy
D. Continent ileostomy (Koch's pouch)
E. None of the above

1065 Which of the following cells do not migrate up the villus axis?

A. Enterocytes
B. Endocrine cells
C. Paneth cells
D. Goblet cells

ANSWERS

745 E. (S&F, ch111)

This patient has typical findings of ischemic colitis. When colonic ischemia is diagnosed and there are no physical examination findings to suggest gangrene or perforation, observation is the recommended therapy, usually with administration of fluids, bowel rest, and broad-spectrum antibiotics. Urgent imaging of any type, including CT or angiography, is not warranted at this time. Because there are no signs of peritoneal disease, laparotomy is not necessary. Mesalamine and glucocorticoid drugs

would not be appropriate in treating ischemic colitis.

746 C. (S&F, ch120)

The liver is the most common site for colon cancer metastases. Patients with liver metastases have a poor prognosis and therefore aggressive treatment is recommended. Resection of liver metastases is considered if the primary tumor has been removed with the intent to cure and no extrahepatic disease is present. Resection could be considered as long as there are no more than four metastases present, even if more than one lobe is involved.

747   **C.** (S&F, ch97)

Triglycerides, cholesterol esters, and phospholipids synthesized in enterocytes are packaged for export in the form of chylomicrons and very-low-density lipoproteins (VLDLs). During fasting, VLDLs are the major triglyceride-rich lipoproteins released from the epithelium; after feeding, chylomicrons predominate. The fatty acids derived from dietary triglycerides are predominantly used in the formation of chylomicrons, whereas those derived from phospholipids appear to be utilized in the formation of VLDLs.

The chylomicron core consists of triglycerides, whereas cholesterol ester and phospholipid form more than 80% of the surface coat. Forming a smaller proportion of the chylomicron surface is the essential component, apolipoprotein. The absence of apolipoprotein B prevents synthesis and secretion of chylomicrons.

Once chylomicrons have formed in the smooth endoplasmic reticulum, they are transferred to the Golgi apparatus, incorporated into the basolateral membrane, and secreted via exocytosis into the lymphatic circulation.

748   **C.** (S&F, ch115)

The Rome II criteria are listed in answer **C**. Answers **A** and **B** list Manning criteria. Gender, age, anal fissures, or hemorrhoids (answers **D** and **E**) are not part of any criteria.1

749   **B.** (S&F, ch121)

Diversion colitis appears to be caused largely by the colonic epithelium suffering luminal nutrient deficiency. The principal nutrient substrates of colonic epithelium are luminal short-chain fatty acids (SCFAs), which are produced in negligible amounts in the excluded segments of colon. The numbers of obligate anaerobes are reduced in the excluded colon, consistent with reduced SCFA production.

750   **B.** (S&F, ch106)

Giardia lamblia is the most common cause of human protozoan infection worldwide. It is also considered a contributory factor in the retardation of growth and development in infants and young children. Infection with *Isospora belli* also causes chronic diarrhea and enteropathy, but the organism is geographically restricted to the tropics and subtropics. *Cyclospora cayetanensis* is a recently recognized intracellular protozoan that has been identified in a number

of tropical and subtropical locations as a cause of chronic diarrhea and enteropathy in immunocompetent and immunocompromised persons. *Cryptosporidium parvum* is a well known cause of chronic diarrhea worldwide in immunocompetent persons, in whom the diarrhea usually is self-limited. It is also a major cause of chronic, intractable diarrhea in patients with human immunodeficiency virus (HIV) infection.

751   **D.** (S&F, ch122)

Pruritus ani is an itch localized to the anus and perianal skin. Pruritus ani is categorized as either idiopathic or secondary. Idiopathic pruritus ani is diagnosed when no underlying etiology is found. Secondary pruritus ani results from an underlying disorder, and specific treatment leads to resolution of symptoms. Leakage of stool or mucus because of fecal incontinence and leakage of mucus because of prolapse of the rectum or hemorrhoids can cause irritation and itching. Other causes include contact dermatitis, infections (such as *Candida*), parasites, systemic diseases (diabetes mellitus), diet (coffee, cola, chocolate, milk, beer, and others), and some medications. It has been said that dietary factors, especially any form of coffee, may be the most common culprit. The exact mechanism whereby coffee acts as an irritant to the perianal skin is unclear, but perhaps for some individuals, one of its metabolites can be irritating.

752   **B.** (S&F, ch99)

The glucose hydrogen breath test probably is the most widely used breath test in clinical practice: the substrate is inexpensive, and the hydrogen meter is economical, portable, and easy to use. Normally, glucose is absorbed entirely in the upper small intestine; if there is bacterial overgrowth, the glucose is cleaved by bacteria into carbon dioxide and hydrogen. The hydrogen is measured in the exhaled breath (at baseline, and every 30 minutes for 2 hours), and an increase of 20 parts per million (ppm) above the baseline is regarded as diagnostic of small intestinal bacterial overgrowth (SIBO). Fasting breath hydrogen levels of more than 20 ppm are also considered positive, but high baseline hydrogen levels are common in patients with untreated celiac disease and normalize after gluten withdrawal. Patient preparation is important for this test: Patients must avoid smoking and eating nonfermentable carbohydrates such as pasta and bread the night before the test because they may increase baseline breath hydrogen values; exercise may induce hyperventilation, thereby reducing baseline breath hydrogen values, and thus should be avoided for 2 hours before the test.

753 **E.** (S&F, ch108)

Although many infectious organisms have been investigated as possible factors in Crohn's disease, the organism that has gained most attention is *Mycobacterium paratuberculosis,* although most investigations in this area have been inconclusive. The other organisms listed have also been investigated, but less extensively; no definite association has been found.

754 **C.** (S&F, ch111)

Almost all patients with acute mesenteric ischemia (AMI) have acute abdominal pain. The pain may be out of proportion to findings on the physical examination. The pain is often severe but the abdomen is usually flat, soft, and nondistended. Nausea, vomiting, and bloody diarrhea would not be common early in an ischemic episode. This is also true of abdominal distention. When abdominal distention does occur, it is usually late and is the first sign of intestinal infarction.

755 **C.** (S&F, ch119)

Sulindac has gained some popularity in treating patients with familial adenomatous polyposis (FAP). It has been shown in controlled and uncontrolled trials to decrease the number and size of adenomas in patients with intact colons as well as those with intact rectums and ileorectal anastomoses. Unfortunately, sulindac does not protect from the development of rectal cancer and the drug's effects in reducing adenomas are reversible upon discontinuation. Sulindac is less successful in controlling upper gastrointestinal (GI) neoplasia.

756 **B.** (S&F, ch93)

Hirschsprung's disease is due to the failure of craniocaudal migration of neural crest cells, resulting in the absence of ganglion cells in both the myenteric and submucosal plexus. This most commonly affects a short segment of the rectosigmoid colon, but disease can extend more proximally and, although rarely, can involve the small intestines. The involved segment fails to relax, resulting in a functional colonic obstruction. Full-thickness or deep-suction biopsies of the distal colon are required to demonstrate an absence of ganglion cells. Superficial mucosal biopsies are inadequate. Several genetic mutations have been identified, including the *RET* proto-oncogene, which may be the cause of half of familial cases of Hirschsprung's disease.

757 **C.** (S&F, ch120)

Fecal occult blood testing has been extensively studied and utilized in practice. It relies on the fact that hemoglobin is a compound that exhibits pseudoperoxidase activity, changing from colorless to colored when it undergoes oxidation. Rehydrating stool specimen slides increases the sensitivity of the test but decreases its specificity. Ascorbic acid may enhance or inhibit oxidation of the dye. The ingestion of red meat should be avoided during the collection of stool for test, because it may cause false-positive results. Peroxidase containing foods should be avoided; these include turnips, cauliflower, broccoli, radishes, and cantaloupe. Nonsteroidal anti-inflammatory drugs may cause frank or occult blood loss and will affect the accuracy of the test. Tocopherol is not known to interfere with fecal occult blood testing.

758 **D.** (S&F, ch93)

Mucosal folds of the small intestine are called plicae circularis. These folds are more numerous in the proximal jejunum and gradually decreased in number in the distal small bowel. Haustra refer to colonic outpouchings between the teniae coli, longitudinal muscular bands that extend the length of the colon. Appendices epiploicae are small peritoneal projections filled with adipose tissue; they are found on the surface of the colon. Columns of Morgagni are longitudinal folds within the anal canal that terminate in the anal papilla. Rugae refer to redundant gastric folds.

759 **B.** (S&F, ch117)

Many drugs affect gastrointestinal motility.

Antiparkinsonian drugs decrease colonic and small bowel motility and can cause pseudo-obstruction.

Opiate analgesics suppress motility throughout the gastrointestinal tract, particularly the colon.

Calcium channel antagonists, especially verapamil, slow colonic transit and can cause constipation, although verapamil does not appear to have an effect on small bowel motility.

Clonidine, an α-2-adrenergic agent, prolongs orocecal transit of liquids but recently has not shown any significant effect on gastric, small bowel, or colonic transit in healthy patients.

Octreotide increases the frequency of migrating motor complexes (MMCs) by shortening the duration of phase II; octreotide was shown in a small group of scleroderma patients with pseudo-obstruction to be able to induce phase III contractions and possibly to decrease the risk of bacterial overgrowth. Octreotide retards small bowel transit in healthy patients when given before a meal.

When given after a meal, intravenous somatostatin interrupts the "fed" pattern of motility and induces bursts of propagated activity similar to phase III, in both healthy and diseased bowels.

760 D. (S&F, ch97)

The terminal products of luminal starch digestion, together with the major disaccharides in the diet (sucrose and lactose), cannot be absorbed intact and are hydrolyzed by specific brush border membrane hydrolases that are maximally expressed in the villi of the duodenum and jejunum. Several types of carbohydrases have been identified, including lactase, maltase, sucrase-isomaltase, α-limit dextrinase, and trehalase.

Lactase hydrolyzes lactose to produce one molecule of glucose and one molecule of galactose.

The three major diet-derived monosaccharides (glucose, galactose, and fructose) are absorbed by saturable carrier-mediated transport systems located in the brush border membrane of enterocytes in the proximal and mid small intestine.

761 B. (S&F, ch113)

Appendicitis is the most common acute abdominal emergency seen in developed countries, whereas the prevalence of appendicitis is as much as 10 times lower in many of the less developed African countries. The incidence of disease peaks between the ages of 15 and 19 years.

762 D. (S&F, ch119)

Duodenal adenomas occur in 60% to 90% of those with familial adenomatous polyposis (FAP), and duodenal cancers occur in 4% to 12%. Additionally, adenomas or adenocarcinomas may occur in the periampullary or ampullary region and thus a side-viewing scope should be used for follow-up endoscopy in these patients. Gastric polyps may occur in 30% to 100% of those with FAP but the polyps are usually in the fundus and non-neoplastic; gastric adenomatous polyps only occur in 5% of those with FAP. Microcarcinoids may occur but are not usually clinically significant. Jejunal and ileal adenomas occur in 40% and 20% of patients, respectively.

763 D. (S&F, ch95)

The vermiform appendix arises from the base of the cecum. It is variable in length, averaging about 6 cm, and is anchored by the mesoappendix. It is most commonly retrocecal (posterior to the cecum). It is rarely retrocolic (posterior to the ascending colon), anterior, medial, or lateral to the cecum. Appendiceal inflammation most often causes pain in the right lower quadrant or right lower flank. Importantly, during pregnancy the appendix may be displaced by the gravid uterus and appendicitis may present in pregnant women with right upper quadrant or midepigastric symptoms.

764 C. (S&F, ch115)

The best accepted risk factor for irritable bowel syndrome (IBS) is bacterial gastroenteritis. Depression and hypochondriasis may increase the risk of postinfectious IBS. Food intolerance is another possible IBS risk factor. Glucocorticoid users may be at a lower risk for IBS.

765 C. (S&F, ch121)

Melanosis coli is a misnomer. Initially the pigment was thought to be melanin, but now it is known that lipofuscin is the pigment responsible for coloration in this condition. This condition develops in more than 70% of persons who use anthraquinone laxatives (*Cascara sagrada*, aloe, senna, rhubarb, and frangula), often within 4 months of use, but on average after 9 months of use. The pigment generally disappears within 1 year of stopping laxatives.

766 D. (S&F, ch98)

Autoimmune gastritis (pernicious anemia) is the most common cause of vitamin B_{12} malabsorption. Cobalamin malabsorption in pernicious anemia is caused both by decreased intrinsic factor secretion due to parietal cell destruction in the stomach and by blockage of autoantibodies, which inhibit intrinsic factor binding to vitamin B_{12}.

767 E. (S&F, ch118)

The lower risk of adenocarcinoma of the small bowel is believed to be due to a lower burden of bacteria in the small bowel (resulting in lower risk of bile acid conversion to carcinogens) and the rapid transit time in the small bowel (which limits contact between carcinogens and the mucosa).

A diet high in animal fat and protein is associated with small bowel adenocarcinoma. DNA adducts are 30 times more common in the colon than in the small intestine. The most frequent cause of death in patients with FAP after colectomy is proximal small bowel cancer, but these cancers can occur in patients without FAP. The min mouse, with predominantly small bowel polyps, is used to study FAP; BDF1 mice are used to study exposure to carcinogens.

768 **E.** (S&F, ch101)

Table 101–1 Extraintestinal Manifestations of Celiac Sprue

Organ System	Manifestation	Probable Cause(s)
Hematopoietic	Anemia	Iron, folate, vitamin B_{12}, or pyridoxine deficiency
	Hemorrhage	Vitamin K deficiency; rarely, thrombocytopenia due to folate deficiency
	Thrombocytosis, Howell-Jolly bodies	Hyposplenism
Skeletal	Osteopenia	Malabsorption of calcium and vitamin D
	Pathologic fractures	Osteopenia
	Osteoarthropathy	Unknown
Muscular	Atrophy	Malnutrition due to malabsorption
	Tetany	Calcium, vitamin D, and/or magnesium malabsorption
	Weakness	Generalized muscle atrophy, hypokalemia
Hepatic	Elevated liver enzymes	Unknown
Nervous	Peripheral neuropathy	Vitamin deficiencies such as vitamin B_{12} and thiamine
	Ataxia	Cerebellar and posterior column damage
	Demyelinating central nervous system lesions	Unknown
	Seizures	Unknown
Endocrine	Secondary hyperparathyroidism	Calcium/vitamin D malabsorption causing hypocalcemia
	Amenorrhea, infertility, impotence	Malnutrition, hypothalamic-pituitary dysfunction
Integument	Follicular hyperkeratosis and dermatitis	Vitamin A malabsorption, vitamin B complex malabsorption
	Petechiae and ecchymoses	Vitamin K deficiency; rarely, thrombocytopenia
	Edema	Hypoproteinemia
	Dermatitis herpetiformis	Unknown

Modified from Trier JS: Celiac sprue and refractory sprue. In Feldman M, Scharschmidt BF, Sleisenger MH (eds): Gastrointestinal and Liver Disease, 6th ed. Philadelphia, WB Saunders, 1997, p 1557.

769 **C.** (S&F, ch102)

Tropical sprue almost never occurs in expatriates in Africa, although there have been sporadic reports from South Africa, Zimbabwe, and Nigeria. Endemic tropical sprue is not found universally in tropical and subtropical regions, a finding that strongly suggests that the etiologic factor or factors are geographically restricted.

770 **D.** (S&F, ch112)

After failure of gluten withdrawal to resolve symptoms, glucocorticosteroid drugs are often tried, with varying degrees of success. Patients who do respond to glucocorticosteroid drugs often remain glucocorticoid-drug dependent. Based on the knowledge that refractory celiac disease and ulcerative enteritis are cryptic T-cell lymphomas, open-label studies using immunosuppressant drug therapy have been undertaken. In patients with refractory celiac disease, prednisone and azathioprine are more promising than cyclosporine, as demonstrated in separate trials.

771 **D.** (S&F, ch94)

The enteric nervous system (ENS) consists of two major ganglia, the myenteric plexus and the submucosal plexus and interneurons. These cells facilitate local communication between the ENS neurons of the same or different class, for example, between intrinsic afferent and efferent neurons. The vagus nerve is part of the autonomic nervous system (ANS) and is not part of the ENS.

772 **B.** (S&F, ch111)

Reperfusion injury has been attributed to many factors, including reactive oxygen radicals. Super oxide, hydrogen peroxide, and hydroxyl radicals are formed. The rate-limiting enzyme is xanthenes oxidase, not thiopurine methyltransferase (TPMT). Leukotriene B4 and platelet aggregating factor are produced. not leukotriene B1. Most injury from *brief* ischemia appears during reperfusion, not after prolonged ischemia.

773 **B.** (S&F, ch95)

Enteric excitatory motor neurons synthesize and secrete acetylcholine (Ach). Enteric inhibitory motor neurons synthesize and secrete various neurotransmitters, including nitric oxide (NO), adenosine triphosphate (ATP), and several peptides (e.g., vasoactive intestinal peptide [VIP]). Epinephrine is not an enteric neurotransmitter.

774 **D.** (S&F, ch117)

Familial causes for chronic intestinal pseudo-obstruction (CIP), such as familial visceral myopathy (FVM), are rare. There are three types of FVM. In type II FVM there are mitochondrial DNA disorders and this condition is also called mitochondrial neurogastrointestinal encephalopathy. Histologically all three types exhibit degeneration and fibrosis of gastrointestinal smooth muscle, not neurons. Hirschsprung's disease is an example of a familial visceral neuropathy characterized by aganglionosis within the internal anal sphincter due to a disorder of colonization by migrating neural crest–derived neurons.

775 **E.** (S&F, ch95)

The outer longitudinal smooth muscle layer of the colon forms three distinct cord-like structures called taenia coli that are spaced evenly around the circumference of the colon. Between the taenia, the muscular wall is thinner. In the cecum, the three taenia converge at the base of the appendix and form a complete outer muscular wall. At the rectosigmoid junction, the three taenia fuse again and intercalate with the internal and external anal sphincters. Mucosal folds of the small intestine are called plicae circularis. These are more numerous in the proximal jejunum and gradually decreased in number in the distal small bowel. Haustra refer to dynamic colonic outpouchings between the teniae coli formed by sustained contractions of the circular muscle. Appendices epiploicae are small adipose filled peritoneal projections found on the surface of the colon. Columns of Morgagni are longitudinal folds within the anal canal; they terminate in the anal papilla.

776 **E.** (S&F, ch120)

The United States Preventative Services Task Force, the Agency for Health Care Policy and Research, and the American Cancer Society are some of the groups that have advocated and published colorectal cancer screening guidelines. It has generally been agreed upon that the choices in answers **A** to **D** are all reasonable for screening. Virtual colonoscopy has not been embraced as a screening method at this time.

777 **B.** (S&F, ch95)

The internal anal sphincter (IAS) is a thickened band of smooth muscle with a relatively high resting tone that is in continuity with the circular smooth muscle of the rectum. The IAS is innervated extrinsically, via the pelvic plexus, by lumbar sympathetic and sacral parasympathetic nerves and it receives inhibitory innervation from enteric inhibitory neurons with cell bodies in the enteric ganglia. In contrast, the external anal sphincter (EAS) is a striated muscle and is located distal to, but partially overlying, the

IAS. Unlike the IAS, the EAS is influenced by voluntary efforts to maintain continence. The EAS and other pelvic floor muscles are innervated via the pudendal nerve (S3 to S4), by motor neurons with cell bodies in the spinal cord.

778 **D.** (S&F, ch109)

In contrast to hemorrhoidal bleeding, bleeding due to ulcerative proctitis usually involves only small quantities of blood and mucus, without fecal matter. Patients with ulcerative proctitis usually complain of frequency and urgency to defecate.

779 **A.** (S&F, ch112)

Enteropathy-type intestinal T-cell lymphoma (ETL) has also been referred to as ulcerative jejunoileitis and idiopathic chronic ulcerative enteritis. It occurs as a complication of chronic celiac disease or it can present de novo with multiple intestinal ulcerations and malabsorption in patients without underlying celiac disease. The abnormal T-cells express intracytoplasmic CD3 but lack cell surface expression of CD3-TCR complexes, CD4, and CD8, thus distinguishing this condition from uncomplicated celiac disease (which is CD3+, CD4–, CD8+). Patients with ETL may also have chromosomal imbalances (in 87% of cases), with 58% showing gains on chromosome 9q and 16% on chromosome 1q. Most patients present in their forties or later. Women are affected slightly more often than men, in a ratio of 1.6:1.0. Typical symptoms are profound weight loss with signs of cachexia, severe malabsorption, steatorrhea, and protein-losing enteropathy.

780 **C.** (S&F, ch114)

Fistulae are thought to develop in fewer than 5% of patients with diverticulitis and they are present in about 20% requiring surgery for diverticulitis. Colovesicular fistulas are most common and account for 65% of fistulae in diverticular disease. The 2:1 male predominance is attributed to protection given the bladder by the uterus. Vaginal fistulas are the next most common internal fistula, accounting for approximately 25% of all fistulae.

781 **B.** (S&F, ch116)

Hernias are the second most common cause of small bowel obstruction (SBO), accounting for 25% of cases. External hernias such as inguinal, umbilical, or femoral hernias, are more common than internal hernias. Inguinal hernias are more prevalent in the elderly. Internal hernias can be either congenital or acquired. SBO from hernias has a particularly high risk for strangulation, failure to resolve, and recurrence when not corrected surgically.

782 **B.** (S&F, ch120)

This family meets the criteria for hereditary nonpolyposis colorectal cancer (HNPCC) syndrome. This syndrome is inherited in an autosomal dominant fashion. There is a predominance of proximal tumors. Germline mutations in the *hMSH2* or *hMLH1* gene are present in 80% of colon cancers. There is an increased frequency of cancers of the female genital tract. This syndrome accounts for about 6% of all reported colorectal cancers, whereas familial adenomatous polyposis (FAP) accounts for fewer than 1%.

783 **D.** (S&F, ch101)

A multicenter study by Fasano et al. of more than 13,000 at-risk and not-at-risk American subjects found the prevalence of anti-endomysial antibodies to be 1:22 among first-degree and 1:39 among second-degree relatives of subjects with celiac sprue. A prevalence of 1:56 was documented among patients with gastrointestinal symptoms of celiac sprue or associated disorders. The prevalence of anti-endomysial antibodies was 1:133 among 4126 not-at-risk individuals.

784 **B.** (S&F, ch104)

Bacterial toxins produce diarrhea by different mechanisms. *Vibrio cholera* produces enterotoxins, which alter intestinal salt and water transport without affecting mucosal morphology. Cholera toxin stimulates adenylate cyclase, which binds to the basolateral membrane. The resultant increase in cAMP activates cAMP-dependent kinase(s), which inhibit NaCl-coupled transport and stimulate chloride secretion. Sodium-coupled nutrient pathways are unaltered by the toxin.

785 **B.** (S&F, ch96)

Decrease in cAMP leads to net absorption. Other proabsorptive pathways include the inhibitor G protein (G_i) cascade and the phosphatidylinositol (PI) cycle. Secretagogues act through signal transduction cascades such as those involving cAMP, cyclic guanosine monophosphate (cGMP), Ca^{2+}, or PI.

786 **D.** (S&F, ch103)

Almost all patients with Whipple's disease suffer from involvement of the intestinal tract by this infection, regardless of whether gastrointestinal symptoms are present. Thus, the primary diagnostic approach to a patient with clinically suspected Whipple's disease is upper endoscopy

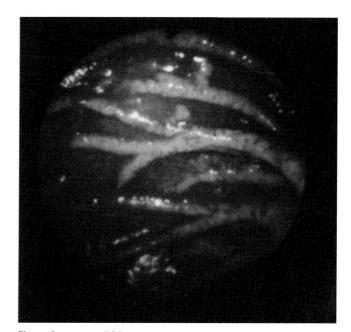

Figure for answer **786**

(see figure) with mucosal biopsy. To avoid sampling errors in patients with patchy lesions, one should obtain approximately five biopsy specimens from regions as far distal as possible within the small intestine. Histologic examination with routine hematoxylin and eosin and periodic acid–Schiff (PAS) stains is usually sufficient to establish a diagnosis. In some cases, findings may be corroborated with silver stains; in contrast, the Gram stain is less useful in identifying the cause of infection. Traditionally, electron microscopy has been used as the "gold standard" for confirming the diagnosis of Whipple's disease, but currently polymerase chain reaction (PCR) analysis is the gold standard.

787 **E.** (S&F, ch99)

SIBO appears to be common in patients with chronic liver disease. SIBO is more common in patients with advanced (Child-Pugh class C) liver disease, and may be an independent risk factor for spontaneous bacterial peritonitis, although this latter association is controversial. There does not appear to be an association with any particular cause of chronic liver disease, but SIBO does not occur in cirrhotic patients if portal hypertension is absent. The etiology of SIBO in patients with chronic liver disease is likely related to disturbances in motility and possibly to the use of antacids, which might permit proliferation of bacteria. Small intestinal dysmotility is more severe in cirrhotic patients with a history of spontaneous bacterial peritonitis, and treatment of SIBO improves motility. Liver transplantation also improves small bowel dysmotility in cirrhotic patients. Both antibiotic and prokinetic drugs are effective in SIBO associated with cirrhosis.

788 **C.** (S&F, ch109)

The risk of colorectal cancer in patients with ulcerative colitis (UC) varies depending primarily on duration and extent of UC, but it has been estimated to be approximately 7% to 10% after 20 years with UC and as high as 30% after 35 years with UC. In general, the risk of colorectal cancer may be estimated to increase within the range of 0.5% to 1.0% per year after 8 or 10 years with extensive UC.

789 **A.** (S&F, ch104)

Diarrhea due to antibiotic treatment for *C. difficile* infection is the most prevalent type of acute diarrhea in hospitalized patients. Diarrhea can be a side effect of other types of medication, can result from ingestion of elixirs containing sorbitol or mannitol, or may occur as a consequence of tube feedings. *Salmonella, Shigella, Campylobacter,* viruses, and parasites are rarely the cause of diarrhea in hospitalized patients.

790 **A.** (S&F, ch111)

"Thumbprinting" as a finding on x-rays of a barium enema examination refers to the appearance of what can be seen at colonoscopy to be hemorrhagic nodules. The colon single-stripe sign (CSSS) is found in 75% of biopsy specimens examined histopathologically in cases of ischemic colon injury and predicts a milder course than if a circumferential ulcer were present. Rectal sparing is typical of ischemic injury and stricture formation is usually a late finding.

791 **A.** (S&F, ch116)

The pathophysiology of postoperative ileus involves a complex interaction of inhibitory neuroenteric reflexes, including increased efferent inhibitory sympathetic activity and inflammation within the bowel wall. Predisposing factors may include the local and systemic release of inhibitory gastrointestinal peptides and endogenous opioids and the use of exogenous opioids for anesthesia and postoperative analgesia. The making of an incision through the abdominal wall activates inhibitory sympathetic reflexes, which leads to the release of norepinephrine, which inhibits acetylcholine release from excitatory neurons in the myenteric plexus, which causes relaxation of the intestinal wall.

Serotonin stimulates peristalsis. Evidence is lacking for a role for somatostatin and nitrous oxide in postoperative ileus.

792 **A.** (S&F, ch117)

The mechanisms proposed for acute pseudo-obstruction include (1) reflex motor inhibition through splanchnic afferents in response to noxious stimuli; (2) excess sympathetic (inhibitory) motor input to the gut; (3) excess parasympathetic (excitatory) motor input to the gut; (4) decreased parasympathetic (excitatory) motor input to the gut; (5) excess stimulation of peripheral μ-opioid receptors, by endogenous or exogenous opioids; and (6) inhibition of nitrous oxide (NO) release from inhibitory motor neurons.

793 **B.** (S&F, ch99)

SIBO is probably second only to celiac disease as the commonest cause of malabsorption in developed countries. Nowadays most patients do not present with the classic features of steatorrhea and megaloblastic anemia, and most patients do not have a blind loop or other predisposing anatomic abnormality. Many patients may have nonspecific symptoms similar to those of IBS. Although the glucose hydrogen and ^{14}C-xylose breath tests are simple and noninvasive, the gold standard for diagnosis is culture of an aspirate of small intestine contents. The aspirate may be collected easily at endoscopy, which usually is performed to obtain biopsies of the small intestine wall during evaluation of malabsorption. Treatment with one of several broad-spectrum antibiotics is recommended and effective.

794 **C.** (S&F, ch95)

Sensation of the colon is mediated by the spinal primary afferent neurons, which have cell bodies located outside the bowel wall in the lumbar dorsal root ganglion. Lumbar spinal afferents project via the lumbar splanchnic nerves, through the prevertebral inferior mesenteric ganglion and via the lumbar colonic nerves to the colon, where they terminate in sensory endings on the mesentery, muscular layers, and mucosa throughout the entire colon.

795 **C.** (S&F, ch99)

The classic association of SIBO is with the "blind loop" resulting from abdominal surgery, such as Billroth II partial gastrectomy; other anatomic abnormalities that may cause SIBO include intestinal strictures and small bowel diverticulosis. Disorders affecting peristalsis in the small intestine, such as diabetes mellitus and scleroderma, are the next most common cause of SIBO after anatomic abnormalities. The ileocecal valve prevents reflux of colonic bacteria into the small intestine and resection of the valve or development of fistulae between the colon and upper gastrointestinal tract may lead to reflux of colonic contents into the small intestine with ensuing bacterial overgrowth. Achlorhydria is known to be a predisposing factor for SIBO, and SIBO has been described in patients after vagotomy, with atrophic gastritis, and in those taking acid-suppressant medication.

796 **C.** (S&F, ch107)

Strongyloides stercoralis is endemic in tropical and semitropical areas but has also been identified in the southeastern United States. It lives in the soil and larvae can penetrate the skin. Larva currens is a serpiginous rash caused by the migrating larvae. Although most patients with this condition have no symptoms relating to the abdomen, some have abdominal pain, nausea, or occult GI bleeding. If the patient is immunosuppressed or taking a glucocorticoid drug, this condition can take a fulminant course, frequently leading to sepsis and death. Intestinal biopsy is very insensitive for this diagnosis but the other methods listed are sensitive for the diagnosis.

797 **E.** (S&F, ch115)

One randomized study measured participants' levels of IgG antibodies to various foods and then excluded from the diet those foods for which there were IgG antibodies. The exclusion of these foods improved both diarrhea- and constipation-predominant IBS. Supplementation with wheat bran has shown no better results than supplementation with placebo. Supplementation with soluble fiber may improve symptoms of constipation-predominant but not diarrhea-predominant IBS; when using this treatment, supplementation should be started at low doses to reduce side effects. In most patients with typical IBS symptoms, reducing lactose does not help.

798 **A.** (S&F, ch98)

Severe steatorrhea has often been noted to occur after total or partial gastric resection. Suggested mechanisms include defective mixing of nutrients with digestive secretions, lack of gastric acid and gastric lipase secretion, decreased small bowel transit time, small intestinal bacterial overgrowth, and pancreatic insufficiency.

Loss of parietal cells after total gastric resection results in diminished intrinsic factor secretion, which in turn leads to malabsorption of vitamin B_{12} and, in about 30% of patients, vitamin B_{12} deficiency. Lack of release of food-bound cobalamin by diminished gastric acid and pepsin secretion has been implicated as an additional pathogenic factor.

Although the mechanisms for iron malabsorption are not fully established, lack of acid secretion and resultant decreased solubilization of iron salts has been suggested as a possible cause. Total and partial gastric resections also can results in significant protein malabsorption, whereas absorption of carbohydrates seems not to be significantly impaired.

799 **B.** (S&F, ch94)

Multichannel intraluminal impedance (MII) is a technique that depends upon the differential conductivities of luminal contents (air versus liquid/solid) to track the movement of the bolus along the intestines. When combined with manometry, this technique can provide real-time information about the pressure-flow relationship.

800 **E.** (S&F, ch108)

Most studies have found breast-feeding to be protective against development of inflammatory bowel disease (IBD; Crohn's disease) in the child. NSAID use has been implicated not only in the exacerbation of IBD, but also as a potential cause for new cases; the mechanism is believed to be NSAID-mediated increases in intestinal permeability. A diet high in refined sugars and low in fresh fruits and vegetables has also been associated with development of Crohn's disease. Smoking is one of the more notable environmental factors predisposing to Crohn's disease but smoking is a negative risk factor for ulcerative colitis. There seems to be an increased risk of Crohn's disease among women who use oral contraceptives.

801 **C.** (S&F, ch115)

Contrary to what many clinicians believe, nighttime symptoms are common in patients with IBS and do not discriminate IBS from organic disease. In contrast, weight loss, rectal bleeding, late age at onset, and dysphagia are alarm symptoms that warrant further investigation.

802 **A.** (S&F, ch104)

Bacillus cereus is an aerobic spore-forming Gram-positive rod that is frequently found in uncooked rice. It causes an acute (usually epidemic) food poisoning syndrome characterized by either profound vomiting or watery diarrhea. It is not invasive, so one would not expect to find leukocytes in a stool sample from a patient with diarrhea due to ingestion of this organism. All of the other organisms cause an acute colitis, characterized by various degrees of leukocyte shedding into the feces.

803 **E.** (S&F, ch107)

D. latum is the largest parasite that affects humans; it may be as long as 40 feet. It is acquired by consumption of undercooked fresh-water, and not salt-water fish. Ivermectin may be effective in treating an infection due to *Strongyloides,* but praziquantel or albendazole would be the drug of choice for treatment of a *D. latum* infestation. The worms absorb nutrients from the intestinal contents of the host and have the ability to cleave vitamin B_{12} from intrinsic factor. Absorption of vitamin B_{12} by the worm can lead to vitamin B_{12} deficiency and thus megaloblastic anemia with neurologic symptoms.

804 **B.** (S&F, ch98)

The most common cause of carbohydrate malabsorption is late-onset lactose malabsorption due to decreased levels of the intestinal brush border enzyme lactase (adult-type hypolactasia, acquired primary lactase deficiency). Depending on ethnic background, lactase is present in fewer than 5% to more than 90% of the adult population. Lactase activity persists in most adults of Western European heritage. Some of the ethnic groups among which lactase deficiency predominates (60% to 100% of adults are lactase-deficient) include Native Americans, African Americans, East Asians, and people of Near Eastern and Mediterranean descent.

805 **D.** (S&F, ch108)

The fertility of women with Crohn's disease is similar to or only slightly lower than the fertility of women in the general population. Decreased fertility generally correlates with increased disease activity, which is accompanied by decreased libido, diarrhea, abdominal pain, and fatigue. In addition, women with perianal disease may have dyspareunia. Another reason why patients with Crohn's disease do not have children is because of a decision not to do so rather than inability to conceive. Men with Crohn's disease rarely have fertility problems unless they are taking sulfasalazine, which causes reversible sperm abnormalities. If a pregnant woman with Crohn's disease has no perianal disease, a cesarean section is not absolutely necessary. Among women with active disease at conception, the one-third rule applies.

806 **D.** (S&F, ch94)

Motor activity in the small intestine is influenced by the presence of luminal contents and their characteristics (i.e., osmolality and pH) and by the autonomic and enteric nervous systems. The interdigestive motor cycle (IDMC), which occurs during fasting, is a complex series of contractions with distinct amplitudes and periodicity. These contractile complexes regularly sweep the small intestines during fasting. Interestingly, IDMC activity remains intact in denervated or transplanted organs, implying that the ENS is important in regulation of this activity. Upon feeding, IDMC activity stops almost immediately and peristalsis begins. The result is both the anterograde and retrograde mixing of chyme to insure adequate absorption of nutrients (rhythmic segmentation). The fasting motor pattern (IDMC) re-emerges about 4 hours after a meal.

807 **A.** (S&F, ch118)

The C-kit mutation is expressed in 60% of GISTs and is associated with higher mortality. The other factors (gastric location, size less than 5 cm, low mitotic and proliferative indexes) are good prognostic factors.

808 **E.** (S&F, ch119)

High intake of vitamin C has not been shown to increase the risk of colonic adenomas. Diets high in fat or low in fiber, obesity, and cigarette smoking have been associated with elevated risk of colonic adenomas.

809 **C.** (S&F, ch104)

E. coli O157:H7 is the cause of acute hemorrhagic colitis in this case. The leading vehicle of infection is hamburger meat. *E. coli* O157:H7 usually causes right-sided colitis. The infection can be complicated by the development of hemolytic uremic syndrome (HUS) or thrombotic thrombocytopenic purpura, especially in children. Antibiotic therapy for diarrhea caused by *E. coli* 0157:H7 may be associated with HUS.

810 **D.** (S&F, ch118)

Carcinoids are multifocal in 30% of patients. Carcinoids are almost always located in the ileum, are more common in patients over the age of 50 years, are the second most commonly diagnosed small bowel malignancy, and are generally less than 1.5 cm at diagnosis.

811 **C.** (S&F, ch101)

A Finnish study of 3654 schoolchildren aged 7 to 16 years screened in 1994 and in 2001 for anti-endomysial and tissue transglutaminase antibodies demonstrated that celiac disease is heterogeneous: the prevalence of biopsy-proven celiac sprue was 1:99, while the prevalence of the HLA-DQ2 or HLA-DQ8 haplotype (both of which are strongly associated with celiac sprue) and antibodies was 1:67. A large multicenter study by Fasano et al. found the prevalence of anti-endomysial antibodies among Americans *not* at risk to be 1:133.

 C. (S&F, ch96)

The total volume of endogenous secretions presented to the gastrointestinal tract daily is 7000 cc. Bile amounts to 500 cc. The small intestine produces 1000 cc of secretions. Of the total volume of fluid secreted daily, 98% of it is absorbed, mostly in the small intestine.

813 **B.** (S&F, ch116)

The epidural administration of a local anesthetic blocks afferent and efferent inhibitory reflexes, including inhibitory sympathetic efferent signals. Studies have shown that bupivacaine hydrochloride significantly reduces the duration of postoperative ileus. Studies have not shown any significant benefit from administration of metoclopramide or erythromycin. NSAIDs have been shown in several experimental and clinical studies to decrease the frequency of postoperative nausea and vomiting and improve gastrointestinal transit, but their effects on the duration of postoperative ileus have not been determined. Several randomized studies have shown that use of a nasogastric (NG) tube for decompression does not shorten the duration of postoperative ileus.

814 **D.** (S&F, ch121)

Inflammatory colitis due to glutaraldehyde remaining on the endoscope after cleaning is the most likely cause of this patient's symptoms. The radiology studies would have ruled out perforation. Colitis due to *C. difficile* infection and ischemic colitis are less likely.

815 **D.** (S&F, ch105)

Toxin A is an inflammatory enterotoxin and toxin B is an extremely potent cytotoxin but has minimal enterotoxin activity in animals. Initial studies suggest that toxin B does not contribute to diarrhea and colitis in human patients. However, both toxins produced by this organism have been found to cause injury and electrophysiologic changes in human colonic explants in vitro, and toxin B was 10 times more potent than toxin A in inducing both of these changes.

816 **C.** (S&F, ch95)

Myenteric potential oscillations (MPOs) are small-amplitude, rapid (12 to 20 per minute) oscillations that originate from the myenteric plexus and spread via gap junctions into both the longitudinal and circular muscular layers. In contrast, slow waves occur with a frequency of 2 to 4 per minute. When the colon is excited by neurotransmitters released from the excitatory enteric motor neurons, each MPO or slow wave will reach the threshold potential for generating an action potential, resulting in powerful contractions lasting seconds. Migrating motor complexes (MMCs) occur in the stomach and small intestines; in the fasting (interdigestive) state, they occur every 60 to 90 minutes. This motor complex sweeps luminal contents along the upper digestive tract. Giant motor complexes (GMCs) are powerful muscular contractile waves that propel luminal contents from the ileum into the colon.

817 **C.** (S&F, ch104)

Listeria infections have a case fatality rate of 27%, the highest among the food-borne pathogens. The vehicles of infection that have been reported include raw and pasteurized milk, soft cheeses, coleslaw, shrimp, rice salad, pork dishes, and raw vegetables. *Listeria* infection usually causes systemic disease due to bacterial seeding of the meninges, heart valves, or other organs. Neurologic sequelae are common in survivors of listeriosis affecting the central nervous system.

818 **B.** (S&F, ch106)

These two organisms share several characteristics. They both stain positive with acid-fast stains. Trimethoprim/sulfamethoxazole readily treats infections with either organism in immunocompetent patients. Protracted illness usually occurs in immunocompromised hosts, but the disease is usually self-limited in immunocompetent hosts. *Isospora* may cause a peripheral eosinophilia with Charcot-Leyden crystals in the stool, but *Cyclospora* does not.

819 **C.** (S&F, ch109)

This patient with longstanding disease refractory to medical treatment has too low a cholesterol level to use cyclosporine and his previous history of TB is a contraindication to the use of infliximab (Remicade). Typical indications for surgery in patients with UC include medically refractory disease, intractable disease with impaired quality of life, and unacceptable side effects of medication (see table). Therefore, the best course of action in this case is a total proctocolectomy with ileal pouch anal anastomosis (IPAA).

820 **C.** (S&F, ch104)

Several antibiotic medications have been used successfully to treat or prevent traveler's diarrhea.

Trimethoprim-sulfamethoxazole (TMP-SMX) or TMP alone reduced the duration of diarrhea from 93 hours to approximately 30 hours in one study. Antibiotics can also prevent traveler's diarrhea in approximately 80% of cases. For healthy individuals, the best prophylaxis is to take measures to avoid ingesting contaminated food or drink. Antibiotic prophylaxis is recommended, however, for persons with severe kidney, liver, or heart disease, achlorhydria, or an immunosuppressive illness. Several studies have shown that the nonabsorbable antibiotic rifaximin is effective.

821 B. (S&F, ch115)

Selective serotonin-reuptake inhibitors (SSRIs) accelerate small bowel transit and may be more beneficial in patients with constipation-predominant IBS. Tricyclic antidepressants are safe and effective even at doses below full antidepressant levels. They are most beneficial for patients with diarrhea-predominant IBS. Octreotide reduces intestinal transit time, secretions, and sensation in patients with IBS but is impractical for those with diarrhea due to IBS. Clonidine may be useful in managing diarrhea-predominant IBS because it enhances rectal compliance and reduces fasting colonic motor activity. Colchicine increases the frequency of spontaneous bowel movements and accelerates colonic transit and has been used to manage constipation-predominant IBS.

822 A. (S&F, ch94)

Small intestinal motility is influenced by multiple factors, including metabolic disturbances (i.e., electrolyte imbalance), underlying disease (i.e., diabetes mellitus, scleroderma), medication use (i.e., sedatives, calcium channel blockers, antidepressants), and pregnancy. Colonic distention does not appear to affect small intestinal motor activity. Because there are few tests to evaluate function of the small intestine, caring for those with suspected small bowel disorders may be frustrating for both the patient and clinician.

823 B. (S&F, ch119)

Gardner's syndrome is a familial adenomatous polyposis (FAP) syndrome with associated osteomas of the mandible, skull, and long bones. Dental abnormalities may be present. The osteomas have no malignant potential. Congenital hypertrophy of the retinal pigmented epithelium (CHRPE) has been reported in some families with FAP and Gardner's syndrome. These lesions are asymptomatic and clinically unimportant. Desmoid tumors (diffuse

mesenteric fibromatoses) are a serious complication with significant morbidity and mortality. There is no generally effective treatment for Gardner's syndrome. The inheritance pattern of Gardner's syndrome is autosomal dominant, as is familial adenomatous polyposis.

824 E. (S&F, ch108)

No single symptom/diagnostic test establishes a diagnosis of Crohn's disease. The diagnosis is based on the results of thorough assessment of the patient's history, physical examination findings, and radiologic, endoscopic, and, in many cases, histopathologic findings.

825 A. (S&F, ch118)

Small bowel obstruction is the most common presentation for benign lesions that occur secondary to either luminal constriction or intussusception. Gastrointestinal bleeding is the second most common symptom. Intestinal perforation is rare.

826 E. (S&F, ch101)

Autoimmune disease is associated strongly with celiac sprue and has a prevalence of approximately 20% in adult patients. There is an established association between celiac sprue and insulin-dependent diabetes mellitus (IDDM). The frequency of celiac sprue in those with IDDM ranges from 3% to 8%, and the frequency of IDDM in patients with celiac sprue is approximately 5%. Celiac sprue also may be associated with a variety of other autoimmune connective tissue diseases, including systemic lupus erythematosus, Sjögren's syndrome, and polymyositis. Evidence also supports associations between celiac sprue and inflammatory bowel disease, particularly ulcerative proctitis, chronic hepatitis, sclerosing cholangitis, primary biliary cirrhosis, IgA nephropathy, interstitial lung disease (including chronic fibrosing alveolitis), idiopathic pulmonary hemosiderosis, and Down syndrome.

827 A. (S&F, ch119)

Age is the single most important independent determinant of adenoma prevalence. Adenomas are more prevalent in those older than 60 years. Adenoma prevalence is also higher in patients with a family history of colon cancer or a family history of colonic adenomas. Race and gender do not appear to be independent determinants of adenoma prevalence.

828 **D.** (S&F, ch104)

Although all of these organisms can cause serious infections in patients with underlying liver disease, infections due to *V. vulnificus* can be lethal. Mortality among those with septicemia due to this organism is 50%. The infection can be acquired as a wound infection in people swimming in salt waters or by consumption of seafood, usually raw oysters. Persons with a history of liver problems should be warned to avoid eating raw seafood, especially oysters.

829 **D.** (S&F, ch101)

An understanding of the nature of the genetic predisposition to celiac sprue began with the observation by Howell and coworkers that celiac sprue was associated with specific human leukocyte (HLA) class II DQ haplotypes. HLA class II molecules are glycosylated transmembrane heterodimers (α- and β-chains) that are organized into three related subregions (DQ, DR, and DP) and encoded within the HLA class II region of the major histocompatibility complex on chromosome 6p. The HLA-DQ (α1*501,β1*02) heterodimer, known as HLA-DQ2, is found in 95% of patients (compared with 30% of controls) and the related DQ (α1*0301,β1*0302) heterodimer, known as HLA-DQ8, is found in most of the remaining patients with celiac sprue. Only a minority of individuals who express DQ2 actually develop celiac sprue. In fact, HLA DQ2 is common in Europeans and is expressed in 25% to 30% of the European population without celiac sprue.

830 **E.** (S&F, ch119)

The coexistence of hyperplastic and adenomatous polyps is quite common in patients with a strong family history of colon cancer and/or HNPCC. The distribution of hyperplastic polyps is mostly in the distal colon and rectum. These polyps show little, if any, intrinsic malignant potential, although their association with adenomatous polyps may suggest a pathogenetic relationship. Diminutive polyps are considered polyps less than 5 mm in diameter. In the rectosigmoid colon, these polyps are usually hyperplastic in nature. Serrated adenomas previously were called mixed hyperplastic and adenomatous polyps. Because they have adenomatous features, they should be considered and treated as adenomas.

831 **B.** (S&F, ch98)

The hydrogen breath test is a noninvasive test that takes advantage of the fact that in most people, bacterial carbohydrate metabolism results in the accumulation of hydrogen, which then is absorbed by the intestinal mucosa and excreted in the breath. The diagnosis of lactose malabsorption is established if there is an increase in breath hydrogen concentration of more than 20 parts per million over baseline after ingestion of 50 g of lactose. An increase within the first 30 minutes after ingestion of lactose must be disregarded, because it may be due to bacterial degradation of lactose in the oral cavity. It may take up to 4 hours for the increase in breath hydrogen concentration to occur.

The lactose tolerance test involves measurement of blood glucose before and 30 minutes after ingestion of 50 g of lactose. It can be used in hydrogen nonexcretors. An increase in glucose concentration of less than 20 mg/dL over baseline is indicative of lactose malabsorption. A stool test to detect a fecal pH lower than 5.5 can serve as a qualitative indicator of carbohydrate malabsorption.

832 **D.** (S&F, ch104)

B. anthracis is an aerobic, Gram-positive, spore-forming, nonmotile bacillus. The primary mode of transmission of gastrointestinal anthrax is consumption of endospore-contaminated meat from infected animals. Nausea, vomiting, abdominal pain, and fever develop approximately 1 to 7 days after the ingestion. There is often rapid progression of symptoms to bloody diarrhea, diffuse abdominal pain with rebound tenderness, and, occasionally, hematemesis. Purulent ascites may develop 2 to 4 days later. More than 50% of episodes are fatal, with death occurring as a consequence of toxemia, intestinal perforation, or shock from hemorrhage and fluid losses. Dysphasia occurs in those with oropharyngeal anthrax. Some strains of *B. anthracis* contain an inducible beta-lactamase. The recommended first-choice antibiotic for this infection is ciprofloxacin.

833 **A.** (S&F, ch115)

A meta-analysis of 23 randomized controlled trials concluded that antispasmodics were superior to placebo in the treatment of abdominal pain in patients with IBS. They are more useful for postprandial abdominal pain when taken before meals. There is no proven advantage for sublingual anticholinergics. Loperamide is effective for diarrhea but not abdominal pain or bloating. Stimulant laxatives are safe for patients with constipation-predominant IBS. Codeine phosphate should be avoided because of its side effects and high risk of inducing drug dependence.

834 **B.** (S&F, ch97)

Salivary and pancreatic amylases are endoenzymes. They cleave the α-1-4 links internal to, or at the second or third bond from, the end of the polysaccharide chain. The products of amylase digestion are maltotriose; maltose; and short-chain, branched oligosaccharides called α-limit dextrins.

The effect of salivary amylase depends on its proximity to the ingested starches and the time they spend within the mouth. Thus, careful, slow chewing affords a good start to digestion, whereas rapid swallowing of poorly chewed foods may result in suboptimal salivary amylase action. Salivary amylase is inactivated rapidly by gastric acid, but some activity may persist within the food bolus.

Pancreatic amylase is the major enzyme of starch digestion. Glucose monomers are not produced. Most of this hydrolysis occurs within the intestinal lumen, but because amylase also attaches itself to the brush border membrane of enterocytes, some digestion may occur at this site as well.

835 **C.** (S&F, ch117)

CIP that occurs in association with small-cell carcinoma of the lung, carcinoid tumor, or epidermoid carcinoma of the lip represents a paraneoplastic syndrome and is due to visceral neuropathy.

836 **C.** (S&F, ch100)

When more than 100 cm of terminal ileum has been resected, fat maldigestion may develop. The bile acid sequestering agent cholestyramine may be useful in decreasing bile salt–related diarrhea in patients who have had less than 100 cm of terminal ileum resected but may worsen steatorrhea in those patients who have undergone resection of a longer segment because cholestyramine binds to dietary lipids. Fat-soluble vitamin deficiency may also develop.

837 **C.** (S&F, ch115)

The Manning criteria are not gender-specific. The criteria are as follows: (1) abdominal pain that is relieved after a bowel movement; (2) looser stool at pain onset; (3) more frequent stools at pain onset; (4) abdominal distension; (5) sensation of incomplete rectal evacuation; and (6) passage of mucus. Only four of these criteria were found to be statistically significant in the initial report. One study reported that the presence of three or more Manning criteria in the absence of alarm features correctly diagnosed 96% of cases of IBS.

838 **C.** (S&F, ch93)

The celiac artery supplies the foregut organs, including the distal esophagus, stomach, spleen, omentum, hepaticobiliary tree, and proximal duodenum. The blood supply to the duodenum is from the superior and inferior pancreaticoduodenal arteries, via branches of the gastroduodenal artery (from the celiac artery) and superior mesenteric arteries, respectively. Ulcers of the lesser gastric curve may penetrate, causing hemorrhage from the left gastric artery, whereas ulcers of the greater curve may penetrate and lead to hemorrhage from the left or right gastroepiploic arteries. Duodenal bulb ulcers may penetrate and cause hemorrhage from the gastroduodenal artery. The remaining regions of the small bowel and the ascending and proximal transverse colon are supplied by the superior mesenteric artery or its branches. The distal transverse, descending, and rectosigmoid colon are supplied by the left colic and superior sigmoid arteries, branches of the inferior mesenteric artery. The distal sigmoid and rectum are supplied by the superior rectal arteries (terminal branch of the inferior mesenteric artery), the middle rectal artery (branches of the internal iliac arteries), and the inferior rectal arteries (branches of the internal pudendal arteries). Given the location of the diverticular bleed in the patient described, the source of bleeding is most likely to be in the right colon, at the hepatic flexure, or in the proximal transverse colon. This territory is supplied by branches of the superior mesenteric artery, specifically the ileocolic, right, or middle colic artery.

839 **D.** (ch118)

GISTs are believed to arise from mesenchymal cells. Carcinoids arise from argentaffin cells. Fibromas or fibrosarcomas arise from fibroblasts. Adenocarcinomas arise from mucosal glands, and leiomyomas arise from smooth muscle cells.

840 **A.** (S&F, ch102)

Therapy for tropical sprue would include parenteral administration of vitamin B_{12}, oral administration of folic acid and iron, and possibly administration of a broad-spectrum antibiotic, although this last treatment is somewhat controversial. The recommendation for tetracycline is based on a report that the condition in travelers from the United Kingdom to Puerto Rico improved on tetracycline, 250 mg four times daily, usually given over a period of several months.

841 **B.** (S&F, ch122)

Anal cancers are infrequent. They account for 1.5% of gastrointestinal cancers in the United States; 3,500 new cases are diagnosed each year. The incidence has increased 2% to 3% every year in the United States since the early 1980s. Almost 80% are squamous cell cancers, 16% are adenocarcinomas, and 4% are other types. Anal bleeding is the most common symptom (45%), followed by the sensation of a mass (30%) or no symptoms (20%). The development of anal cancer has been associated with infection with human papillomavirus, history of receptive anal intercourse, HIV infection, history of sexually transmitted diseases, history of cervical cancer, and use of immunosuppressive medication after solid-organ transplantation.

842 **D.** (S&F, ch102)

The patient's symptoms, radiologic findings, and recent history of travel to Southeast Asia are consistent with a diagnosis of tropical sprue. The same symptoms and radiologic findings in a patient with a recent history of travel to Africa would be consistent with tropical enteropathy. The radiologic image shown in the question shows an increase in the caliber of the small intestine and thickening of the folds. These changes are present throughout the small intestine, and usually there is slow transit of the barium column through the gut.

843 **C.** (S&F, ch97)

Although many enzymes and hormones are secreted by the gastrointestinal tract in response to the presence of food in the lumen, only a few are able to influence food intake directly. Cholecystokinin (CCK), gastrin-releasing peptide, and apolipoprotein A IV (apo A IV) have all been implicated as transmitters of the satiety signal to the central nervous system. They potentiate each other's actions, and a combination of these agents may participate in the satiety signal. Additional peptides, known as the anorectic peptides, including peptide tyrosine-tyrosine (PYY), pancreatic polypeptide (PP), glucagon-like peptide 1 (GLP-1), and oxyntomodulin, also have been shown to decrease appetite and promote satiety in both animal and human models.

Leptin, a hormone released from fat cells, is an important peripheral signal from fat stores that modulates food intake. Leptin deficiency and leptin receptor defects produce massive obesity.

Only one gastrointestinal signaling substance, ghrelin, has been shown to increase appetite.

844 **C.** (S&F, ch119)

The activation of oncogenes, the inactivation of tumor suppression genes, and participation of the stability genes are involved in the development of colon cancer. *K-ras* is an oncogene, not a tumor suppressor gene. The tumor suppressor genes include the *APC* gene, which is located on chromosome 5, the *DCC* gene, located on chromosome 18, and the *p53* gene, located on chromosome 17. Mutation or loss of these oncogenes and tumor suppressor genes will promote the progression to adenoma/carcinoma. The stability genes may play a role in the development of cancer in patients with HNPCC, but not usually in the development of sporadic cases of colorectal cancer.

845 **A.** (S&F, ch94)

As a rule, the parasympathetic nervous system (PNS) input is supplied by cranial nerves and consists of cholinergic activity, and the sympathetic nervous system (SNS) input is supplied is by spinal (thoracic) nerves and consists of adrenergic activity. Sympathetic nervous system input to the autonomic nervous system (ANS) is inhibitory, resulting in decreased smooth muscle activity, with an opposite effect on sphincter tone. PNS input to the ANS can be either inhibitory or excitatory, depending on whether parasympathetic input activates a stimulatory or inhibitory ANS neuron. As a result, parasympathetic efferents can inhibit or excite smooth muscle.

846 **B.** (S&F, ch93)

As a result of embryonic folding during the third and fourth weeks of development, the primitive gut is formed from a portion of the yolk sac. Initially, the gut tube communicates with the yolk sac through the vitelline duct, but this communication eventually narrows and then disappears. As a consequence of this folding, endoderm lines the digestive tract and ultimately gives rise to many of the digestive glands. The gastrointestinal organs may be connected to, or suspended from, the body wall by mesenteries, a derivative of the mesoderm. By the end of the fourth week of fetal life, the primitive gut has divided into the foregut (which gives rise to the tracheobronchial tree, esophagus, stomach, proximal duodenum, and hepaticopancreaticobiliary tree), midgut (which gives rise to the distal duodenum, jejunum, ileum, and ascending and proximal transverse colon), and hind gut (which gives rise to the remaining gastrointestinal tract). Organogenesis is complete by 12 weeks.

847 **A.** (S&F, ch116)

The classic radiologic feature of sigmoid volvulus is a distended, ahaustral sigmoid loop (which has the appearance of a bent inner-tube), the apex of which often is directed toward the patient's right shoulder. The classic features of cecal volvulus include a massively dilated cecum located in the epigastrium or left upper quadrant; a coffee bean appearance of the distended cecum; distended loops of small bowel suggestive of SBO; and a single, long air-fluid level present on upright or decubitus films. A colon cut-off sign is seen in patients with pancreatitis.

848 **C.** (S&F, ch104)

Norwalk and Norwalk-like viruses are members of the calcivivirus family and are a major cause of outbreaks of gastroenteritis among camp, cruise ship, nursing home, and hospital populations. *C. difficile* has not been reported to cause gastroenteritis in cases such as the one described. Generally the symptoms of illness due to this virus include nausea, abdominal cramps, vomiting, diarrhea, and muscle aches and they last no longer than 24 to 48 hours. No specific treatment is available.

849 **B.** (S&F, ch116)

Neoplasms of the small intestine are a relatively unusual cause of SBO and account for only about 5% to 10% of cases. In patients who present with symptoms of SBO who have no history of laparotomy or evidence of a hernia, about 50% will have malignant neoplasms as the cause. Usually the small bowel has become obstructed by extrinsic compression or local invasion or by an advanced gastrointestinal (usually colorectal) or gynecologic (usually ovarian) malignancy.

850 **B.** (S&F, ch120)

Several morphologic and histologic characteristics of the primary tumor may correlate with the prognosis. The depth of invasion in the bowel wall and the presence of regional lymph node spread are most important. Lymphatic, perineural, and venous invasion have all been associated with local recurrence and decreased survival. The more poorly differentiated the tumor, the worse the prognosis. Additionally, it appears that tumors with diploid DNA content have a better prognosis than those that are nondiploid or aneuploid. Unlike most cancers, with a primary colon cancer, size does not correlate with prognosis.

851 **B.** (S&F, ch97)

Digestion of proteins begins in the stomach with the action of pepsins secreted by gastric mucosa. Pepsins form from their precursor pepsinogens by the splitting off, in an acid (low pH)

environment, of a small, basic (alkaline) peptide. The release of pepsinogen from chief cells is stimulated by gastrin and histamine and cholinergic stimulation. The rate of pepsinogen release closely mirrors the rate of acid secretion.

Pepsins remain active as long as the gastric contents are acidic, producing a mixture of peptides and small amounts of amino acids. The completeness of gastric proteolysis depends, in part, on the rate of gastric emptying, the pH of gastric contents, and the types of protein ingested. Subjects who are achlorhydric or who have lost control of gastric emptying as a result of pyloroplasty or partial gastrectomy do not appear to have a problem with assimilation of protein, suggesting that gastric proteolysis is not an essential component of digestion.

852 **E.** (S&F, ch116)

In a study reviewing the association with SBO of 12 abdominal radiologic findings, the combination of air-fluid levels of different heights in the same bowel loop and a mean air-fluid level diameter of greater than or equal to 2.5 cm were found to be predictive of high-grade partial or complete SBO. The clinical and physical findings are not sufficiently reliable to predict the presence of a complete SBO.

853 **D.** (S&F, ch100)

D-lactic acidosis is a rare complication of short bowel syndrome that is only seen in patients with a preserved colon. Episodes of acidosis are usually precipitated by increased oral intake of refined carbohydrates. Malabsorbed carbohydrates are metabolized by colonic bacteria, short-chain fatty acids, and lactate, which lowers colon pH. Lower pH inhibits the growth of predominant *Bacteroides* species and promotes the growth of acid-resistant Gram-positive anaerobes such as *Bifidobacterium* and others that have the capacity to produce d-lactate. D-lactate is absorbed from the colon and is only metabolized to a limited extent in man, because of d-lactate dehydrogenase is lacking. Absorption of d-lactate results in the development of metabolic acidosis and the neurologic symptoms described in this case. Blood tests can be used to confirm the presence of metabolic acidosis with a normal lactate level; however, the laboratory should be notified that the concentration of d-lactic acid rather than the concentration of l-lactic acid is to be measured. The finding of the specific neurologic complaints described in this case in a patient with metabolic acidosis and short bowel syndrome should raise the suspicion of possible d-lactic acidosis. The diagnosis is confirmed by finding a significantly elevated d-lactate concentration in a specimen of whole blood (level greater than 3 mmol/L; normal, less than 0.5 mmol/L).

854 **A.** (S&F, ch94)

The primary neurotransmitter of the parasympathetic nervous system is acetylcholine.

855 **B.** (S&F, ch104)

Yersinia enterocolitica is the most likely diagnosis. *E. coli, Salmonella, Shigella,* and *Campylobacter* can cause bloody diarrhea but not ileitis. Enterocolitis occurs most frequently in children younger than 5 years of age. The presenting signs are nonspecific, including fever, abdominal cramps, and diarrhea. Abnormal radiographic findings may be identified when symptoms have been present for some time; in these cases, abnormalities are usually located in the terminal ileum and may resemble those seen in patients with Crohn's disease.

856 **E.** (S&F, ch117)

Most patients with small intestine dysmotility have similar clinical manifestations regardless of the underlying causes for the dysmotility. Both neuropathic and myopathic forms can cause postprandial abdominal pain, the appearance of air-fluid levels and colonic dilatation on radiographic series, and bacterial overgrowth. Bowel sounds tend to be subdued in patients with smooth muscle dysfunction but are hyperactive and high-pitched in patients with neuropathic dysfunction.

857 **D.** (S&F, ch104)

Most bacterial pathogens are highly susceptible to low pH and thus exposure to gastric acid significantly reduces the number of ingested bacteria that survive. Gastric mucus may act in conjunction with gastric acidity as the first line of enteric defense. Mucus, in concert with intestinal motility, acts as a nonspecific physical barrier to bacterial proliferation and mucosal colonization. Secretory antibody (immunoglobulin A, IgA) appears in the intestine prior to serum antibody (immunoglobulin G, IgG) in response to intestinal infection with *Shigella*. Breast-feeding also serves as a defense mechanism against infection by bacterial enteropathogens, as indicated by the finding that bacterial diarrhea is less prevalent among breast-fed infants than formula-fed infants.

858 **D.** (S&F, ch119)

Turcot's syndrome is a polyposis syndrome characterized by adenomatous polyposis and brain tumors. Due to the adenomatous nature of the tumors, there is an increased risk of colon cancer. Peutz-Jeghers syndrome is an autosomal dominant–inherited polyposis syndrome with hamartomas. One of the hallmarks of this disease is mucocutaneous pigmentation that may be noted on the mouth, nose, lips, and buccal mucosa. These polyps may cause intestinal obstruction, intussusception, and acute or chronic bleeding. Cancer of the colon, duodenum, jejunum, and ileum has been reported, and adenomatous epithelium may also develop within these hamartomatous polyps.

Juvenile polyposis syndrome may also occur and is associated with an increased risk of colon cancer. Youngsters with single polyps without the polyposis syndrome are generally not at increased risk for cancer.

Cronkhite-Canada syndrome is an acquired, nonfamilial syndrome with diffuse gastrointestinal polyposis, dystrophic changes in the fingernails, alopecia, cutaneous hyperpigmentation, diarrhea, weight loss, abdominal pain, and malnutrition. The polyps are hamartomatous but there may be foci of adenomatous tissue. However, malignant degeneration is the exception rather than the rule. The malabsorption syndrome is progressive in most cases and the prognosis is poor.

Cowden's syndrome is a syndrome of multiple hamartomatous polyps of the stomach, small intestine, and colon, along with orocutaneous hamartomas and fibrocystic disease and cancer of the breast. Nontoxic goiter and thyroid cancer may also occur. Cowden's syndrome is inherited in an autosomal dominant fashion. There does not appear to be an increased risk of gastrointestinal cancer.

859 **A.** (S&F, ch106)

This patient is infected with *Entamoeba histolytica*. The diagnosis may be made by serologic testing; 75% to 85% of blood specimens from patients with this infection test positive for the organism. Colonoscopy and biopsy can also be helpful in diagnosis, but examination of a stool specimen for ova and parasites is not reliable for diagnosis. Although 90% of infected individuals are asymptomatic, 10% will develop invasive disease. Acute necrotizing colitis and toxic megacolon is a severe form of invasive disease and only occurs in 0.5% of individuals infected with this organism. All patients in whom the organism is found should be treated, even if asymptomatic.

860 C. (S&F, ch99)

Most human enteric bacteria cannot be cultured because of a lack of truly selective growth media. Nonetheless, molecular profiling has shown that although different individuals have different flora, the population in each individual is relatively stable after weaning. Environmental factors such as diet and sanitation appear to have a profound effect on early intestinal colonization with bacteria. In adulthood, dietary fluctuations appear to induce changes in bacterial enzymes and metabolic activity rather than changes in the population of flora.

861 C. (S&F, ch118)

Primary tumors in all of the locations listed can metastasize to the small bowel, but 60% of patients with melanoma have metastasis to the GI tract, making melanoma by far the most common source of secondary GI cancer.

862 E. (S&F, ch98)

Chronic diarrhea is common in patients with longstanding diabetes mellitus. Mild steatorrhea often is present in patients with diabetic diarrhea and in patients who do not complain of diarrhea. Although the pathophysiologic mechanism of malabsorption in patients with diabetes mellitus is unknown, poor glycemic control is an important cofactor. Most of these patients have signs of autonomic neuropathy. Therefore diarrhea and malabsorption have been attributed in some patients to rapid gastric emptying and rapid intestinal transit, causing impaired mixing of nutrients with digestive secretions and decreased contact time between nutrients and the intestinal mucosa. Certain treatable diseases, like celiac disease, small intestinal bacterial overgrowth, and pancreatic insufficiency, can be associated with diabetes mellitus.

863 B. (S&F, ch120)

The incidence and mortality of colorectal cancer have decreased in the United States since 1985 by annual rates of 1.6% and 1.8%, respectively. Both the incidence and mortality of colorectal cancer are higher in African American than in white populations. There is a rapid rise in the colorectal cancer risk in populations that move from areas of low risk to areas of high risk.

864 A. (S&F, ch101)

Dermatitis herpetiformis (DH) is closely associated with celiac disease. In fact, most, if not all, patients with DH have at least latent celiac

sprue, whereas fewer than 10% of patients with celiac sprue have DH.

865 A. (S&F, ch104)

Enteritis necroticans is caused by strains of C. *perfringens* type C that produce a β-toxin that can cause transmural intestinal wall necrosis in malnourished patients. Intestinal perforation, sepsis, and hemorrhage may occur, and when they do, the risk of death is 40%. In the uncomplicated case described here, treatment should be supportive. Enteritis necroticans is encountered rarely in the United States.

866 C. (S&F, ch100)

Postoperative adaptation is more prominent in the ileum than in the jejunum. Digested food, bile, and pancreatic secretions are believed to be trophic for crypt cells.

867 A. (S&F, ch116)

Complete SBO necessitates early laparotomy. The rationale for early laparotomy in patients with complete SBO is based on three factors: (1) the low likelihood of resolution with nonoperative management; (2) the risk of strangulation in these cases; and (3) the difficulty in detecting strangulation due to obstruction by clinical parameters until very late in the course of the disease.

868 C. (S&F, ch121)

Malakoplakia is a rare chronic granulomatous disease characterized by abdominal pain, diarrhea, hematochezia, fever, and rectal mass. On colonoscopy, yellowish, sessile, ulcerated plaques may be seen. Histologic examination of a biopsy specimen will reveal characteristic von Hansemann bodies and Michaelis-Gutmann bodies. These histologic features are absent in the other three conditions listed.

869 E. (S&F, ch105)

Risk factors for development of pseudomembranous enterocolitis (PMC) in the absence of C. *difficile* infection include intestinal surgery (postoperative *Staphylococcus aureus* infection is the second most common cause of PMC), intestinal ischemia, and other enteric infections. PMC is associated with a wide variety of other intestinal disorders, including *Shigella* infection, Crohn's disease, neonatal necrotizing enterocolitis, intestinal obstruction, and Hirschsprung's disease.

870 E. (S&F, ch119)

Fecal occult blood testing and sigmoidoscopy have been shown in many studies to decrease mortality related to colorectal cancer. The removal of colonic adenomas from patients enrolled in the National Polyp Study led to a decreased risk of colon cancer. Polyps less than 1 cm in size generally do not bleed and therefore fecal occult blood testing is not an accurate technique for their diagnosis. Sigmoidoscopy may be accurate for diagnosis of cancer in the left colon only. Barium enema has never been studied as a screening tool for colorectal cancer. There is about a 5% to 10% false-positive and about a 10% false-negative detection rate for colonic adenomas by barium enema. Adenomas between 6 and 10 mm were identified in approximately 53% of patients by barium enema in the National Polyp Study. There has been controversy in the literature regarding the accuracy of CT colonography for identifying polyps of less than 1 cm. Colonoscopy is the overall preferred method for diagnosis of colonic adenomas and is probably the most accurate method for detecting adenomas of less than 1 cm, even though about 6% of adenomas less than 1 cm are not detected by this method.

871 **E.** (S&F, ch105)

The first step in the management of *C. difficile* diarrhea and colitis is to discontinue the precipitating antibiotics, if possible. Anti-motility agents are best avoided because they may impair clearance of toxin from the colon and worsen toxin-induced colonic injury, precipitating ileus of the colon. Metronidazole is generally recommended as the drug of choice for acute *C. difficile* diarrhea and colitis because it is inexpensive and highly effective. Metronidazole may potentiate the action of warfarin, resulting in prolongation of the prothrombin time, so this combination should be avoided. Vancomycin doses of 125 mg 4 times a day are as effective as vancomycin doses of 500 mg 4 times a day; this medication should be administered by mouth, because effective colonic luminal concentrations are not achieved when it is given intravenously. Vancomycin is generally recommended for infections that fail to respond to metronidazole, for patients intolerant of metronidazole, and for patients with fulminant pseudomembranous colitis.

872 **C.** (S&F. ch119)

Patients with ureterosigmoidostomies, when the ureter has been implanted into the sigmoid colon, are at elevated risk for colonic adenomas and carcinomas at the anastomosis site. Other conditions associated with adenomatous polyps include acromegaly, *Streptococcus bovis* bacteremia, skin tags, atherosclerosis, breast cancer, and history of cholecystectomy. The

other choices mentioned do not have a strong or known relationship to colonic adenomas.

873 **C.** (S&F, ch104)

Salmonella infection is most often acquired from flies, food, fingers, feces, or fomites. Eggs and poultry are the major sources of food-borne *Salmonella* infection. The two most common serotypes in the United States are *S. enteritidis* and *S. typhimurium*. The most common condition caused by *Salmonella* infection is gastroenteritis. Sickle cell anemia predisposes to *Salmonella* osteomyelitis. Several other hemolytic anemias, neoplastic diseases, immunosuppressive conditions, and gastric surgery predispose to this infection.

874 **C.** (S&F, ch93)

In about 2% of the population, a small remnant of vitelline duct remains and forms what is called a Meckel's diverticulum. This outpocketing most commonly occurs in the distal ileum and may contain functional gastric or pancreatic tissue. Acid production by this ectopic tissue may cause ulceration and bleeding, resulting in anemia or maroon stools. Intestinal obstruction caused by either intussusception with the diverticulum as a lead point, or herniation through or volvulus around the fibrous remnant of the vitelline duct, are less common but have been reported. Meckel's diverticulum is more common in male patients and is usually diagnosed before the third decade of life.

875 **B.** (S&F, ch93)

The best initial diagnostic test is colonoscopy with terminal ileum intubation. This will exclude other diagnostic possibilities and potentially localize the source of bleeding to the small intestines. A Tc-99 scan to detect ectopic gastric mucosa may be helpful in evaluation of Meckel's diverticulum, but not as the initial test. Cimetidine has been used to enhance the diagnostic usefulness of a Tc-99 scan by minimizing uptake of radiotracer by the duodenum, which could give false-positive results for Meckel's diverticulum. Visceral angiography and surgical exploration are not suitable initial studies in a patient with suspected Meckel's diverticulum.

876 **A.** (S&F, ch117)

Intestinal pseudo-obstruction is a syndrome of impaired intestinal propulsion that causes symptoms that resemble those of intestinal obstruction but without a mechanical cause. It may involve the small or large bowel and presents in acute, subacute, or chronic form.

There are both myopathic and neuropathic forms. The pathophysiologic processes underlying this condition are unclear.

877 **B.** (S&F, ch109)

None of the 5-ASA agents is approved for treating Crohn's disease; however, they are utilized for this purpose. There have been no well-designed large randomized double-blind placebo-controlled trials in which an 5-ASA compound in doses equivalent to mesalamine proved superior to another 5-ASA compound. Because the 5-ASA agents are generally thought *not* to be effective for severely active disease, they are often discontinued when patients require hospital admission for intravenous administration of glucocorticoid medications. There does appear to be a dose-dependent response when 5-ASA medications are used as induction therapy for patients with UC. Doses between 4 and 4.8 grams a day of mesalamine (Asacol), for example, may be needed before remission is noted in cases of mild to moderate UC. There are limitations with sulfasalazine, including inability to give high doses because of toxicity of the active moiety.

878 **E.** (S&F, ch104)

Several diseases present with a mass in right lower quadrant. The primary diseases to consider include intestinal tuberculosis, Crohn's disease, *Yersinia enterocolitica,* cecal carcinoma, and amebiasis. Syphilis and lymphogranuloma venereum should be considered as well, but intestinal involvement with these infections is now uncommon.

879 **B.** (S&F, ch121)

Selective mesenteric angiography is the diagnostic study of choice. Colonoscopy can identify the lesion in some cases, but it is often difficult or impossible to perform, especially when bleeding continues or thorough cleansing of the colon cannot be accomplished. Exploratory laparotomy with resection of the colonic segment is needed to control the bleeding.

880 **E.** (S&F, ch99)

Many patients with celiac sprue who have persistent symptoms despite adherence to a gluten-free diet have SIBO. A motility disturbance seems the most likely explanation. SIBO is common in those with Crohn's disease, particularly in patients who have a history of intestinal resection. Positive results of a glucose hydrogen breath test are particularly associated with the presence of a small bowel stricture. SIBO is also common among patients with chronic pancreatitis. It may be caused by small bowel

dysmotility resulting from chronic opioid use. Furthermore, pancreatic juice may have an antibacterial effect and so its absence might allow enteric bacteria to proliferate more freely.

More recently, there have been reports of SIBO in patients with rheumatoid arthritis, specifically those with high disease activity. SIBO occurs late in the course of radiation enteritis, and in these cases it appears to be related to intestinal dysmotility. SIBO is common among patients with chronic renal failure, which is associated with neuropathic-like abnormalities of small intestinal motility.

881 **E.** (S&F, ch106)

Only 10% of infected individuals have invasive disease, in which invasion of the colonic epithelium leads to spread of organisms through the bloodstream and infection at distant sites (i.e., liver abscess). The other 90% of individuals remain asymptomatic. The two-stage life cycle of this organism includes the cyst stage, during which the infection is acquired by ingesting food or water contaminated with cyst-infected feces. The other stage is the trophozoite stage, which is responsible for tissue invasion. Amebic colitis may present like other colitides, which most often affect the cecum and right colon. Immigrants from endemic areas, institutionalized patients, and male homosexuals are at greatest risk for this disease. Infants, the elderly, pregnant women, and those receiving glucocorticoid drugs are at increased risk of fulminant disease, but persons with AIDS are not at increased risk for invasive disease.

882 **E.** (S&F, ch114)

Acute diverticulitis often presents with left lower quadrant abdominal pain, reflecting the propensity for this disorder to occur in the sigmoid colon in Western populations. In contrast, Asian patients with diverticulitis have predominantly right-sided symptoms, corresponding to the typical location of diverticula in these populations. Examination may disclose tenderness or a mass, particularly in patients with a deep pelvic abscess. Fever is present in most patients, whereas hypotension and shock are unusual symptoms. The white blood cell count frequently is elevated, although in one study normal white blood cell counts (less than $11,000/mm^3$) and no left shift were found in 46% of patients.

883 **B.** (S&F, ch101)

Celiac sprue is characterized by malabsorption in the small intestine of wheat gluten or related proteins in rye and barley. The reason why oats may be tolerated by patients with celiac sprue is that oats contain a relatively smaller proportion of a toxic prolamin moiety compared to other gluten-containing cereals.

884 **E.** (S&F, ch117)

Intestinal pseudo-obstruction is a well-described complication of scleroderma. The small bowel is the second most frequently involved gastrointestinal organ, after the esophagus. An uncommon but potentially serious finding is pneumatosis cystoides intestinalis, which usually signifies a poor prognosis. Degeneration of smooth muscle and its replacement by collagen is responsible for the small bowel dysmotility seen in patients with scleroderma. The circular muscle is involved more often than is the longitudinal muscle layer. Small bowel dysmotility leads to bacterial overgrowth, resulting in steatorrhea, malabsorption, and weight loss. The hallmark dysmotility is absence of the interdigestive migrating motor complex, low-amplitude clusters of propagated and nonpropagated contractions, abnormally prolonged MMC cycle, diminished activity of phase III, hypomotility of the fed pattern, and antral hypomotility.

885 **B.** (S&F, ch122)

An anal fissure is a longitudinal cut in the anoderm. More than 90% of anal fissures are located in the midposterior portion of the anus. It has been shown that the posterior area of the anoderm is less well perfused than other areas of anoderm. There is speculation that increased tone in the internal sphincter muscle further reduces the blood flow to this area. Based on these findings, fissures are thought to represent ischemic ulceration. Trauma during defecation, especially with passage of a hard stool, is believed to initiate the formation of a fissure.

Fissures usually are exquisitely tender. The history is classically one of *severe* pain during defecation. Bright red blood may be seen on the toilet tissue. On examination, simply spreading the buttocks usually increases the pain and leads to anal sphincter muscle spasm. *A digital examination causes inhumane pain, increases the spasm, and should be avoided.* Once the fissure is healed or the pain has lessened, an examination can be performed to exclude associated problems. If the diagnosis is in doubt or the patient does not respond to treatment, an examination under anesthesia is indicated.

886 **D.** (S&F, ch109)

Perinuclear antineutrophilic cytoplasmic antibody (p-ANCA) is present in 60% to 85% of patients with UC, not 100%. There is no evidence that patients who test positive for p-ANCA have more aggressive disease. Patients who test positive for p-ANCA are at increased risk of pouchitis.

887 **C.** (S&F, ch122)

Unexplained anal pain refers to pain in the anorectal region in the absence of an underlying anatomic abnormality. Diagnosis is based almost entirely on the patient's symptoms. Levator ani syndrome affects women younger than 45 years of age. Episodes of pain are chronic or recurring. Each episode typically lasts 20 minutes or more. The discomfort is described as a vague tenderness or aching sensation high in the rectum. Discomfort usually does not awaken the patient from sleep, and usually it is worse after defecation and with sitting. Walking or lying down seems to relieve the pain. Symptoms have been attributed to spasm of the levator muscles. On rectal examination the levator muscle may feel like a tight, tender band.

Proctalgia fugax occurs in young men and "perfectionists." It is seen in early adulthood and subsides by middle age. The pain lasts seconds or minutes and then disappears. Pain is described as a sharp cramp or stabbing pain and may awaken the patient from sleep. The results of a physical examination will be normal.

Coccygodynia is a pain or ache in the tailbone and typically results from trauma to the coccyx or arthritis involving this bone. Movement of the coccyx on digital rectal examination can reproduce the pain.

888 **A.** (S&F, ch95)

Sympathetic activation inhibits colonic motor activity, reduces colonic blood flow, and inhibits secretion to minimize fluid loss. The major sympathetic colonic inputs arise from the inferior mesenteric ganglion. Parasympathetic activation plays a central role in the propulsive activity of the distal colon prior to evacuation. The colon receives parasympathetic inputs via the vagus and spinal nerves.

889 **E.** (S&F, ch105)

Elderly patients and patients undergoing cytotoxic chemotherapy for malignancy are at increased risk for *C. difficile*–associated diarrhea and colitis. HIV-infected patients are also at increased risk due to factors such as prophylactic or therapeutic use of antibiotic medications, hospitalization, and immunocompromised status. *C. difficile* is the most frequently identified specific pathogen among patients with IBD living in North America or Europe, and in some case series it was present in as many as 5% to 19% of patients who experienced relapse. The fact that many patients with IBD have *C. difficile* infection but no other risk factors such as a history of recent antibiotic drug use suggests that IBD itself may cause sufficient alteration of the colonic microenvironment to impair the ability of normal colonic microflora to resist infection.

890   B. (S&F, ch97)

Several steps in lipid digestion and absorption depend on intraluminal pH. Pancreatic lipase activity is greatest in the presence of bile salts and at pH 6 or above. This enzyme therefore has good activity at the pH of the lumen of the duodenum, where most lipid digestion occurs. Most dietary lipid is absorbed by the upper two thirds of the jejunum, although the rate and extent of absorption are influenced by the presence of other foods, particularly dietary fiber, which reduces the rate of absorption.

891   D. (S&F, ch112)

The most effective treatment for solitary rectal ulcer syndrome is biofeedback. It has been associated with an increase in local blood flow. Other treatments include local agents (although topical glucocorticoid drugs and sulfasalazine are not effective), improving bowel habits, and surgery. Sucralfate enemas and human fibrin sealant have been effective in small studies. The addition of fiber to the diet (acting as a bulking agent) along with habit training to reduce straining may result in symptomatic improvement in patients with mild disease.

Behavioral therapy or biofeedback is the first line of therapy for patients with more severe disease, and it improves symptoms in more than 50% of patients, although ulcer healing is seen in a minority. This therapy aims at bowel habit training to normalize (coordinate) contractions of pelvic floor muscles. Jarrett and associates demonstrated that biofeedback resulted in improved rectal blood flow, which was associated with a successful clinical outcome.

Surgery is indicated in patients with severe disease that has not responded to medical or biofeedback therapy. Surgical procedures include operations for rectal prolapse, excision of the ulcer, or colostomy.

892   E. (S&F, ch113)

The perforation rate for appendicitis is between 10% and 30% in most series. Perforation is most common in patients at the extremes of age; rates as high as 90% have been reported in children younger than 2 years. Adults older than 70 years have perforation rates between 50% and 70%. Perforation is often the result of delay in diagnosis; however, the delay in diagnosis is often due to a delay in presentation to medical attention rather than a delay in medical decision-making.

893   C. (S&F, ch112)

Although not necessary for the diagnosis of celiac disease, the presence of HLA-DQ2 and HLA-DQ8 is typical for patients with celiac disease. Tests for these markers are most helpful in ruling out celiac sprue.

894   A. (S&F, ch104)

The most common cause of traveler's diarrhea is enterotoxigenic *Escherichia coli* (which causes 40% to 60% of cases). The highest-risk destinations include Latin America, Africa, the Middle East, and Asia, where 25% to 50% of travelers are affected. Younger travelers, particularly those between 20 and 29 years of age, are at highest risk. The national origin of the traveler is another important factor in traveler's diarrhea. The attack rate is higher for people from developed countries.

895   E. (S&F, ch111)

The most common presentation of focal segmental ischemia (FSI) is chronic small bowel obstruction with intermittent abdominal pain, distention, and vomiting. Bacterial overgrowth in the more proximal dilated loops may produce a "blind loop syndrome." Radiologic studies typically reveal a smooth, tapered stricture of variable length with an abrupt change to normal bowel distally and dilated bowel proximally. Treatment of FSI is resection of the involved bowel.

896   D. (S&F, ch113)

The results of many epidemiologic studies suggest that appendectomy may protect against the development of ulcerative colitis, a relationship not seen in Crohn's disease. Researchers have also suggested that appendectomy may attenuate the course of active ulcerative colitis. Although appendiceal tumors are rare (they have been found in fewer than 1% of specimens), the vast majority of appendiceal tumors are carcinoid tumors. Common types of epithelial malignancies include mucinous and cyst adenocarcinoma. The lifetime risk of appendicitis is about 1 in 12 at birth and declines to 1 in 35 by age 35 years. The greatest risk of appendicitis in a given year is during the second decade of life, when the risk is about 0.25% per year.

897 **B.** (S&F, ch119)

The optimal treatment is to perform a total proctocolectomy with either a conventional ileostomy or an ileoanal pouch. These procedures remove all colonic tissue and thus the risk for adenomatous transformation of colon polyps and carcinoma. Other procedures that may be performed, depending on patient preference, include subtotal colectomy with ileorectal anastomosis; if this is performed, the remaining rectal segment is at risk for carcinoma and therefore periodic surveillance is required. A colectomy with creation of a Hartmann's pouch is not the optimal treatment because the rectum remains and surveillance examinations will be needed.

898 **C.** (S&F, ch122)

In the past, the standard treatment for anal canal cancer was abdominal-perineal resection with a permanent colostomy. In 1974, Nigro and colleagues presented the results of a trial of combined radiation and chemotherapy and showed that cure was possible without abdominal-perineal resection. This led to a regimen of external beam radiation with 5-fluorouracil and mitomycin as the treatment of choice; surgery was reserved for cases in which residual cancer is identified in the scar after treatment. In recent treatment trials, cisplatin was substituted for mitomycin and this combination treatment led to complete response in 94% of patients. Patients with persistent or recurrent squamous cell carcinoma of the anal canal are treated with abdominal-perineal resection. About 50% of patients who undergo surgery can be cured. Success has also been reported with an additional boost of radiation therapy combined with cisplatin-based chemotherapy.

899 **C.** (S&F, ch95)

In response to distention of the rectum, there is simultaneous activation of the enteric descending inhibitory pathway. This causes relaxation of the IAS and of the extrinsic pathway, which leads to contraction of the EAS. This rectoanal inhibitory reflex allows entry of a small amount of feces into the proximal rectum while continence is maintained by the EAS. This allows the rectum to temporarily store material until defecation is convenient.

900 **D.** (S&F, ch105)

Approximately 15% to 30% of patients successfully treated with vancomycin or metronidazole suffer a relapse after completion of their initial course of antibiotic therapy. The infection may recur as long as 2 months after stopping the antibiotic. Reoccurrence of *C. difficile* colitis and diarrhea is confirmed by stool toxin assay. Patients with recurrence typically are treated with a second course of the same antibiotic, at the same daily dose but for 14 days; the cure rate in these cases is about 40%.

901 **B.** (S&F, ch96)

E. coli heat-stable enterotoxin (STa) causes diarrhea by increasing intracellular levels of cyclic guanosine monophosphate (cGMP). *Vibrio cholerae* releases cholera toxin that binds to the GM1-ganglioside receptor, leading to increase in cytosolic cyclic adenosine monophosphate (cAMP), which ultimately results in the inhibition of Na^+Cl^--coupled transport and increased Cl^- secretion. Rotavirus releases the enterotoxin NSP4, which leads to an increase in intracellular calcium levels, thereby affecting calcium-sensitive anion channels. *Salmonella typhimurium* infection causes increased membrane permeability to calcium influx. The resulting increase in intracellular Ca^{++} might ultimately activate secretion of the cytokines necrosis factor (NF)-kappaB and interleukin (IL)-8. *Clostridium difficile* toxins A and B modify the Rho family of guanosine triphosphatases (GTPases) that are critical for maintaining cell cytoskeletal architecture.

902 **D.** (S&F, ch100)

Short bowel syndrome is defined as malabsorption due to insufficient intestinal surface area such that a person is unable to absorb sufficient fluid, energy, or nutrients to sustain life in the absence of specialized nutritional support. Short bowel syndrome, also known as "intestinal failure," occurs when there is less than 200 cm of intestine.

903 **E.** (S&F, ch105)

Pseudomembranous colitis occurs in only 3% to 5% of patients with *C. difficile* infection but has mortality of up to 65%. Diarrhea may be minimal or absent because of ileus, or diarrhea may be present with abdominal pain or peritoneal signs. Vancomycin is often used as the first-line agent in critically ill patients. In the presence of ileus, vancomycin may be administered via a nasogastric tube with intermittent clamping of the tube.

904 **D.** (S&F, ch111)

A normal white blood cell count does not exclude early AMI, just as a high white blood cell count is not diagnostic of the condition. No serum markers (such as changes in phosphate, amylase, or d-lactate levels) have been shown to be adequately sensitive or specific for AMI. In addition, serum markers, when elevated, usually indicate late-stage disease. In patients with AMI, an elevated amylase level is not secondary to pancreatitis but rather to rapid absorption of intraluminal amylase secondary to a defect in barrier function.

905 **D.** (S&F, ch114)

Administering barium to a patient with an intestinal perforation carries a risk of barium peritonitis. Only water-soluble contrast enemas, i.e., Gastrografin, should be used in patients in whom acute diverticulitis is suspected.

Computed tomography is more sensitive and specific than a barium enema and is the best choice for identifying diverticulitis.

Endoscopy should generally be avoided in the initial evaluation of suspected acute diverticulitis, although rigid or flexible sigmoidoscopy with minimal insufflation may be helpful to exclude alternative diagnoses such as inflammatory bowel disease, carcinoma, or ischemic colitis. When the acute stage of the illness has passed, however, colonoscopy should be performed to confirm the presence of diverticuli and to exclude competing diagnoses, particularly neoplasia.

Ultrasound and MRI may be helpful but not as helpful as CT.

906 **B.** (S&F, ch117)

Mortality due to acute colonic pseudo-obstruction varies from 0% to 32%. The diameter of the colon may be a risk factor for mortality. When surgical decompression is performed in patients with a mechanical obstruction and cecal diameter of 9 cm or less, there is a dramatic reduction in mortality. This is the basis for the use of the 9 cm cut off as a sign of "impending perforation" in patients with acute colonic pseudo-obstruction.

907 **A.** (S&F, ch119)

Adenomas with "advanced pathology" are those that are more than 1 cm in diameter, have villous architecture, and manifest high grades of dysplasia or characteristics of carcinoma. Flat adenomas are also considered to be high-risk lesions because they tend to have higher grades of dysplasia.

Serrated adenomas have features of both adenomas and hyperplastic polyps; serrated adenomas were originally categorized as mixed hyperplastic adenomatous polyps but are now classified as adenomas due to the presence of nuclear atypia. These polyps may exhibit high-grade dysplasia depending on their size.

A tubular adenoma with mild dysplasia is not considered to have advanced pathology.

908 **D.** (S&F, ch111)

CT has for the most part replaced plain radiographic studies of the abdomen for diagnosis of intestinal ischemia because it can identify arterial and venous thrombosis as well as ischemic bowel. CT findings in cases of intestinal ischemia may include colonic dilatation, bowel wall thickening, abnormal bowel wall enhancement, lack of enhancement of arterial vasculature with timed venous contrast injections, arterial occlusion, venous thrombosis, engorgement of mesenteric veins, intramural gas, mesenteric or portal gas, infarction of other organs, ascites, and signs related to the cause of the infarcted bowel (e.g., hernia). Tagging red blood cells would be of little use for making this diagnosis. Duplex ultrasound may have some utility, but CT is the best choice.

909 **D.** (S&F, ch106)

Nitazoxamide has been shown to be consistently effective in the treatment of cryptosporidiosis in immunocompetent hosts. The other three medications listed are not effective.

910 **B.** (S&F, ch104)

The diagnosis of shigellosis should be suspected in this patient with acute onset of the triad of lower abdominal pain, rectal burning, and diarrhea. Dysentery that presents subacutely, with bloody diarrhea, cramps, and rectal pain for 2 to 4 weeks, can masquerade as ulcerative colitis. Sigmoidoscopic findings in patients with shigellosis are indistinguishable from those of with idiopathic ulcerative colitis but a colonic biopsy may be helpful in differential diagnosis. Rotavirus causes secretory diarrhea.

911 **B.** (S&F, ch101)

Celiac sprue affects the mucosa of the small intestine; the submucosa, muscularis propria, and serosa usually are not involved. The mucosal lesion of the small intestine in celiac sprue may vary considerably in both severity and extent.[9] This spectrum of pathologic involvement helps explain the striking variability of the clinical manifestations of the disease. Gross examination with an endoscope reveals scalloping, as seen in Figure 1 (see figure). Examination, by hand lens or dissecting microscope, of the mucosal surface of biopsy specimens from patients with untreated celiac sprue with severe lesions reveals a flat mucosal surface with complete absence of normal intestinal villi. Histologic examination of tissue sections confirms this loss of normal villous structure (see Figure 2). Sparing of the proximal intestine with involvement of the distal small intestine does not occur.

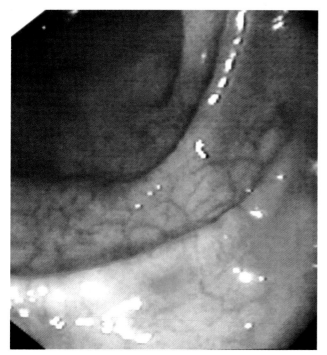

Figure 1 for answer **911**

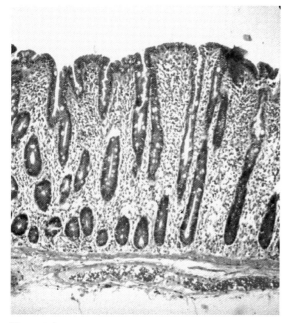

Figure 2 for answer **911**

912 **A.** (S&F, ch112)

Solitary rectal ulcer syndrome (SRUS) is an uncommon disorder of evacuation. Patients may be of any age. SRUS is characterized by the presence of rectal ulceration or erythema in association with straining at defecation, rectal prolapse, a feeling of incomplete evacuation, and typical histologic features. It is also associated with occult or overt rectal prolapse with paradoxical contraction of the pelvic floor.

913 **C.** (S&F, ch117)

Neuropathic causes of chronic intestinal pseudo-obstruction (CIP) include amyloidosis, diabetes mellitus, and Parkinson's disease. Scleroderma is an example of a myopathic form of CIP.

914 **D.** (S&F, ch108)

Infliximab is the first biologic response modifier shown to be effective in Crohn's disease. It is a chimeric monoclonal anti–tumor necrosis factor (TNF) antibody. It has been shown in multiple trials to be effective for patients with moderate to severe Crohn's disease and perianal disease. It is also useful for maintenance therapy. Of all the regimens listed, giving a series of three infusions, one every 6 weeks is most often recommended, since delayed hypersensitivity appears to be less common when the induction regimen is a series of three infusions. This is also the regimen used for fistulous disease. Careful patient selection is key (see figure).

915 **B.** (S&F, ch117)

Familial visceral neuropathies are a group of genetic diseases characterized by degeneration of the myenteric plexus. There are two distinct phenotypes, types I and II. Both forms are generally symptomatic and there is no effective medical or surgical therapy available. Type I may involve both the large and small intestine and type II is associated with hypertrophic pyloric stenosis.

916 **D.** (ch106)

The patient has Chagas' disease, which is caused by an organism from Central and South America that is now, with more people immigrating to the United States and the discovery of large reservoirs in animals in the southern United States, becoming a more common health problem in the United States. The organism, *Trypanosoma cruzi,* is transmitted by the bite of a reduviid bug. Acute Chagas' disease most often affects children. Symptoms of acute disease are fever and edema, mostly periorbital. Chronic Chagas' disease most often affects the heart,

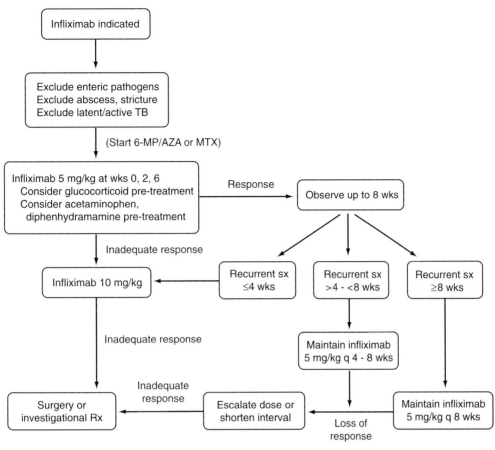

Figure for answer **914**

esophagus, and or colon. The symptoms of chronic disease relate to the organ(s) affected and can include arrhythmias, heart failure, constipation, and achalasia-type symptoms. Manometrically, the disease is indistinguishable from achalasia. The diagnosis is made by finding the trypanosome on blood smears. Treatment with nifurtimox or benznidazole is effective.

917 **B.** (S&F, ch99)

SIBO classically causes a combination of megaloblastic anemia (due to vitamin B_{12} deficiency) and steatorrhea (due to fat malabsorption). Vitamin B_{12} deficiency is caused by bacterial consumption of the vitamin within the intestinal lumen before it can be absorbed across the mucosa. Deficiencies of thiamine and nicotinamide also have been reported in patients with SIBO. Folate levels tend to be high in those with SIBO because the bacteria synthesize folate, which is then absorbed and utilized by the host.

Malabsorption of fat and fat-soluble vitamins mainly results from deconjugation of bile acids, and administration of conjugated bile acids has

been reported to reverse steatorrhea in human and animal studies. Deficiencies of vitamins A, D, and E have been reported, but vitamin K deficiency is uncommon because of production of vitamin K by luminal bacteria.

918 **C.** (S&F, ch112)

The barium radiograph in the question shows diffuse small intestinal ulcerations in a patient with refractory celiac disease (ulcerative enteritis). There is diffuse involvement of the small intestine with multiple ulcerations and separation and thickening of the loops of jejunum and ileum.

919 **A.** (S&F, ch116)

Although intussusception is most often recognized as a cause of SBO in children, about 5% of cases occur in adults. In children there is rarely an anatomical abnormality, whereas in adults an underlying pathologic process is present in more than 90% of cases. The most common cause is small bowel neoplasm. Inflammatory lesions and Meckel's diverticula account for most other cases.

920 **B.** (S&F, ch119)

Familial adenomatous polyposis is a syndrome that is inherited in an autosomal dominant fashion; there is 80% to 100% penetrance. Polyps usually develop by the time the individual is 10 to 12 years old and may be tubular, villous, or mixed. Patients generally have hundreds to thousands of polyps, and the risk of carcinoma is essentially 100%. Patients inherit one mutated *APC* allele as a germline mutation. However, they subsequently develop adenomatous polyps when the second allele undergoes mutation or is lost.

921 **B.** (S&F, ch121)

Pneumatosis cystoides intestinalis (PCI) seems to be most likely diagnosis in this case. Numerous conditions have been associated with PCI, including appendicitis, IBD, diverticular disease, necrotizing enterocolitis, pseudomembranous colitis, ileus, and sigmoid volvulus. Some nongastrointestinal conditions associated with PCI include emphysema (as in this case), collagen vascular disease, AIDS, glucocorticoid use, chemotherapy, and certain medications.

922 **A.** (S&F, ch107)

The patient has been infested by the liver fluke *Clonorchis sinensis,* which is endemic to China, Hong Kong, Taiwan, and North Vietnam. *Opisthorchis* species are closely related and endemic to Thailand, Laos, Russia, and the Ukraine. Both species cause a marked increased risk of cholangiocarcinoma. Most infections are asymptomatic unless the worm burden is heavy. Peripheral eosinophilia does occur. Diagnosis is made by finding parasite eggs in the stool. Additionally, ultrasound, and endoscopic retrograde cholangiopancreatography (ERCP) may reveal evidence of the organism. The treatment of choice is praziquantel. Although albendazole is an alternate treatment, it is teratogenic and is not used in pregnant women.

923 **C.** (S&F, ch115)

5-Hydroxytryptamine (5-HT) is released from enteroendocrine cells of the intestine after a meal. 5-HT then acts on primary intrinsic afferent neurons to initiate the peristaltic reflex mechanism. There is some evidence that an exaggerated release of 5-HT can occur after a meal in those with IBS. A leading hypothesis is that in individuals with IBS, increased availability of mucosal 5-HT can induce diarrhea, but if there is desensitization of 5-HT receptors this can lead to constipation or an alternating bowel pattern.

924 **C.** (S&F, ch104)

Diarrhea, fever, abdominal pain, and bloody stools are present in between 50% and 90% of

individuals with *Campylobacter* gastroenteritis. Constitutional symptoms such as headache, myalgia, backache, malaise, anorexia, and vomiting often occur. Infections rarely may be complicated by gastrointestinal hemorrhage, toxic megacolon, pancreatitis, cholecystitis, HUS, bacteremia, meningitis, and purulent arthritis. Postinfectious complications include reactive arthritis, Guillain-Barré syndrome, and immunoproliferative small intestinal disease.

925 **C.** (S&F, ch122)

Rubber band ligation (RBL) has become the most frequently performed office procedure for the treatment of second- and third-degree hemorrhoids. Patients usually are asked to refrain from taking aspirin or NSAIDs for approximately 5 days before and after the treatment, to reduce the risk of bleeding. Rubber bands are placed on the rectal mucosa just proximal to the internal anal cushion.

Patients may experience discomfort after RBL; soaking in a sitz bath and taking acetaminophen usually are sufficient to relieve the discomfort. Immediate severe pain usually signals that the band has been placed too close to the dentate line and that it must be removed. Bleeding when the band and necrotic hemorrhoidal tissue slough in 4 to 7 days may be severe and even life-threatening. Severe bleeding occurs in about 1% of patients; it usually can be controlled by tamponade by a large-caliber Foley catheter placed in the rectum. If this approach fails, epinephrine can be injected at the bleeding site.

926 **C.** (S&F, ch107)

*Ascaris lumbri*coides can be seen on direct examination of a stool sample from an infected patient. Patients may see the worms on passage of stool. If the worms are being harbored in the pancreaticobiliary tree, they may be seen during ERCP. When an upper GI barium contrast study is performed, *Ascaris* worms will retain barium after the gastrointestinal tract is cleared of the barium. Most patients do not have peripheral eosinophilia.

927 **D.** (S&F, ch102)

The presence of nutritional deficiencies that result in anemia (vitamin B_{12}, folate), stomatitis (iron), glossitis (vitamin B_{12}), pigmentation of the skin (vitamin B_{12}), and edema caused by hypoproteinemia are all consistent with tropical sprue.

928 **D.** (S&F, ch103)

Central nervous system (CNS) findings in patients with Whipple's disease include progressive dementia and cognitive changes (28% to 71% of cases), supranuclear ophthalmoplegia (32% to 51% of cases), and altered level of consciousness (27% to 50% of cases). Less frequent signs are psychiatric symptoms, hypothalamic manifestations (e.g., polydipsia, hyperphagia, insomnia), cranial nerve abnormalities, nystagmus, seizures, and ataxia. Two signs are considered to be characteristic of Whipple's disease affecting the CNS: oculomasticatory myorhythmia and oculofacial skeletal myorhythmia; these have not yet been documented in other CNS diseases. Both consist of slow rhythmic and synchronized contractions (at a rate of about 1/second) of ocular, facial, or other muscles; both occur in fewer than 20% of patients with Whipple's disease affecting the CNS.

929 **C.** (S&F, ch116)

All of the conditions listed can cause small bowel obstruction. The three most common causes, in order of incidence, are intra-abdominal adhesions, hernias, and neoplasms. Adhesions cause 50% to 75% of all cases.

930 **B.** (S&F, ch106)

Giardia lamblia is ubiquitous in the United States. A course of metronidazole, 250 mg/day for 5 days, is 80% to 95% effective in treating this infection. Tinidazole, furazolidone, and quinacrine are alternatives. Paromomycin is the treatment of choice in pregnant women because it is not absorbed. Prolonged lactose intolerance may occur after infection.

931 **A.** (S&F, ch116)

The most common cause of ileus is abdominal or retroperitoneal surgery. Other causes of ileus include inflammatory, metabolic, neurogenic, and drug-related conditions.

932 **B.** (S&F, ch96)

Flagyl is not used to treat chronic diarrhea in those with diabetes mellitus. Autonomic and possibly enteric neuropathy in those with diabetes is likely to impair the neural regulation of salt and water transport. When routine anti-diarrheal medications fail to adequately control chronic diarrhea in those with diabetes, an α-2-adrenergic receptor agonist such as clonidine or a somatostatin analogue such as octreotide should be considered.

933 **A.** (S&F, ch101)

The mainstay of treatment for celiac sprue is avoidance of gluten and gluten containing foods, such as wheat, rye, and barley. Although refractory celiac sprue can be treated with glucocorticoid drugs, the effect rarely persists once treatment is stopped. Therefore, glucocorticoid drugs are not indicated in the routine management of celiac disease. Cyclosporine, azathioprine, and 6-mercaptopurine can be used to minimize the dose or as an alternative to glucocorticoid therapy in diabetic patients with treatment-refractory sprue.

934 **A.** (S&F, ch116)

A Richter's hernia is a herniation of the intestinal wall through a laparoscopic trocar site. This hernia can result in bowel obstruction. The incidence of this hernia following laparoscopic fundoplication or cholecystectomy is 1% to 3%. When a patient develops SBO shortly after a laparoscopic procedure, a Richter's hernia should be suspected as the cause.

935 **B.** (S&F, ch101)

Malignancy, ulcerative jejunoileitis, and collagenous sprue are the major complications of celiac sprue. In the past, patients with celiac sprue or dermatitis herpetiformis (DH) had been reported to have a 10-fold increased risk for certain gastrointestinal tract malignancies and a 40- to 70-fold increased risk for non-Hodgkin's lymphoma (NHL). Recent studies, however, indicate that the risk of malignancy and particularly lymphoma is much lower than initially thought. Small intestinal lymphoma, often multifocal and diffuse, accounts for half to two thirds of malignancies that occur in those with celiac sprue, and this malignancy typically occurs after 20 to 40 years of disease (see Chapter 28, 112). Whereas most small intestinal lymphomas identified in the general population are of B-cell origin, intestinal lymphomas in those with celiac sprue are typically of T-cell origin, and the term enteropathy-associated T-cell lymphoma (ETL) was coined to describe both the intestinal and extraintestinal lymphomas that can occur in those with celiac sprue. Carcinoma, particularly of the oropharynx, esophagus, or small intestine, can also occur in those with celiac sprue.

936 **E.** (S&F, ch99)

Although much remains to be learned about the metabolites of indigenous bacteria, these bacteria apparently benefit the host in several ways. In addition to producing regulatory signals for mucosal homeostasis, these flora have important metabolic functions not possessed by the host. These include biotransformation of bile acids; degradation of oxalate; breakdown of otherwise indigestible dietary components, such as plant polysaccharides; and production of short-chain fatty acids, a major energy source for colonic epithelia, from fermentable carbohydrates. Other activities include synthesis of biotin, folate, and vitamin K. Clinicians also have exploited enteric bacterial enzymes such as azoreductase to convert pro-drugs such as sulfasalazine to active drug metabolites e.g., aminosalicylate. Other examples of drug bioavailability due to the actions of bacterial flora include the metabolism of L-dopa to dopamine and degradation of digoxin.

937 **A.** (S&F, ch98)

Hartnup disorder is an autosomal recessive disorder in which there is decreased intestinal absorption of free neutral amino acids, including tryptophan. The amino acids affected by the transporter defects still can be absorbed as oligo- and dipeptides and, therefore, protein malnutrition can be avoided. The manifestations of Hartnup disorder are therefore mainly due to amino acid transport defects in the kidney. Most patients are asymptomatic. In some patients photosensitive skin rash, intermittent ataxia, psychotic behavior, mental retardation, and diarrhea occur. Oral administration of nicotinamide and a high-protein diet have been shown to improve symptoms to some extent.

938 **D.** (S&F, ch113)

It remains controversial whether a laparoscopic appendectomy is superior to open appendectomy. Both procedures are safe and effective in the treatment of nonperforated appendicitis. Patients who have undergone laparoscopic appendectomy require less pain medication and return to normal activity one week sooner than those who have undergone open appendectomy.

939 **B.** (S&F, ch116)

The risk of adhesive small bowel obstruction is greatest following operations involving resection and re-anastomosis of intestine. The risk of adhesive small bowel obstruction after partial or subtotal colectomy is as high as 18%. Appendectomy and gynecologic surgery such as tubal ligation have a risk of only 1%. Upper abdominal surgery such as cholecystectomy and Heller myotomy have lower risks than lower abdominal or pelvic surgery.

940 **E.** (S&F, ch109)

A course of daily doses of 40 to 60mg of prednisone is effective first-line therapy for

moderate to severe flares of UC. Doses greater than 60mg are not associated with increased efficacy but only increased side effects. None of the other drugs mentioned would be adequate. Mesalamine suppositories and enemas would only take care of distal disease and this patient has documented pancolitis. Balsalazide is a 5-ASA compound and none of the 5-ASA drugs is likely to lead to remission of moderate to severe disease. Azathioprine and 6-mercaptopurine do not show an effect until 2 to 4 months after the start of therapy; therefore, they are not useful for acute exacerbations.

941 **A.** (S&F, ch103)

The symptoms in this case are all clinical manifestations of Whipple's disease. Arthralgias can precede intestinal symptoms by several years. Polyarthralgias are a common complaint. Skin hyperpigmentation can be found in 17% to 66% of those with Whipple's disease. The predominant signs of Whipple's disease include diarrhea, weight loss, and abdominal pain.

942 **D.** (S&F, ch117)

Both mechanical obstruction and chronic intestinal pseudo-obstruction (CIP) can be associated with constipation. Urinary retention, dysphagia, and cachexia are features of CIP as opposed to mechanical obstruction. Mechanical obstruction is characterized by symptom-free periods between attacks whereas CIP is characterized by more persistent symptoms of abdominal pain, nausea, vomiting, and dysphagia.

943 **C.** (S&F, ch108)

Diseases of the ileum and cecum can present insidiously. Patients often present with symptoms and signs of small bowel obstruction, especially after eating indigestible food such as popcorn or raw fruits and vegetables. Patients may have a long history of intermittent colicky abdominal pain, sometimes associated with nausea and vomiting. A tender mass can also be felt in the right hypogastrium. Many have lost weight and have frequent, loose bowel movements. Acute appendicitis does not usually present with the classic symptoms of early partial small bowel obstruction. Ulcerative colitis usually presents with bloody diarrhea, as does *E. coli* 0157-H7 infection.

944 **A.** (S&F, ch104)

Typhoid fever is the most likely diagnosis. The causative organism is *S. typhi*. The *incubation period* is generally 7 to 14 days. During the *first week,* high fever, headache, and abdominal pain are common. The patient has relative bradycardia, a finding referred to as Faget's sign. Abdominal pain is localized to the right lower quadrant in most cases but can be diffuse. Near the end of the first week, enlargement of the spleen is noticeable, and a classic, evanescent "rose spots" rash becomes manifest, most commonly on the chest.

The main presenting sign of cholera, amebiasis, and travelers diarrhea is diarrhea.

945 **B.** (S&F, ch118)

According to literature reports, the results of upper GI radiography with small bowel follow-through (SBFT) are abnormal in 50% to 80% of patients with small bowel neoplasms and the neoplasm can be identified from these results in 30% to 44% of cases. CT and MRI are useful for detecting extraluminal disease but are suboptimal in detecting intraluminal or mucosal disease. Barium enemas may demonstrate lesions in the distal ileum only. Angiography is of limited value.

946 **A.** (S&F, ch108)

Inflammation in the gut is kept in check through an active process called "immune tolerance." This type of tolerance is mediated in part by the subset of CD4-positive helper T-cells that are generated in the intestinal mucosa and secrete the down-regulating cytokines, transforming growth factor (TGF)-beta-1 and interleukin (IL)-10.

947 **C.** (S&F, ch107)

Schistosomiasis can be acquired by skin contact with contaminated water. Different species are endemic to Africa, the Middle East, Central and South America, and parts of the Caribbean. The worms reside in the mesenteric vessels and can eventually reach the liver.

Chagas' disease is transmitted by a reduviid bug. Praziquantel is the effective treatment for this infection.

Katayama fever is an acute infection. An early immune response to the eggs leads to fever, malaise, arthralgias, myalgias, diarrhea, and cough. Eggs that lodge in the portal veins cause presinusoidal portal hypertension. Synthetic function of the liver is intact, cirrhosis does not develop, and liver biopsy is not sensitive for the diagnosis.

948 **A.** (S&F, ch104)

Infection with *Bacillus cereus* causes acute-onset diarrhea. Chronic diarrhea due to an infection acquired during travel could be caused by

bacteria, protozoa, parasites, or postinfectious complications.

949 **C.** (S&F, ch103)

Positive periodic acid–Schiff (PAS) staining reflects the presence of glycoprotein residue of the degraded cell walls of bacteria. This sign is associated with infection by *Tropheryma whippelii*, *Mycobacterium avium* complex, or *Histoplasma* or with macroglobulinemia, intestinal xanthelasmas, or pseudomelanosis duodeni.

950 **D.** (S&F, ch100)

All of the choices mentioned are complications of short bowel syndrome. Interruption of the intrahepatic circulation of bile acids by ileal resection results in decreased hepatic bile acid secretion and altered composition of hepatic bile. Hepatic bile becomes supersaturated, which leads to formation of cholesterol crystals and gallstones in gallbladder bile. After 5 years of total parenteral nutrition (TPN), more than 50% of patients in one study developed severe liver disease. Fat malabsorption secondary to bile acid deficiency in patients with extensive ileal resections and intact colons is associated with the presence of calcium oxalate kidney stones.

951 **C.** (S&F, ch111)

It is the weight loss in relation to abdominal pain with meals that characterizes this syndrome. The cardinal clinical feature of chronic mesenteric ischemia (CMI) is abdominal cramping discomfort that occurs within 30 minutes after eating, gradually increases in severity, and then fully resolves over 1 to 3 hours. This usually progresses over weeks to months. Nausea, bloating, episodic diarrhea, malabsorption, or constipation may occur.

952 **D.** (S&F, ch112)

The anterior wall of the rectum, 7 to 10 cm from the anal verge, is the most common area of prolapse into the anal canal and this area corresponds to the usual location of ulceration in patients with solitary rectal ulcer syndrome.

953 **E.** (S&F, ch107)

A. lumbricoides has a worldwide distribution but is most prevalent in underdeveloped countries and areas of poor sanitation. Most patients infected are asymptomatic. Disease occurs when the worm burden is heavy. These worms can cause intestinal obstruction. Migration into the biliary or pancreatic ducts may cause jaundice, cholangitis, biliary colic, acalculous cholecystitis, or pancreatitis. A self-limited pneumonia can occur as the larvae migrate into the alveoli.

954 **A.** (S&F, ch102)

Tropical enteropathy has been detected in most tropical regions of Asia, the Middle East, the Caribbean, Central and South America, and Africa.

955 **A.** (S&F, ch115)

IBS is associated with a 3-fold increased risk of ischemic colitis. IBS is not known too be associated with an increased risk of these other illnesses.

956 **E.** (S&F, ch109)

Although the results of small trials show some efficacy for antibiotics, probiotics, or methotrexate, none has proveneffective in well-designed large randomized controlled trials. Antibiotics do seem to be effective for Crohn's disease but not for ulcerative colitis (UC). The primary role of antibiotics in the treatment of UC is the management of suppurative complications.

957 **C.** (S&F, ch107)

Trichinosis is acquired by ingestion of undercooked contaminated meats, usually pork. The enteral phase occurs first, with typical symptoms of nausea, vomiting, diarrhea, abdominal pain, and low-grade fever; in this stage, the infection is often misdiagnosed as food poisoning or viral gastroenteritis. The parenteral phase starts 1 week later as the larvae migrate into muscle, including that of the heart, or the nervous system. This leads to myalgias, headache, high fever, dysphagia, paresthesia, and periorbital edema. Eosinophilia and an elevated level of creatinine phosphokinase (CPK) are present. The diagnosis can be made by finding larvae on muscle biopsy or by serology. *Trichinella* are not found in the stool. Albendazole or mebendazole can be used for treatment.

958 **B.** (S&F, ch104)

S. dysenteriae 1, also known as the *Shiga bacillus,* produces the most severe form of dysentery. By contrast, *S. sonnei* produces the mildest disease. *S. flexneri* is the most common serotype in tropical countries, whereas in the United States and Europe, *S. sonnei* is the most common serotype.

959 **C.** (S&F, ch115)

Decision analysis has shown that testing for celiac disease is cost-effective if the prevalence of

celiac disease in the population is greater than 1%. Bile salt malabsorption can occur in patients with IBS but a therapeutic trial of cholestyramine is more useful than SeCAT testing for this complication. Routine testing for IBD, chronic pancreatitis, or lactose tolerance is not recommended.

960 **A.** (S&F, ch108)

Patients with the *NOD-2/CARD-15* mutation have a 40-fold relative risk of Crohn's disease compared to those lacking variant *NOD-2/CARD-15* genes. Heterozygous individuals only have a 7-fold relative risk of Crohn's disease. This gene is associated with younger age of onset, ileal (not colonic) location, and increased likelihood of stricture formation. The gene product of *NOD-2/CARD-15* is a *cytosolic* protein, not a mitochondrial protein, and it functions as an intracellular sensor of bacteria.

961 **D.** (S&F, ch109)

The diagnosis of ulcerative colitis can usually be made by flexible sigmoidoscopy without preparation. Colonoscopy is not recommended for patients with severe active disease, because of the greater risk of perforation. Serologic tests are not sensitive enough to confirm the diagnosis and their specificity is controversial. CT may be helpful to rule out complications but cannot confirm a diagnosis of IBD. Once the active disease has been completely controlled in a patient with newly diagnosed UC, a full colonoscopy should be performed to establish the extent of disease and to exclude Crohn's disease. Multiple biopsies should be taken throughout the colon to confirm the diagnosis histologically and map the extent of disease.

962 **A.** (S&F, ch101)

The laboratory findings in cases of celiac sprue, like the symptoms and signs, vary with the extent and severity of the intestinal lesion. Serum tests for celiac sprue include tests to identify IgA to endomysial antibodies (EMAs) or tissue transglutaminase (tTG) antibody. However, the gold standard for confirmation of the diagnosis remains biopsy of the small intestine. Several biopsy specimens should be obtained from the distal duodenum (second or third parts) to avoid the mucosal architectural distortion produced by Brunner's glands and changes caused by peptic duodenitis, both of which can cause difficulty in histopathologic diagnosis.

963 **C.** (S&F, ch116)

SBO in the early postoperative period may be very difficult to distinguish from normal postoperative ileus. The most important clinical feature differentiating early postoperative SBO from postoperative ileus is the occurrence of obstructive symptoms after an initial return of bowel function and resumption of oral intake. Abdominal distention, pain, nausea and vomiting can occur with both conditions. The type of surgery performed or the cumulative dose of narcotic drugs administered do not help to distinguish between ileus and mechanical SBO.

964 **C.** (S&F, ch108)

Discriminating features for Crohn's disease include the presence of small bowel disease, predominantly right-sided colonic disease, rectal-sparing fistulization, and major perineal complications. Once the patient develops perianal disease, Crohn's disease is a more likely diagnosis than ulcerative colitis.

965 **E.** (S&F, ch108)

The mechanisms of action of 5-ASA agents include all of those listed. Many of the therapeutic effects of these agents appear to be mediated through down-regulation of NF-kB activity.

966 **B.** (S&F, ch115)

A history of sexual, physical, or emotional abuse is reported more often by those with IBS than by those without IBS. Abuse does not alter rectal sensation. Patients with IBS are more likely to report more lifetime and daily stressful events. Childhood stress may be even more important than stress during adulthood. In rat studies, stress accelerated colonic transit.

967 **B.** (S&F, ch103)

Several studies indicate a statistically significant increase in recent decades in the age of patients at diagnosis. Presently, the mean age at diagnosis is 56 years, and approximately 80% of those diagnosed with this condition are male.

968 **B.** (S&F, ch116)

In two series, partial SBO resolved in 65% and 81% of patients with nonoperative treatment, and 85% to 95% of patients whose partial SBO ultimately resolved had substantial improvement within the first 48 hours of treatment. Gangrene of the bowel can occur and patients need to be monitored closely for signs of this complication. Partial SBO cannot always be distinguished from complete SBO radiographically. Oral Gastrografin administration may enhance resolution of partial SBO but is not the treatment of choice.

969 **B.** (S&F, ch119)

Short-term follow-up colonoscopy is indicated in this case. Approximately 10% of patients with malignant colorectal polyps will experience an adverse outcome, defined as residual cancer in the bowel wall or positive lymph nodes. If unfavorable features are found within a malignant polyp, the chance of an adverse outcome rises to about 10% to 25% and in these cases surgery is usually recommended. The unfavorable features include adenocarcinoma in the submucosa of a sessile polyp, adenocarcinoma within 2 mm of the resection margin, poorly differentiated carcinoma, and vascular or lymphatic involvement. This patient has no unfavorable features and, therefore, surgical resection is not appropriate. Chemotherapy is also not appropriate because the risk of an adverse outcome is low. However, short-term colonoscopy is recommended to rule out polyp recurrence or residual cancer. Colonoscopy in 3 years would be too long an interval in this situation.

970 **A.** (S&F, ch103)

The current recommendation for treatment of Whipple's disease is to begin with an induction phase using either penicillin G plus streptomycin or a third-generation cephalosporin, such as ceftriaxone, followed by treatment with at least one drug that efficiently crosses the blood-brain barrier (e.g., trimethoprim-sulfamethoxazole), for at least 1 year.

971 **A.** (S&F, ch117)

In patients with smooth muscle dysfunction, manometry demonstrates a decrease in amplitude of contractions in the affected bowel segment. This pattern generally is found during both fasting and fed periods. Antral and duodenal contraction amplitudes are usually reduced. MMCs are usually present but with diminished amplitudes.

972 **D.** (S&F, ch120)

Patients with a family history of HNPCC should undergo colonoscopy, because other screening methods are not as accurate in this high-risk group. Colonoscopic surveillance has been suggested every 2 years starting at age 25 or at 5 years younger than the index case. Genetic testing can also be performed.

Sigmoidoscopy is not an adequate screening method in this population.

973 **A.** (S&F, ch122)

Almost all anorectal suppurative disease results from infection of the anal glands. Abscesses are classified according to their extent and may be perianal, ischiorectal, intersphincteric, or supralevator. The most common type is the perianal abscess (present in 40% to 50% of cases), and the least common type is the supralevator abscess (present in 2% to 9% of cases).

The diagnosis of anorectal abscess is based on typical symptoms and signs. Swelling, throbbing, and continuous pain are the most common symptoms. On examination, erythema or swelling may be seen. If the abscess is in the intersphincteric space, however, there may be no abnormal findings on the external skin. An ischiorectal abscess may produce pain in the buttock, but no abnormality may be appreciated on examination. Symptoms of a supralevator abscess may be intra-abdominal and patients may have no anorectal findings. If no abnormality can be found on examination, the patient should undergo an examination under anesthesia.

Treatment of an abscess in the perineal region requires incision and drainage. *Antibiotics alone are not adequate.* Failure to drain an abscess promptly can result in spread to adjacent spaces. Some necrotizing infections can be mutilating and life-threatening.

974 **C.** (S&F, ch98)

Measurement of the serum concentration of β-carotene has been suggested as a useful screening test for steatorrhea, with values below 100 mg/100 mL suggesting the presence of steatorrhea and values less than 47 mg/100 mL strongly indicative of steatorrhea. Low levels of serum β-carotene, cholesterol, triglycerides, and calcium and a prolonged prothrombin time suggest malabsorption of fat and fat-soluble vitamins. Low levels of vitamin B_{12}, folate, iron, and albumin suggest malabsorption of water-soluble substances and, therefore, may be seen in patients with intestinal disease but not in those with pancreatic or biliary disease.

975 **E.** (S&F, ch109)

The figure in the question shows classic histologic features of chronic quiescent UC. These include changes in size, space, and shape of the crypts, for example, branching or bifid glands, widespread separation among glands, and shortened glands that do not extend down to the muscularis mucosa. Another characteristic feature of chronic colitis and UC is Paneth cell metaplasia, with Paneth cells being found beyond the hepatic flexure where they typically are absent.

976 **C.** (S&F, ch110)

Patients with ulcerative colitis have a much higher rate of pouchitis than those with FAP. In addition, patients with preoperative extraintestinal manifestations of chronic UC have significantly higher rates of pouchitis. Although metronidazole is often the first choice in antibiotics, it is not the only effective antibiotic.

Forty percent of patients with a pouch will never have pouchitis, 40% will have a single episode, 15% will have intermittent recurring episodes, and 5% or fewer will develop chronic pouchitis. Histopathologic study of healthy and diseased pouches has shown that chronic inflammation is usual, even when the patient is asymptomatic. Villous architecture changes such as those described in this patient are often noted.

977 **E.** (S&F, ch109)

Inheritance of ulcerative colitis cannot be described by a simple Mendelian model. There are multiple genes involved. These include susceptibility genes for ulcerative colitis on chromosomes 2, 3, 6, 7, and 12. The IBD-2 locus on chromosome 12 appears to have the strongest linkage.

C3435T relates to human multidrug resistance 1 gene (MDR 1). The MDR 1 gene product, P-glycoprotein, is highly expressed in intestinal epithelial cells and serves as an important barrier to xenobiotic infection.

Certain other genes appear to influence disease behavior. These include the HLA alleles. HLA-DR1, 2, and 3 have all been identified in patients with ulcerative colitis, and their presence is related to greater severity of disease; in some studies, this relationship to extensive colitis was especially strong in women.

978 **B.** (S&F, ch116)

In adults the imaging modality of choice for evaluating intussusception is CT. A typical finding is an intraluminal mass with the density of soft tissue (representing the intussusception) with an eccentrically placed fatty area (an area of CT attenuation) that represents the intussuscepted mesentery.

979 **B.** (S&F, ch119)

A low-carbohydrate diet has not been shown to decrease the risk of colonic adenomas. Factors that have consistently been shown to protect against adenoma development include a diet high in dietary fiber, a higher level of physical activity, high calcium intake, high folate intake, use of nonsteroidal anti-inflammatory drugs, hormone replacement therapy, and selenium supplementation. A significant lower risk for colorectal adenomas or cancers and lower cancer-associated mortality have been found for users of Aspirin and nonsteroidal anti-inflammatory drugs.

980 **C.** (S&F, ch109)

Cyclosporin A is a potent inhibitor of cell-mediated immunity. It is primarily used in patients with UC that is severe and refractory to treatment with glucocorticoid drugs. The response to cyclosporine is generally rapid, with onset a mean of 7 days after the start of therapy. Cyclosporine cannot be used as monotherapy, however. Imuran, 6-mercaptopurine (6-MP), and glucocorticoid medications need to be added to the cyclosporine regimen. Patients will also need prophylaxis against pneumocystic pneumonia (PCP). Due to the severe adverse events associated with cyclosporine therapy, it is critical that the blood levels of this medication be monitored. Patients with a serum cholesterol of less than 120 mg/dL should receive nutritional support to improve their cholesterol level before initiating cyclosporine therapy, because at this level, there is an increased risk of seizures.

981 **A.** (S&F, ch115)

In the United States, 12% of patients seen by primary care physicians have IBS. In gastrointestinal practices more than one third of patients have functional gastrointestinal disorders, with IBS being the most frequent diagnosis. IBS is associated with abdominal pain relieved with defecation, noncolonic symptoms, and younger age. Patients with inflammatory bowel disease can also suffer from IBS.

982 **D.** (S&F, ch98)

Patients with cobalamin deficiency have elevated serum concentrations of methylmalonic acid and total homocysteine. Folate deficiency results only in an increase in serum homocysteine concentration. In patients with slightly low or borderline serum cobalamin levels, determination of methylmalonic acid and homocysteine levels may therefore be helpful in establishing the diagnosis of cobalamin deficiency. Levels of these metabolites tend to normalize within 1 to 2 weeks after the start of cobalamin replacement therapy, and some authors have suggested that measuring methylmalonic acid and total homocysteine levels can be used to distinguish between cobalamin and folate deficiency.

983 **D.** (S&F, ch109)

In the majority (80%) of patients with UC the disease is characterized by intermittent flares and periods of remission. These relapses vary among

patients. More than 50% of patients present with mild disease at their first attack and 6% to 19% of patients have severe disease at presentation.

Following the initial flare, 40% to 65% of patients have an intermittent course and 5% to 10% of patients have a chronic continuous course. Up to 10% of patients have a severe attack that ultimately requires colectomy.

984 **E.** (S&F, ch113)

In 50% to 60% of cases the diagnosis of appendicitis will require no imaging studies and can be made on clinical grounds alone. Plain abdominal radiography often is the initial imaging test for patients with acute abdominal pain, although CT is considered the imaging study of choice in nonclassic cases of appendicitis. With the development of rapid helico and multi detector CT, CT is increasingly being used to evaluate acute abdominal pain. Findings consistent with appendicitis include inflamed distended (greater than 6 mm) appendix that fails to fill with contrast or air, often accompanied by an appendiceal colith or wall thickening. Periappendiceal inflammation, cecal apical thickening, and pericecal fluid collections are associated findings in appendicitis.

985 **A.** (S&F, ch120)

Testing for *APC* gene mutations is available for patients with FAP. If HNPCC is suspected, genetic testing for mutations in the *hMSH2* and *hMLH1* genes can be explored. In families with HNPCC, there is a high probability of microsatellite instability in their tumors and testing to identify this can be performed. Genetic testing for those at risk for sporadic colorectal cancer is not available at the current time.

986 **D.** (S&F, ch94)

The interstitial cells of Cajal (ICCs) are cells that are interspersed within and between the muscular layers of the small intestine. These cells generate the electrical slow wave that determines the basic rhythm of small intestine contractions. This "intestinal pacemaking," by modulating the neurologic input to the smooth muscle cells, alters the myocyte membrane potential and regulates contractile activity. There are three distinct functional groups of ICCs: ICCs-MY (myenteric), ICCs-IM (intramuscular), and ICCs-DPM.

987 **D.** (S&F, ch109)

Answers **A**, **B**, and **C** are all autoimmune diseases seen in association with ulcerative colitis (UC).

988 **B.** (S&F, ch115)

Women are more likely to have IBS than men, by a ratio of 2:1. African-American and white populations have similar prevalences of IBS. Hispanic groups have a lower prevalence. IBS is commonly seen in China and Japan. Women have slower colonic transit and smaller stool output than men.

989 **B.** (S&F, ch102)

Roughly 90% of patients with tropical sprue in India and most patients in Asia and the Caribbean have impaired fat absorption. Absorption of micronutrients, particularly folic acid, is impaired, and as the enteropathy progresses to involve the ileum, vitamin B_{12} malabsorption often develops.

990 **B.** (S&F, ch93)

Intestinal atresia and stenosis may occur anywhere throughout the gastrointestinal tract but are most common in the duodenum. Most duodenal atresias are contiguous with or distal to the ampulla of Vater. Colonic atresia is rare. These abnormalities may be due to a failure of recanalization following a solid stage of duodenal development or they may result from a transient period of low blood flow (intestinal ischemia) during a crucial period in development, in which case the atresia may be mild and there may be no detectable evidence of a vascular accident. Most children with intestinal atresia have other congenital abnormalities.

991 **E.** (S&F, ch114)

Culture specimens of most diverticular abscesses grow mixed aerobic and anaerobic organisms. The most frequently cultured single organisms are *E. coli, Streptococcus* spp., and *Bacteroides fragilis*. Small pericolic abscesses can often be treated conservatively with broad-spectrum antibiotics and bowel rest. Percutaneous drainage of abdominal abscesses is now performed as often as surgery because it offers rapid control of sepsis and stabilization of the patient's condition without the disadvantages of the effects of general anesthesia; in addition, percutaneous drainage often obviates the need for multiple-stage procedures with colostomy. Urgent surgical procedures are required in 20% to 25% of patients because the abscess is multiloculated, inaccessible to percutaneous management, or does not resolve after percutaneous drainage.

992 **C.** (S&F, ch118)

Two thirds of small bowel neoplasms are malignant. The most common small bowel malignancy is adenocarcinoma. Small bowel neoplasms are more common in male patients and the elderly. Small bowel neoplasms are the least common GI malignancy; they are less common than malignancies of the colon, esophagus, or stomach.

993 **E.** (S&F, ch109)

Thiopurine methyltransferase (TPMT) is one of the key enzymes involved in the biotransformation of 6-mercaptopurine (6-MP) to its inactive metabolite 6-MMP and 6-MMPR. The *TMPT* gene shows population polymorphism. Most of the population (89%) are homozygous for wild-type *TPMT*, whereas 11% and 0.3% of the population are heterozygous or homozygous for *TMPT* mutations. Those who are homozygous for the mutated gene (0.3% of the population) are at marked increased risk for myelosuppression. It is probably reasonable to identify these patients before initiating therapy with azathioprine or 6-MP, to decrease the risk of myelotoxicity.

994 **B.** (S&F, ch98)

The Schilling test is used clinically to distinguish between gastric and ileal causes of vitamin B_{12} deficiency and to evaluate the function of the ileum in patients with diarrhea or malabsorption. It is performed by administering a small oral dose of radiolabeled vitamin B_{12}. Simultaneously, a large intramuscular "flushing dose" of non-radiolabeled vitamin B_{12} is administered. The latter saturates vitamin B_{12} carriers; thus, radioactive vitamin B_{12} absorbed by the intestine is excreted in the urine. If less than 7% to 10% of the administered dose is recovered in urine within 24 hours, vitamin B_{12} malabsorption is confirmed. To specify the site of vitamin B_{12} malabsorption, a second phase of the test must be performed. This phase involves oral administration of intrinsic factor. In patients with pernicious anemia, the results of the Schilling test normalize after oral administration of intrinsic factor. In those with ileal disease or who have undergone resection, abnormal results persist despite administration of intrinsic factor. Results of the Schilling test are normal in patients with dietary vitamin B_{12} deficiency. Patients with pancreatic exocrine insufficiency may have an abnormal results of a Schilling test, but results normalize if they are administered pancreatic enzymes.

995 **B.** (S&F, ch117)

Patients with paraneoplastic visceral neuropathy often test positive for anti-neuronal nuclear (anti-Hu) antibody, which can be detected by immunofluorescence. This antibody is postulated to be directed toward an epitope that is shared between the neuronal elements within the enteric nervous system and the underlying malignancy.

996 **B.** (S&F, ch108)

Up to 75% of patients with Crohn's disease and spondylitis may test positive for HLA-B27. Iritis, but not uveitis, may occur in association with spondylitis. Most patients with spondylitis are asymptomatic. Spondylitis is *less* common than peripheral arthropathies and occurs in 3% to 6% of patients with IBD.

997 **A.** (S&F, ch103)

The histopathologic features of intestinal Whipple's disease are quite distinctive. Upon gross inspection, the mucosa of the distal duodenum and jejunum appears abnormal in most patients. Whitish to yellow plaque-like patches are observed in approximately three quarters of patients (see the figure in the question); alternatively, the mucosa may appear pale yellow.

998 **A.** (S&F, ch122)

Internal hemorrhoids are treated differently, depending on their grade. Grade 1 and some early grade 2 internal hemorrhoids usually respond to manipulation of the diet and avoidance of medications that promote bleeding, such as nonsteroidal anti-inflammatory drugs. A high-fiber diet that includes 25 to 30 g of fiber daily should be introduced gradually and accompanied by 6 to 8 glasses of fluid daily. Fiber supplementation with psyllium or hydrophilic colloid may be added to achieve the optimal amount of daily fiber, if the amount of dietary fiber is not sufficient. When diet manipulation does not work, more aggressive treatment may be needed.

999 **B.** (S&F, ch106)

The two important species of microsporidia are *Enterocytozoon bieneusi* and *Encephalitozoon intestinalis*. The former causes 90% of cases of microsporidiosis but responds poorly to albendazole, whereas the latter accounts for 10% of cases and responds well to albendazole. Disease due to these organisms primarily occurs in patients with impaired cell-mediated immunity (i.e., AIDS or immunosuppression after undergoing solid organ transplantation). Some studies suggest that up to 50% of HIV-positive patients with diarrhea will test positive for microsporidiosis. Microsporidiosis, like cryptosporidiosis, can be associated with sclerosing cholangitis. Restoration of immune system function is essential in the treatment of microsporidiosis.

1000 **C.** (S&F, ch111)

Alesetron was taken off the market for general use because of its association with increased risk of colon ischemia. This increased risk seems to be related to serotonergic (5-HT antagonist) drugs and not to serotonin (5-HT) agonist drugs, although a few cases have been reported of colon ischemia in patients taking 5-HT agonist medications. Reducing the dosage of Alesetron is not adequate to manage drug-induced colon ischemia; the medication must be stopped immediately. Because IBS is more common in girls and women than in boys and men, the incidence of colonic ischemia would also be higher among female patients.

1001 **A.** (S&F, ch99)

SIBO classically causes a megaloblastic anemia due to vitamin B_{12} deficiency that is not reversible by intrinsic factor. Vitamin B_{12} deficiency is caused by bacterial consumption of the vitamin within the intestinal lumen before it can be absorbed across the mucosa. Anaerobic organisms mainly are responsible for the vitamin B_{12} deficiency. Unlike aerobic bacteria, anaerobes can use vitamin B_{12} in both its free form or as a complex with intrinsic factor. Anaerobic bacteria deprive the host of ingested vitamin B_{12} and exacerbate its deficiency by using ingested vitamin B_{12} to produce inactive cobamides that then compete with dietary vitamin B_{12} for ileal binding sites, thereby decreasing absorption of the vitamin.

1002 **C.** (S&F, ch109)

The figure in the question shows high-grade dysplasia. In one study, 15 (32%) of 47 patients with high-grade dysplasia who underwent colectomy were found to have synchronous cancer. The magnitude of risk for patients with low-grade dysplasia versus more advanced lesions varies among studies. However, most studies have suggested a high risk of developing more advanced lesions. Most authorities recommend annual or biannual colonoscopy with biopsies in patients with UC extending beyond proctitis who have disease for 8 or 10 years.

It is important to know that examinations should be performed during periods of inactive disease, to avoid the difficulty of differentiating between inflammation or reactive changes and malignant transformation. Four-quadrant biopsies should be obtained every 10 cm and from any potentially dysplastic lesions. Therefore, multiple biopsies (up to 64) are required to detect the highest rates of dysplasia anywhere in the colon with 95% confidence. Colectomy is recommended for flat dysplasia, whether low-grade or high-grade, or invasive cancer. Focal low-grade dysplasia may be managed by surveillance colonoscopy, while colectomy is recommended for patients with multifocal low-grade dysplasia. All biopsy findings should be confirmed by a second opinion from a pathologist with experience in analyzing biopsy specimens from patients with IBD.

1003 **B.** (S&F, ch97)

The delivery of chyme from the stomach to the duodenum is controlled so that the rate allows efficient mixing with pancreaticobiliary secretions. The characteristics of gastric contents that determine this rate of emptying include their consistency, pH, osmolality, and lipid and calorie content. Meals of high viscosity empty more slowly than do those of low viscosity. Duodenal mucosal receptors for pH and osmolality trigger a delay in gastric emptying when the gastric effluent is acidic or hyper- or hypotonic. The total caloric content of meals also controls gastric emptying rates. An increase in the size or energy density of a meal leads to a corresponding increase in the rate of delivery.

Gastric emptying is also controlled by a mechanism involving the ileum and colon. If much nutrient escapes digestion and absorption in the jejunum, its presence in the ileum and colon delays gastrointestinal transit, and this again provides more time for digestion and absorption.

1004 **B.** (S&F, ch106)

The intracellular protozoan *Cryptosporidium* is of note because it can cause severe debilitating disease if it infects those with AIDS prior to the start of HAART therapy. It is now recognized as a cause of self-limited diarrhea in the immunocompetent host. It causes more severe disease in those with immunoglobulin deficiency, lymphocytic malignancy, or low CD4 counts due to HIV disease. Women of childbearing age, teenagers, and HIV-positive patients with adequate CD4 counts generally have a milder, self-limited disease.

1005 **B.** (S&F, ch108)

Loss of haustra is a finding in ulcerative colitis. Aphthous ulcers are difficult to find on x-rays of the small bowel. Cobblestoning is a late, and not an early, finding. Cobblestoning is the result of edema and inflammation of the relatively spared islands of the mucosa separated by intersecting longitudinal and transverse knife-like clefts of ulceration.

1006 **B.** (S&F, ch111)

When vasoconstriction occurs due to occlusion of a major blood vessel, collateral vessels open immediately in response to the drop in arterial pressure distal to the obstruction. After several hours, however, vasoconstriction develops in the obstructing bed, and the elevation in pressure reduces collateral flow. Vasoconstriction that is sustained for a prolonged period can persist even after correction of the cause of the ischemic event and can become irreversible.

1007 **D.** (S&F, ch109)

This patient has PSC, which occurs in approximately 3% of those with UC. It is a chronic inflammatory disease of the biliary tree resulting in fibrosis and eventual cirrhosis and hepatic failure. Radiologic studies will show beading and irregularity and strictures in the bile ducts. PSC can be diagnosed by ERCP or MRCP. PSC must be excluded in patients who have persistently abnormal levels of liver enzymes, especially alkaline phosphatase. PSC is independent of the underlying colitis. Ursodeoxycholic acid may slow disease progression. Patients with a dominant stricture in the extrahepatic biliary tree may benefit from endoscopic dilation, possibly with stent placement. Patients who develop end-stage liver disease (manifested as poor synthetic function, ascites, etc.) would require liver transplantation. Patients with PSC are at significantly increased risk for cholangiocarcinoma.

1008 **D.** (S&F, ch111)

Colonic ischemia (CI) usually presents with sudden, crampy, mild left lower quadrant abdominal pain and an urge to defecate. This usually occurs within 24 hours of the precipitating event and is associated with bright red or maroon bloody diarrhea. Bleeding is not significant enough to require transfusion. It is not likely that this patient's symptoms are secondary to recurrence of the previous viral infection or a new viral infection. The endoscopic findings are not typical of ulcerative proctitis. Rather, the figure in question 1008 shows hemorrhagic nodules typically seen during sigmoidoscopy that represent bleeding into the submucosa and are equivalent to "thumbprinting" that can be seen on barium enema studies.

1009 **A.** (S&F, ch104)

Diarrhea and abdominal pain in this pregnant patient may be due to malaria, amebiasis, or *Giardia* infection or to another pathogen. A *Campylobacter* infection in a pregnant woman may cause spontaneous abortion, fetal prematurity, neonatal sepsis, neonatal enterocolitis, and fetal death. *S. sonnei* cause septicemia in neonates more often than in adults. Fluoroquinolones or trimethoprim-sulfamethoxazole (TMP-SMX) are *not* recommended in pregnant women; ampicillin and ceftriaxone are the drugs of choice in these patients.

1010 **E.** (S&F, ch114)

There is no clear indication for any therapy or follow-up protocol for patients in whom diverticulosis is diagnosed incidentally. Diverticuli are increasingly being found in people undergoing endoscopic screening for colon cancer. A high-fiber diet has been suggested for prophylaxis against diverticulosis. Conversely, diets high in fat and red meat have been associated with an increased risk of diverticular disease. Prospective randomized trials have yet to be performed, but some studies suggest that patients with asymptomatic diverticulosis may benefit from increasing fruit and vegetable (fiber) intake while decreasing their fat and red meat consumption.

1011 **A.** (S&F, ch120)

The first statement is true. Colorectal cancer will develop in 6% of the U.S. population. The incidence of colorectal cancer is equal in men and women in the United States. However, worldwide there is a slight male predominance. The incidence and mortality of colorectal cancer have declined in the United States since 1985.

1012 **A.** (S&F, ch104)

Ciguatera poisoning presents with a combination of gastrointestinal, neurological, and cardiovascular symptoms and findings. The illness is caused by the consumption of fish containing toxins produced by dinoflagellates. Scombroid poisoning presents with flushing, warmth, erythematous skin rash, pruritus, palpitations, and tachycardia.

1013 **D.** (S&F, ch93)

Paneth cells are flask-shaped, usually located at the crypt base, and contain abundant cytoplasmic eosinophilic granules. These cells secrete lysozyme, zinc, and other antimicrobial peptides. Brunner's glands are submucosal glands found primarily in the duodenum, into the lumen of which they secrete a thin alkaline mucus to neutralize acidic chyme and facilitate small intestinal absorption. M cells are a distinct population of immune cells that process and present antigens to other immune cells. Parietal cells are the primary cell type of the acid-producing gastric oxyntic glands. Peptic (chief) cells synthesize and secrete the zymogen, pepsinogen. Parietal and chief cells are not found in the intestines.

1014 **B.** (S&F, ch111)

Most patients with acute mesenteric venous thrombosis (MVT) initially are believed to have some form of acute myenteric ischemia (AMI) and are treated as discussed and outlined in the algorithm (see figure). Immediate initiation of a 7- to 10-day course of heparin therapy has been shown to diminish recurrence and progression of thrombosis and improve survival. If peritonitis is present, laparotomy is necessary. Thrombolytic agents are not commonly utilized in this situation.

1015 **A.** (S&F, ch112)

Avoidance is the most effective therapy for NSAID enteropathy. Experimental studies have also demonstrated that metronidazole reduces inflammation and occult blood loss without changing intestinal permeability. Sulfasalazine has also been shown to reduce inflammation. Healthy individuals taking COX-2 inhibitors compared to individuals taking naproxen had less small bowel injury noted on capsule endoscopy.

1016 **B.** (S&F, ch108)

This patient's history and physical examination findings are most consistent with a psoas abscess. Of the imaging studies listed, the only one that is likely to elucidate that diagnosis would be CT. There is no problem with the hip or thigh, but rather this is referred pain due to the abscess. A colonoscopy would not be useful. Patients with entrapment of the ureter can present with noncalculous hydronephrosis and can have thigh pain and a limping gait. An intravenous pyelogram (IVP) certainly may have yielded that information; however, CT is still the best to assess for both of these diagnoses.

1017 **A.** (S&F, ch109)

Ankylosing spondylitis affects 1% to 2% of those with ulcerative colitis and 80% of affected individuals have HLA B27 phenotype. The natural history of spondylitis is completely independent of colitis and spondylitis may present years before or long after the onset of colitis.

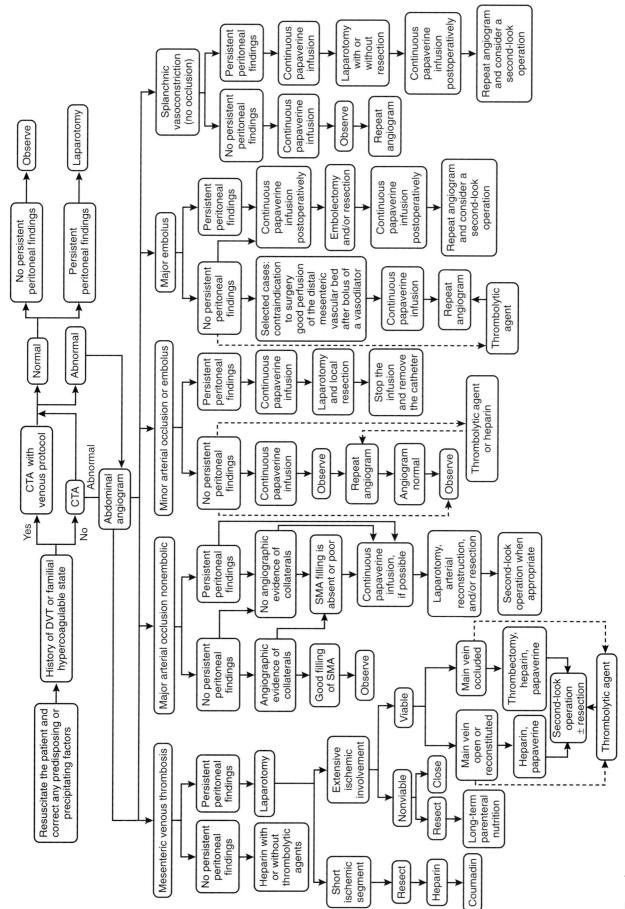

Figure for answer **1014**

1018 B. (S&F, ch95)

The interstitial cells of Cajal (ICCs) are interspersed within and between the muscular layers of the colon. These cells generate an oscillatory membrane potential and therefore modulate the motor activity of the colon. There are three distinct ICC types, which are named according to their location: (1) ICCs within the myenteric plexus (ICC-MP), (2) ICCs within the submucosal plexus (ICC-SM), and (3) ICCs located between the circular and longitudinal muscular layers (ICC-IM). The ICC-MPs and ICC-SMs are probably the pacemakers for the small, rapid oscillations in membrane potential (MPOs) of longitudinal and circular smooth muscle layers. ICC-SMs are probably the pacemakers for the large-amplitude, slow waves originating in the submucosal plexus. The exact mechanisms underlying the oscillating membrane potential and resulting rhythm in ICCs is not well understood.

1019 E. (S&F, ch120)

Advanced colorectal cancer has a high recurrence rate. Therefore, those with positive regional lymph nodes or whose primary tumor has extended into the serosa should consider adjuvant therapy. The standard regimen for stage 3 disease has been 5-FU and leucovorin, which prolongs overall and disease-free survival. Additionally, this regimen is more convenient and efficacious than 5-FU and levamisole. However, there is controversy about the appropriateness of any adjuvant therapy in stage 2 disease.

1020 A. (S&F, ch106)

ELISA of a stool sample to identify *Giardia* is the first test that should be performed, because this test is more than 90% sensitive and nearly 100% specific for giardiasis. Because cysts and trophozoites are only present in the stool intermittently, testing a routine stool for ova and parasites is only about 50% sensitive. Duodenal aspiration or biopsy are accurate tests but more invasive. Modified trichrome or iodine stains are used to detect *Giardia*, not acid-fast stains.

1021 C. (S&F, ch101)

Scalloping or absence of duodenal folds (shown in the figure in question 1021) has been noted in some patients with celiac sprue; however, scalloping is not specific for celiac sprue. Other conditions that can cause duodenal scalloping include eosinophilic enteritis, giardiasis, amyloidosis, tropical sprue, and human immunodeficiency virus enteropathy. In

addition to scalloping or atrophy of the mucosal folds, the duodenal mucosa in untreated celiac sprue may be marked by multiple fissures. A mosaic appearance also has been described in which the fissures circumscribe areas of mucosal nodularity in a manner similar to the grouting around mosaic tile. These mucosal features (atrophy and scalloping of the folds, fissures, nodularity, or a mosaic appearance) should alert the endoscopist to the need for small intestinal biopsy to evaluate for possible celiac sprue. The mucosa of patients with celiac sprue, however, often appears normal at endoscopy. Thus, absence of the macroscopic features just described does not obviate the need for biopsy and histologic examination if celiac sprue is suspected based on clinical grounds or positive results of serologic tests.

1022 E. (S&F, ch113)

Patients with appendicitis, like those with peritonitis, tend to lie still rather than moving about. Right lower quadrant tenderness and rigidity, both voluntary and involuntary, are common findings on abdominal palpation. Additional findings that may be helpful in accurately diagnosing appendicitis include the psoas and obturator signs. The psoas sign is elicited by having a supine patient flex the right hip against resistance or passively flex and extend the right hip in left lateral decubitus position. The obturator sign is elicited by internally and externally rotating the flexed right hip. The pain elicited by either of these maneuvers is thought to arise from an inflamed pelvic appendix irritating the obturator internus muscle.

1023 C. (S&F, ch104)

The organism causing this patient's symptoms is *Vibrio cholerae*. This organism is noninvasive, and therefore it does not cause bacteremia or bloody diarrhea. Its toxin causes an increase in cyclic AMP level, which results in massive fluid loss by intestinal epithelial cells. This patient's osmolar gap of less than 50 suggests secretory diarrhea. This leads to the clinical findings of profound dehydration and hypovolemic shock.

1024 A. (S&F, ch115)

Cases of ischemic colitis have been reported associated with both 5-HT-4 receptor agonists and 5-HT-3 receptor antagonists. Tegaserod has been approved by the U.S. Food and Drug Administration (FDA) for use in women only and should not be used in patients with alternating constipation and diarrhea. Alosetron is indicated in patients with diarrhea-predominant IBS and is available in the United States under a restricted prescribing program.

1025 **C.** (S&F, ch107)

A single oral dose of ivermectin 200 micrograms/kg is the best treatment and better tolerated than thiabendazole. The other drugs listed are not useful for treatment of *Strongyloides* infections.

1026 **B.** (S&F, ch94)

Splanchnic afferent nerve fibers are thought to mediate visceral distention via their connections with mural mechanoreceptors. Vagal afferent fibers are believed to be more important for physiologic homeostasis, for example the regulation of water and nutrient absorption or secretion, than for pain perception.

1027 **A.** (S&F, ch108)

Erythema nodosum is much more frequently seen in women than in men. The classic appearance is that of a tender subcutaneous nodule with an erythematous or dusky appearance. It is most often noted in the pretibial region, as shown in the figure in question 1027. There is also a strong association with arthropathy. There seems to be an association with psoriasis. Pyoderma gangrenosum appears typically as a pustule or nodule, most often on the leg. This can progress after minor trauma. Pyoderma may appear virtually anywhere on the body. It has a violaceous rim and craterlike holes in the base. Metastatic Crohn's is quite rare and not consistent with the rash shown.

1028 **B.** (S&F, ch117)

Demyelination of the proximal vagus nerve and sympathetic nerves supplying the bowel may occur in those with diabetes mellitus. The intrinsic nervous system of the bowel appears not to be affected because no morphologic abnormalities of the myenteric or submucosal plexuses have been observed. In animal studies and in a single case report there was degeneration of the interstitial cells of Cajal. Most authorities believe that myopathy is not a cause of gastrointestinal dysmotility in patients with diabetes mellitus.

1029 **C.** (S&F, ch111)

Henoch-Schönlein purpura typically affects children 4 to 7 years of age. It is characterized by formation of IgA (not IgG) immune complexes that are deposited within the small vessels of the skin, gastrointestinal tract, joints, and kidneys. It

is often preceded by an upper respiratory infection. The classic symptom triad of this disease is palpable purpura (usually seen below the waist), arthritis (knees and ankles), and abdominal pain. Abdominal pain and bleeding occur secondary to mucosal and submucosal hemorrhage. Submucosal hematomas may act as lead points for development of intussusception.

1030 **C.** (S&F, ch121)

Collagenous colitis is usually diagnosed in women between the ages of 50 and 70 years. The female predominance is strong, and there is frequent association with arthritis, celiac disease, and autoimmune disorders. Remicade has not been used for treatment of this condition. About one third of cases respond to antidiarrheal agents, such as loperamide or diphenoxylate with atropine. Bismuth subsalicylate has also been effective. Other treatments studied include 5-aminosalicylate (mesalamine) compounds, glucocorticoid drugs, and bile acid resins, alone or in combination; trials have shown mixed results.

1031 **E.** (S&F, ch97)

In addition to nutrient protein hydrolysis, pancreatic proteases have other functions. Trypsin activates the other proteases from proenzymes and splits more trypsin from trypsinogen. Pancreatic proteases split vitamin B_{12} from the R protein to which it is linked, so that it can then bind intrinsic factor. They increase the turnover of brush border membrane hydrolytic enzymes, and they initiate the final steps in the processing of the sucrase-isomaltase brush border membrane carbohydrate complex. Finally, they may have a role in the inactivation of some organisms.

1032 **A.** (S&F, ch109)

Risk factors for colorectal cancer in those with UC include long duration and extent of UC. PSC is a risk factor for colorectal cancer, and its diagnosis requires immediate institution of yearly colonoscopy with biopsies for early detection of cancer. A family history of colon cancer, an early age at diagnosis of PSC, and pancolitis are other risk factors for colorectal cancer.

1033 **A.** (S&F, ch115)

In individuals with IBS, diarrhea may occur due to a variety of colon-related mechanisms, including increased high-amplitude propagated contractions (HPACs), an enhanced gastrocolonic response, and rectal hypersensitivity. Constipation may occur secondary to increased segmental (nonpropulsive) contractions. A hypertensive internal rectal sphincter may be seen in those with Hirschsprung's disease.

1034 **D.** (S&F, ch93)

Omphalocele is a congenital anomaly that results from the failure of the abdominal viscera, including, liver, gallbladder, stomach, spleen, and small or large intestines, to return to the abdominal cavity following physiologic herniation. The hernia sac is covered by fused layers of amnion and peritoneum and involves the umbilicus. Although it is rare (the occurrence rate is 2.5 per 10,000 births), it is frequently associated with other congenital abnormalities and has a high mortality.

Gastroschisis, which is less common than omphalocele (1 per 10,000 births), involves herniation of the abdominal viscera through the body wall, usually to the right of the umbilicus in an area weakened by regression of the right umbilical vein. Importantly, this herniation does not involve the umbilicus and the excluded bowel is not covered by a sac. As a result, the herniated viscera may be damaged by vascular compromise and extended exposure to amniotic fluid. The morbidity and mortality of omphaloceles in children are related to the extraintestinal anomalies, while the morbidity and mortality of gastroschisis is largely related to the degree of intestinal atresia. Retrocecal appendix and inguinal hernia are not consequences of an abnormality of the physiologic umbilical herniation.

1035 **F.** (S&F, ch119)

Juvenile polyps usually are single, often occur in the distal rectum, and are classified as hamartomatous in nature. These generally should be removed because they often have a generous blood supply and should they prolapse, as often occurs, bleeding will result. Juvenile polyps have essentially no malignant potential when single. However, when there are multiple polyps the risk of cancer may be significantly elevated because of coexisting adenomatous polyps or coexisting adenomatous tissue within juvenile polyps. This is generally thought to occur in juvenile polyposis syndrome.

1036 **D.** (S&F, ch108)

Granulomas, although highly characteristic of Crohn's disease, are not unique nor universally found in those with this disease. The prevalence of granulomas in those with Crohn's disease varies from 15% to as high as 75% in surgical specimens. Granulomas can also, although rarely, be found outside of the intestinal tract such as in

the skin, eye, and liver. TNF, not leukotriene B4, is the key cytokine in the formation of granulomas.

1037 **D.** (S&F, ch111)

The bowel can tolerate 75% reduction of mesenteric blood flow and oxygen consumption for 12 hours with no change in the appearance of mucosa on light microscopy. This is because only one fifth of the mesenteric capillaries are open at any time and when oxygen delivery is decreased, the bowel adapts by increasing oxygen extraction. However, below a critical level of blood flow, these compensatory mechanisms will be overwhelmed.

1038 **D.** (S&F, ch98)

In healthy people, between 2% and 20% of ingested starch escapes absorption in the small intestine. Carbohydrates that reach the colon cannot be absorbed by the colonic mucosa, but they can be metabolized by the bacterial flora. Anaerobic bacterial metabolism results in the breakdown of oligosaccharides and polysaccharides to mono- and disaccharides, which are metabolized further to lactic acid and short-chain (C2-C4) fatty acids, such as acetate, propionate, and butyrate, and to odorless gases, like hydrogen, methane, and carbon dioxide. Approximately 90% of these short-chain fatty acids are absorbed by colonic mucosa.

1039 **D.** (S&F, ch112)

In the Mayo Clinic series of 59 cases of small intestinal ulcers, Boydstun and associates found that the ileum was the most common location of nonspecific ulceration (78%), whereas perforation (13 cases) occurred most commonly in the jejunum.

1040 **B.** (S&F, ch109)

Pancreatitis, fever, rash, and hepatitis are all believed to be idiosyncratic reactions. However, bone marrow suppression occurs in 2% to 5% of patients. Bone marrow suppression is dose-dependent and primarily manifests as leukopenia, although all three cell lines can be affected.

1041 **D.** (S&F, ch111)

If the patient does not have signs of peritonitis, laparotomy is not usually indicated early in the course of acute mesenteric ischemia (AMI). Papaverine infusion currently is the mainstay of diagnosis and initial treatment for both occlusive and nonocclusive forms of AMI and should be performed promptly if AMI is suspected or diagnosed based on the results of imaging tests. Intravenous heparin and hyperbaric oxygen have no role in managing AMI. Prompt laparotomy is indicated in patients with suspected AMI if angiography cannot be performed expeditiously.

1042 **A.** (S&F, ch116)

The most common causes for colonic obstruction are malignancy, volvulus, and strictures secondary to diverticulitis. Less frequent causes include Crohn's disease, endometriosis, intussusception, extrinsic tumors, and fecal impaction. Adenocarcinoma of the colon accounts for more than 50% of all cases of colonic obstruction.

1043 **D.** (S&F, ch112)

Clinical presentations vary with the location and degree of intestinal involvement and range from anemia and hypoproteinemia to abdominal pain, hemorrhage, obstruction, and perforation. Patients with nonspecific ulcers of the small intestine present most commonly with symptoms of intermittent small bowel obstruction (63%), but they may also present with abdominal pain, symptoms of perforation, or signs of acute or chronic gastrointestinal blood loss. Symptoms may be present from a few days to many years prior to diagnosis. The average patient age at presentation is between the fifth and sixth decades of life, and no gender predominance has been noted.

1044 **C.** (S&F, ch119)

All colorectal adenomas, whether tubular or villous, are considered to be dysplastic. However, the degree of dysplasia is related to various histological and morphologic factors. Larger polyps tend to have higher grades of dysplasia. Villous architecture is seen more often in larger adenomas and tends to be associated with higher degrees of dysplasia than tubular architecture. Intramucosal carcinoma and carcinoma in situ are considered noninvasive lesions because they are limited to the mucosal layer of the bowel wall and do not invade the lymphatics or metastasize.

1045 **A.** (S&F, ch111)

Patients older than 50 years old who have longstanding congestive heart failure (CHF), cardiac arrhythmias such as atrial fibrillation, recent myocardial infarction, or hypotension are at particular risk for superior mesenteric arterial embolus. Mesenteric venous thrombosis is far more indolent. Nonocclusive mesenteric ischemia (NOMI) is responsible for 20% to 30% of cases of acute mesenteric ischemia and is usually due to

splanchnic vasoconstriction consequent to a preceding cardiovascular event. The event may have occurred hours to days earlier than the presentation. Superior mesenteric arterial emboli (SMAE) are responsible for 40% to 50% of acute mesenteric ischemic episodes. Emboli usually originate from the left atrium or a ventricular mural thrombus. Focal segmental ischemia (FSI) is due to vascular insults in short segments of the small intestine. The causes include arterial emboli, strangulated hernias, immune complex disorders, vasculitis, blunt abdominal trauma, segmental venous thrombosis, radiation therapy, and oral contraceptives. Patients with FSI typically present with signs and symptoms of an acute abdomen.

1046 **C.** (S&F, ch108)

Perinuclear antineutrophil cytoplasmic antibody (pANCA) and anti-saccharomyces cerevisiae antibody (ASCA) correlate with the diagnosis of ulcerative colitis and Crohn's disease, respectively. The *specificity* of these markers is approximately 85%, but their *sensitivity* is considerably lower. ASCA-positive patients have a higher rate of surgery and require surgery earlier in the course of the disease, independent of disease location and the patient's history of smoking.

1047 **C.** (S&F, ch103)

One remarkable finding in an analysis by Dobbin was the strong relationship between increased risk of Whipple's disease and working in the farming or building trades, working outdoors, or frequent contact with animals or soil; of 191 patients for whom data were available, 43 (22%) were farmers and 10 (5%) were carpenters. Patients in all farming-related trades accounted for 34% of the total. By comparison, the proportion of farm workers among the total workforce in the countries studied was approximately 10%.

1048 **A.** (S&F, ch120)

Both yearly and biennial fecal occult blood testing has been shown in large-scale randomized, controlled studies to decrease mortality from colorectal cancer. The other choices may be options for screening but have not been shown to decrease colorectal cancer mortality. A decrease in colorectal cancer mortality has been demonstrated for proctosigmoidoscopy. Results in the National Polyp Study suggest that removal of adenomatous polyps reduces the mortality from colorectal cancer. Thus, it has been inferred that colonoscopy should have the same effect.

1049 **E.** (S&F, ch114)

Diverticulosis shows striking geographical variability. The disorder is extraordinarily rare in rural Africa and Asia; its highest prevalence rates are in the United States, Europe, and Australia. "Westernization" of diet, such as may occur when Asians migrate to Australia, the United States, or Europe, increases the risk of diverticulosis. Diverticuli do not involve the muscle itself but are rather herniations of mucosa and submucosa through a defect in the muscularis. Common diverticula strictly speaking are pseudo diverticuli. In western countries diverticula occur mainly in the left colon; in these populations, up to 90% of patients have involvement of the sigmoid and only 15% have right-sided involvement. In contrast, right-sided involvement is predominant in Asian countries.

1050 **D.** (S&F, ch109)

In terms of epidemiology, the gradient is typically North-South not South-North. The overall incidence of ulcerative colitis has remained stable over the last three decades. The incidence of ulcerative colitis among Jews is 13 cases per 100,000 person-years compared to 3.8 per 100,000 person-years among non-Jewish white populations. Although ulcerative colitis had been believed to be uncommon amongst minorities, by the late 1970s, the incidence for white and nonwhite populations in the United States were believed to be comparable.

1051 **C.** (S&F, ch117)

The enteric nervous system consists of vast ganglionated plexuses located in the wall of the GI tract. The most important for function are the myenteric and submucosal plexuses. The interstitial cells of Cajal are the intestinal pacemakers, activating neuromuscular function.

1052 **A.** (S&F, ch106)

In HIV-positive patients with cryptosporidiosis, boosting immune function with highly active antiretroviral therapy (HAART) is the most important treatment. Nitazoxamide is effective in immunocompetent hosts. Paromomycin, with or without azithromycin, is another option in immunocompromised patients.

1053 **D.** (S&F, ch109)

A patient with longstanding ulcerative colitis treated with glucocorticoid drugs and immunosuppressant medications can develop superimposed cytomegalovirus (CMV) colitis.

Although they may have diffuse colitis, often they have deep discrete ulcerations. The mucosa and the ulcer bed should be biopsied and the specimens should be examined histologically with care for the presence of giant cells with intranuclear inclusions.

1054 **E.** (S&F, ch111)

Vascular insults of the short segments of the small bowel produce a broad spectrum of clinical features without the typical life-threatening complications of more extensive ischemia. With focal segmental ischemia (FSI), there is usually adequate collateral circulation to prevent transmural infarction. The most common lesion is partial bowel wall necrosis with translocation of intestinal bacteria. FSI may present as acute enteritis, chronic enteritis, or a stricture. In the acute pattern, abdominal pain often seems like acute appendicitis and the physical examination findings are those of an "acute abdomen." An inflammatory mass may be palpated. Chronic forms may resemble Crohn's disease, with symptoms of crampy abdominal pain, diarrhea, fever, and weight loss. FSI must be considered in patients with chronic small bowel obstruction with intermittent abdominal pain, distention, and vomiting.

1055 **D.** (S&F, ch106)

Effective treatment for amebiasis is either a luminal or tissue amebicide. Luminal amebicides include iodoquinol, diloxanide furoate, and paromomycin. The last is preferred because it is the safest, most effective medication and a shorter course is required. The tissue amebicides include metronidazole, tinidazole, nitazoxanide, erythromycin, and chloroquine. The first two are most efficacious.

1056 **B.** (S&F, ch100)

Crohn's disease accounts for 60% to 75% of the cases of short bowel syndrome found in adults. The other conditions listed are less frequent causes of short bowel syndrome in adults. In children, congenital abnormalities account for two thirds of cases of short bowel syndrome and the remainder are caused by necrotizing enteric infections.

1057 **D.** (S&F, ch107)

Patients colonized with these tapeworms are usually asymptomatic. However, ingested *T. solium* eggs cause cysticercosis when the eggs disseminate. Local inflammation occurs in the nervous system and the heart and can be fatal. In endemic areas, neurocysticercosis is a common cause of epilepsy. The diagnosis can be made by finding eggs or proglottids in the stool, although multiple samples may be needed. A single oral dose of praziquantel 10 mg/kg is effective.

1058 **C.** (S&F, ch102)

Acute infectious diarrhea in travelers is most commonly caused by enterotoxigenic *Escherichia coli,* although chronic diarrhea and malabsorption also occur as a result of specific infections and tropical sprue.

1059 **D.** (S&F, ch112)

Symptoms of NSAID-induced ulceration of the small bowel include hypoalbuminemia, anemia, and diaphragm-like strictures. In an autopsy study performed by Allison and associates, 8.4% of NSAID users had ulcerations of the small intestine compared to only 0.6% of NSAID nonusers. Three of the NSAID-using patients had died of a small bowel perforation.

1060 **E.** (S&F, ch109)

E. coli O157:H7 infections can mimic IBD. They can be quite severe in children and the elderly, often presenting with bloody diarrhea. Special culture techniques are necessary to make this diagnosis, along with a high clinical index of suspicion. Children may develop hemolytic uremic syndrome and thrombotic thrombocytopenic purpura. *C. difficile* infection must always be considered in the differential diagnosis of IBD in patients taking antibiotics or who might have been exposed to the organism. The identification of pseudomembranes on sigmoidoscopy is helpful in the differential diagnosis, as is testing for toxins and antigens to the organism. *Aeromonas* and *Listeria* can also mimic ulcerative colitis but less often than *E. coli* O157:H7.

1061 **A.** (S&F, ch105)

The "gold standard" diagnostic test to identify *C. difficile* toxin in the stool is a tissue culture cytotoxicity assay. The enzyme immunoassays are used widely for the detection of toxin A or toxins A and B of *C. difficile* in stool specimens. Although they have high specificity (75% to 100%) for toxins, the immunoassays are less sensitive than the cytotoxicity test (63% to 99%). Stool culture is sensitive (89% to 100%) but is not specific for toxin-producing strains of the

bacterium. Sigmoidoscopy findings of colonic pseudomembranes are virtually pathognomonic for *C. difficile* colitis but can be seen in other diseases.

1062 **B.** (S&F, ch111)

Although poorly sensitive (30%) and nonspecific, plain films of the abdomen still are obtained in evaluating patients with suspected acute myenteric ischemia (AMI). Most plain films are normal before infarction. Subsequently, formless loops of small intestine and ileus "thumbprinting" of the small bowel or right colon can be seen. Even later in the course, pneumatosis and portal or mesenteric vascular gas may be seen. Free air under the diaphragm would suggest perforation and would generally not be an early finding.

1063 **C.** (S&F, ch106)

Infants are infected more often than adults worldwide. In the United States, children in daycare and sexually active homosexual men are at greatest risk. Other risk factors include drinking untreated surface water, a shallow well as a water source, swimming in natural fresh water, and contact with a person infected with *Giardia.*

1064 **A.** (S&F, ch110)

Ileal pouch anal anastomosis (IPAA) is now the procedure of choice for most patients who require proctocolectomy for chronic ulcerative colitis (CUC) or familial adenomatous polyposis (FAP). IPAA is not now considered suitable for patients with Crohn's disease, although the usefulness of IPAA surgery for these patients is being investigated. Ileal rectal anastomosis can be performed; however, this procedure does not remove all diseased mucosa. Although Brooke ileostomies and continent ileostomies can be performed, they are less acceptable to patients than IPAA, which restores bowel function.

1065 **C.** (S&F, ch96)

There are four major types of epithelial cells of the intestinal mucosa: enterocytes, endocrine cells, goblet cells, and Paneth cells. All cells originate from the proliferative zone near the base of the crypt. With the exception of Paneth cells, they migrate up the villus axis, maturing during this process.